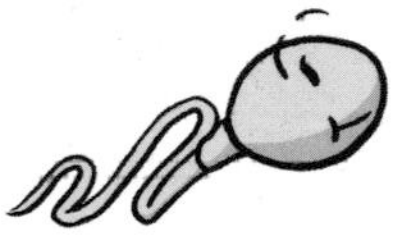

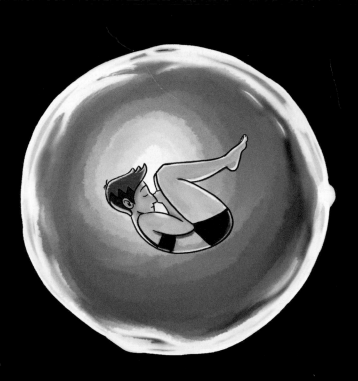

Catalogue Baby

A MEMOIR OF INFERTILITY

MYRIAM STEINBERG

ILLUSTRATIONS BY **CHRISTACHE**

●● **PAGE TWO** BOOKS

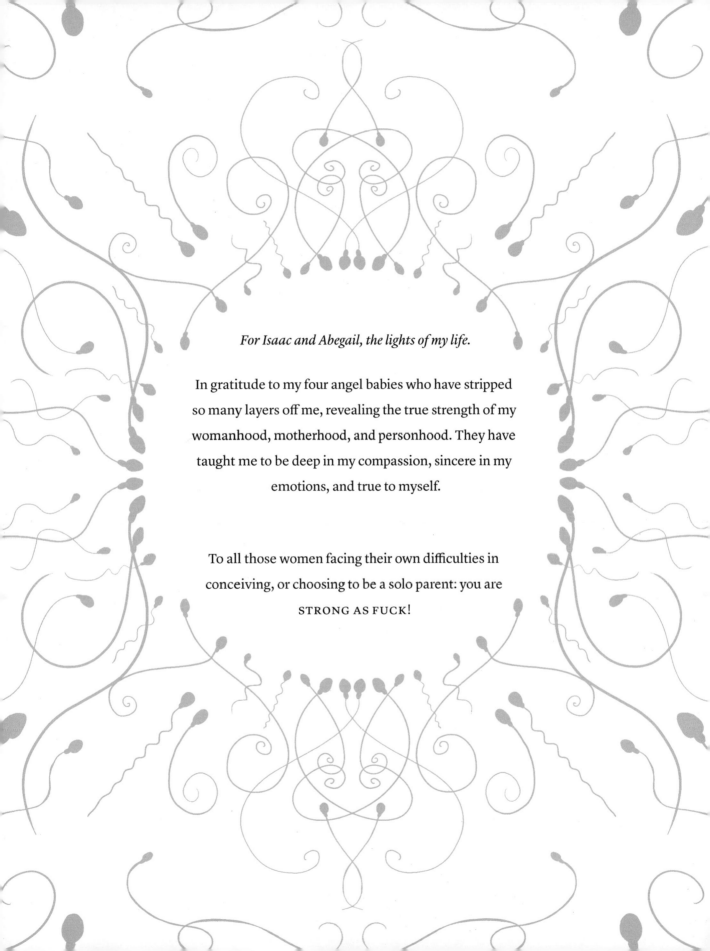

For Isaac and Abegail, the lights of my life.

In gratitude to my four angel babies who have stripped so many layers off me, revealing the true strength of my womanhood, motherhood, and personhood. They have taught me to be deep in my compassion, sincere in my emotions, and true to myself.

To all those women facing their own difficulties in conceiving, or choosing to be a solo parent: you are STRONG AS FUCK!

Preface

This book was hard to write. At times, I felt as if I was going in circles of life and death, life and death, life and death—on repeat without respite.

So many parts of the story were still raw for me, and will likely be so for the rest of my life. At the same time, I didn't want to pull any punches. This story is real, glorious, and brutal. Baby-making is messy business. Sex is messy. Un-sex is just as infinitely messy. As I was writing, I often wondered what readers' reactions would be. How shocked (or not) would they be by the graphic portrayals of emotional and physical realities? Would they laugh or cry? Be horrified or engaged? Find truth or disbelief? Share the book or throw it away after the first page?

There is so much silence around the pain that can accompany miscarriage and difficulties in conceiving. I hope this book will help de-stigmatize a terribly lonely experience, and address a void in materials that cover not only these issues but also the devastating decision-making process around fetal genetic anomalies.

My story is just one of the countless examples out there. There are as many pregnancy stories as there are pregnancies. They are all unique, and dictated by the personality, biology, medical access, and social, financial, and relational circumstances of the people involved.

The tale would not be complete without showing all the emotional aspects. Side by side with the moments of deep grief are incredibly hilarious moments, intense joys, soaring hopes, and the life-saving love of friends, acquaintances, and family. Where there was despair, there was also courage, determination, and stamina that only a woman trying to conceive is privy to (her partner—if she has one—comes a close second).

My hope is that *Catalogue Baby* will be a source of solidarity, compassion, understanding, ideas, and inspiration for those women, and their friends and families.

A little something about the characters in the book: Dozens of people make up this story. Unfortunately, I wasn't able to include absolutely everyone who offered support. Please know, all of you who have been my rocks, that it's not for my lack of love and appreciation for you, and that you are indeed represented in the book. For the sake of clarity and brevity, I had to create composites of some of the characters. One of the things I was hyper-aware of throughout this journey was the reality of compassion fatigue. I didn't want to burn anyone out by depending solely on one or two people for all the emotional and practical support I needed, nor did I want to impose a lot (or at all) on folks who were already bogged down by their own personal lives, work, and/or child-rearing duties. Whether it was taking me to the clinic or hospital, going for walks in the forest, listening to my story and offering emotional support, giving me injections, bringing me food, or infusing me with hope and laughter, I spent a fair amount of time "analyzing" who might have the time, emotional capacity, or personality type to deal with whatever I was going through at any given time. I feel so incredibly blessed and lucky to have a wide-enough community that I was able to reach out to a multitude of people. It was important to me to show that in the book, which is why some friends only appear once or twice (despite often being there for me multiple times in real life). The main takeaway is that no matter how often or to what extent someone helped me, their actions were invaluable and will stick with me forever.

Finally, there are many terms and acronyms in the book that are bandied about in the TTC (Trying To Conceive) world. I didn't want to interrupt the flow of the narrative with footnotes or too many explanations, so I've included a glossary at the back of the book.

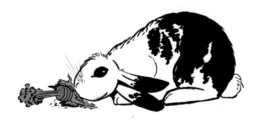

YEAR ONE
JANUARY 2014–APRIL 2015

Tick-Tock

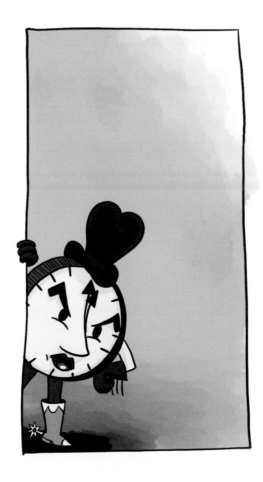

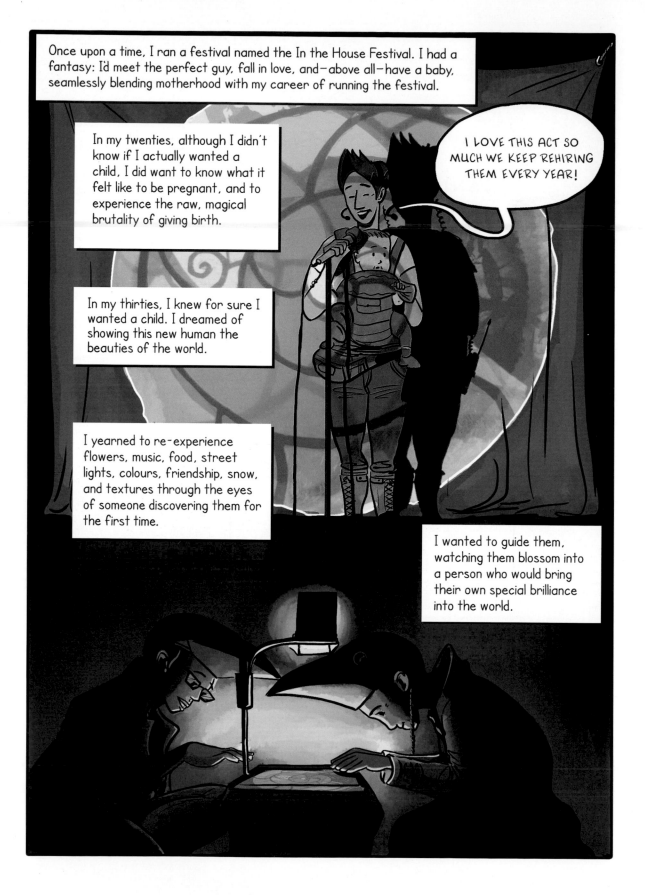

Once upon a time, I ran a festival named the In the House Festival. I had a fantasy: I'd meet the perfect guy, fall in love, and—above all—have a baby, seamlessly blending motherhood with my career of running the festival.

In my twenties, although I didn't know if I actually wanted a child, I did want to know what it felt like to be pregnant, and to experience the raw, magical brutality of giving birth.

I LOVE THIS ACT SO MUCH WE KEEP REHIRING THEM EVERY YEAR!

In my thirties, I knew for sure I wanted a child. I dreamed of showing this new human the beauties of the world.

I yearned to re-experience flowers, music, food, street lights, colours, friendship, snow, and textures through the eyes of someone discovering them for the first time.

I wanted to guide them, watching them blossom into a person who would bring their own special brilliance into the world.

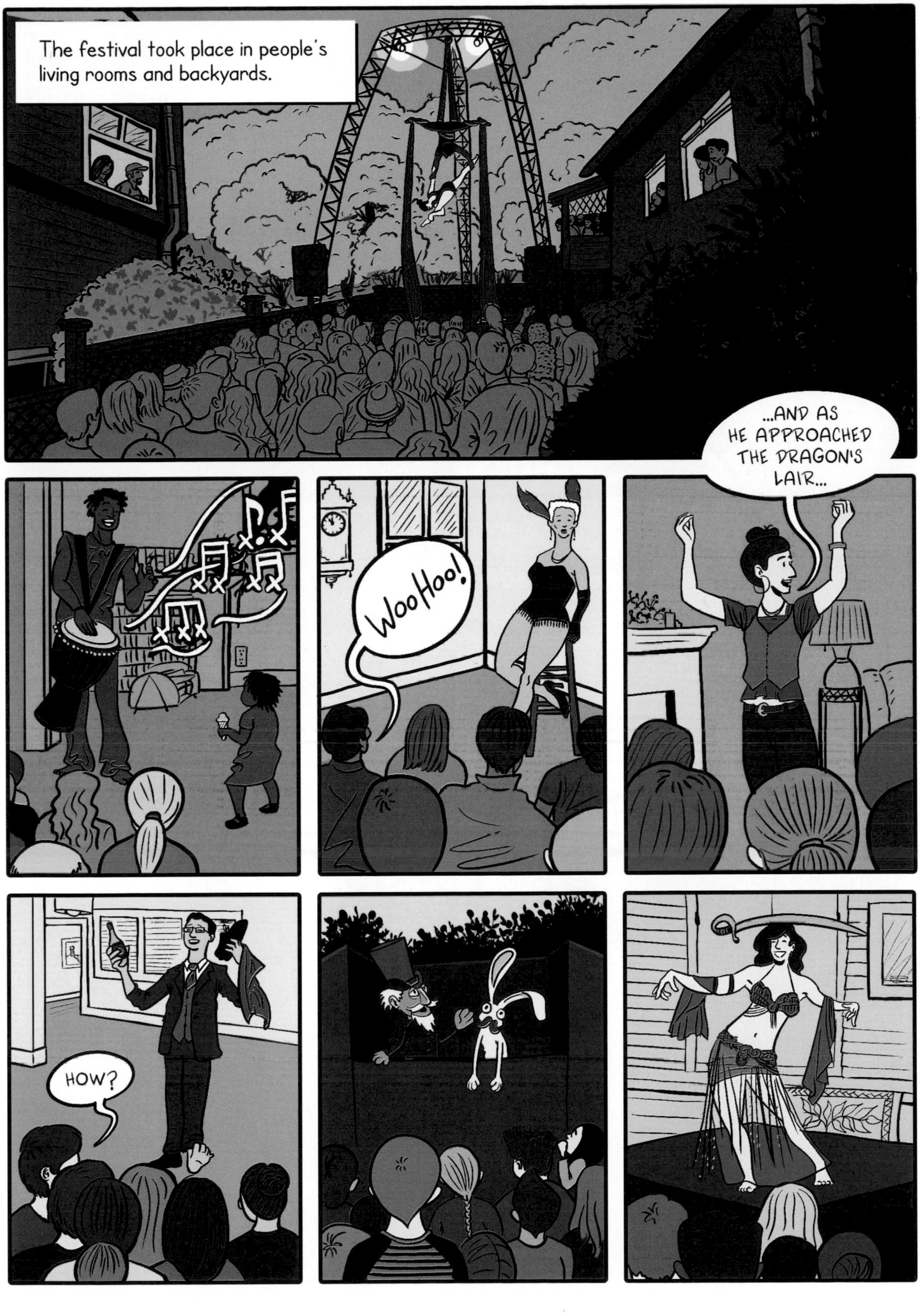

The festival took place in people's living rooms and backyards.
WooHoo!
...AND AS HE APPROACHED THE DRAGON'S LAIR...
HOW?

I ran the festival for 11 years, spending significantly more time organizing it than organizing my personal life. My loneliness and unrequited motherhood flowed along through it all, occasionally reminding me that my life was not quite what I wanted it to be. So when I met Steve on New Year's Eve 2014, I didn't want to mess up the chance to fulfill my dreams.

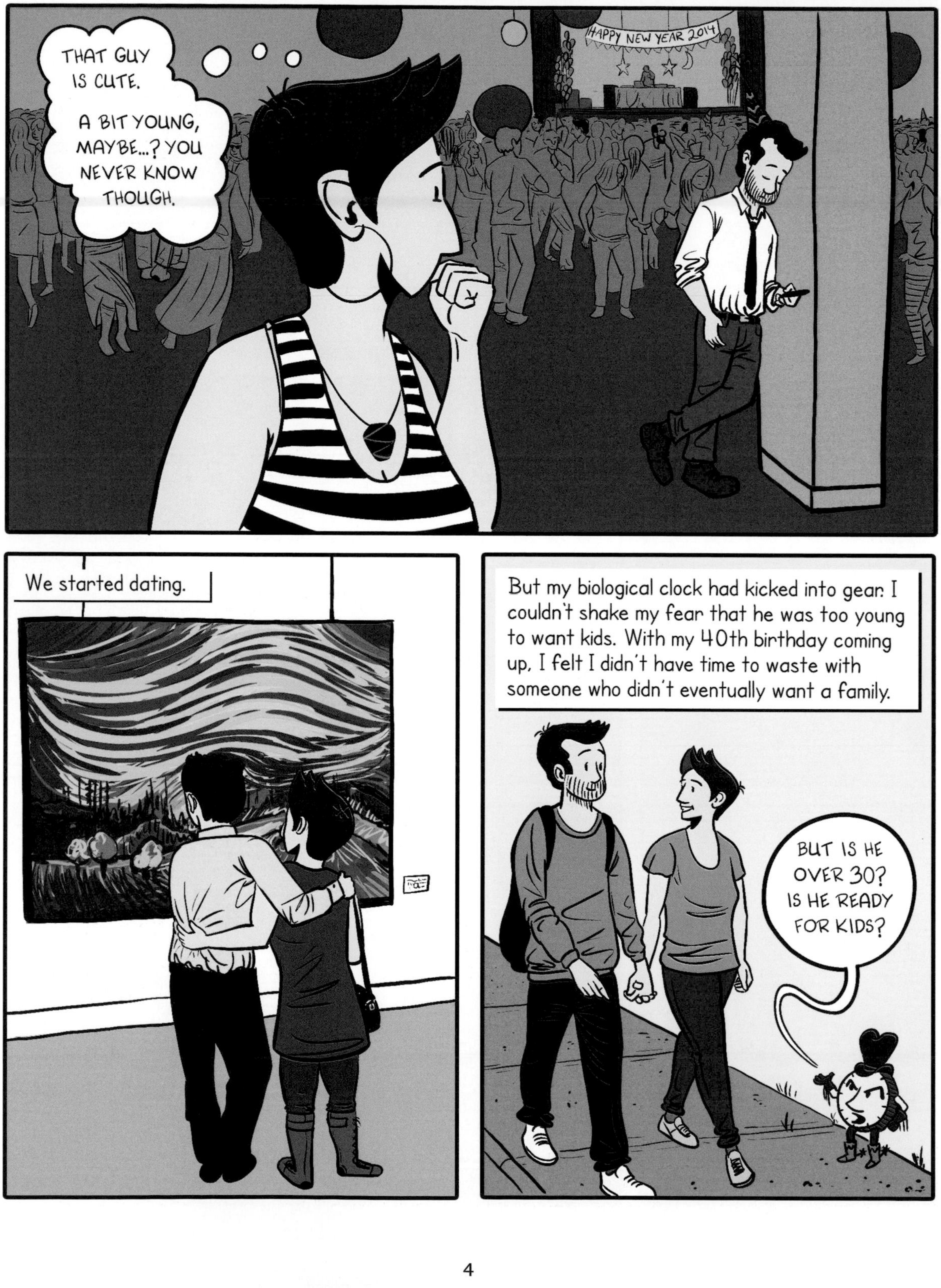
HAPPY NEW YEAR 2014
THAT GUY IS CUTE.
A BIT YOUNG, MAYBE...? YOU NEVER KNOW THOUGH.
We started dating.
But my biological clock had kicked into gear. I couldn't shake my fear that he was too young to want kids. With my 40th birthday coming up, I felt I didn't have time to waste with someone who didn't eventually want a family.
BUT IS HE OVER 30? IS HE READY FOR KIDS?

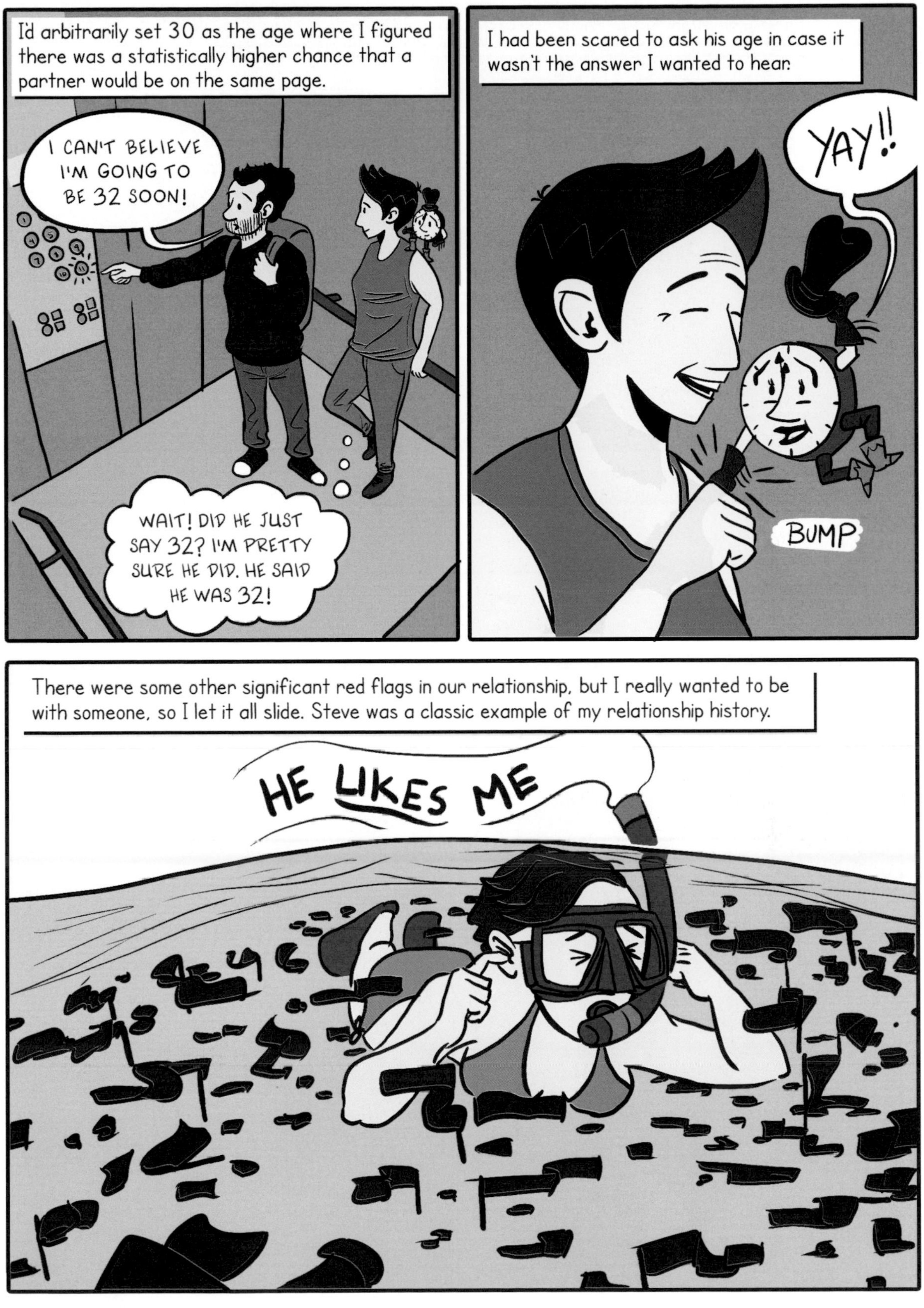
I'd arbitrarily set 30 as the age where I figured there was a statistically higher chance that a partner would be on the same page.
I CAN'T BELIEVE I'M GOING TO BE 32 SOON!
WAIT! DID HE JUST SAY 32? I'M PRETTY SURE HE DID. HE SAID HE WAS 32!
I had been scared to ask his age in case it wasn't the answer I wanted to hear.
YAY!!
BUMP
There were some other significant red flags in our relationship, but I really wanted to be with someone, so I let it all slide. Steve was a classic example of my relationship history.
HE LIKES ME

As the relationship went on, I kept compromising my deepest wish to eventually have a baby.

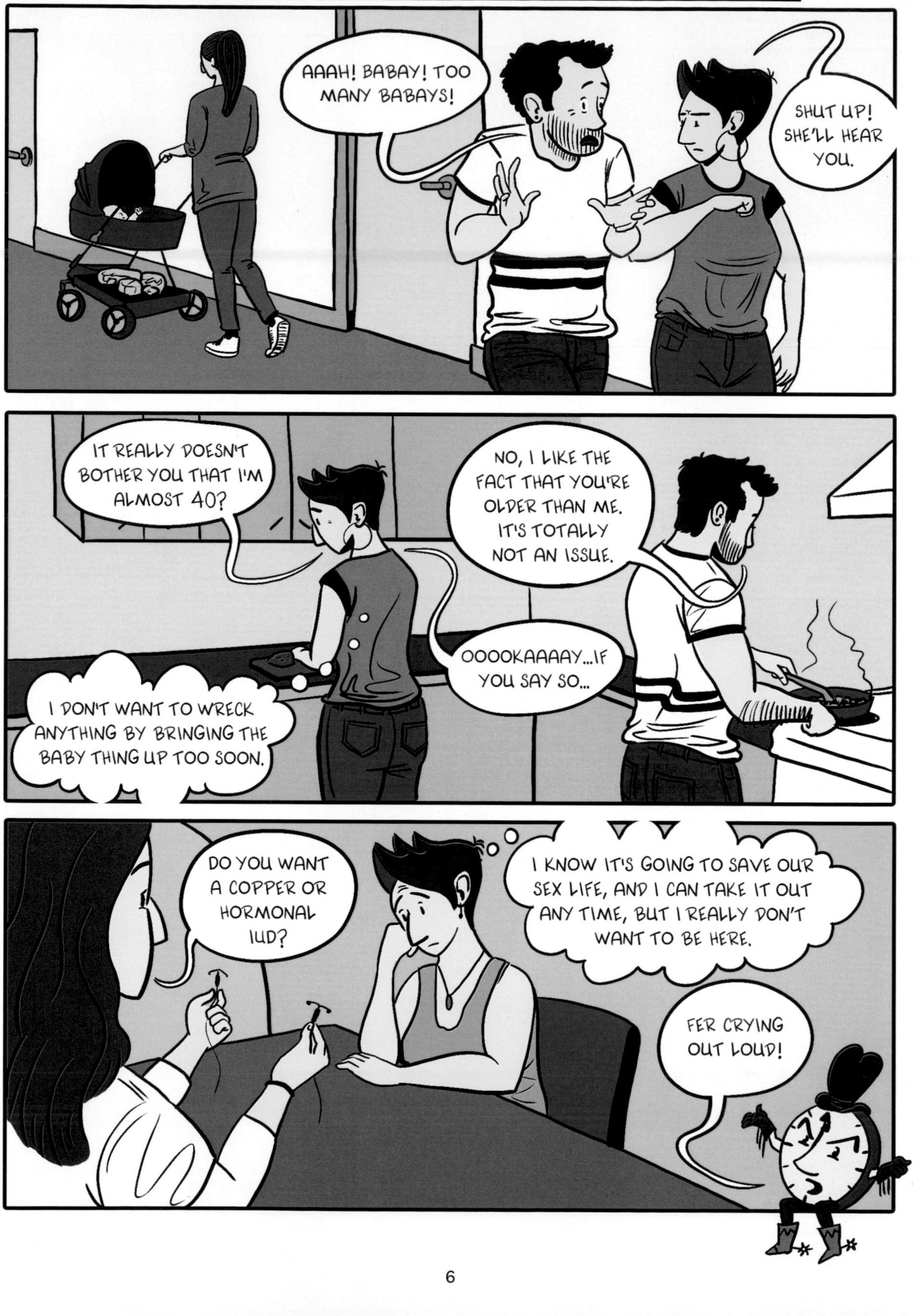
AAAH! BABAY! TOO MANY BABAYS!
SHUT UP! SHE'LL HEAR YOU.
IT REALLY DOESN'T BOTHER YOU THAT I'M ALMOST 40?
NO, I LIKE THE FACT THAT YOU'RE OLDER THAN ME. IT'S TOTALLY NOT AN ISSUE.
OOOOKAAAAY...IF YOU SAY SO...
I DON'T WANT TO WRECK ANYTHING BY BRINGING THE BABY THING UP TOO SOON.
DO YOU WANT A COPPER OR HORMONAL IUD?
I KNOW IT'S GOING TO SAVE OUR SEX LIFE, AND I CAN TAKE IT OUT ANY TIME, BUT I REALLY DON'T WANT TO BE HERE.
FER CRYING OUT LOUD!

I tried bringing up the baby topic a couple of times. Pretty sure I won 1st Prize for Most Bumbling Broaching of a Topic.

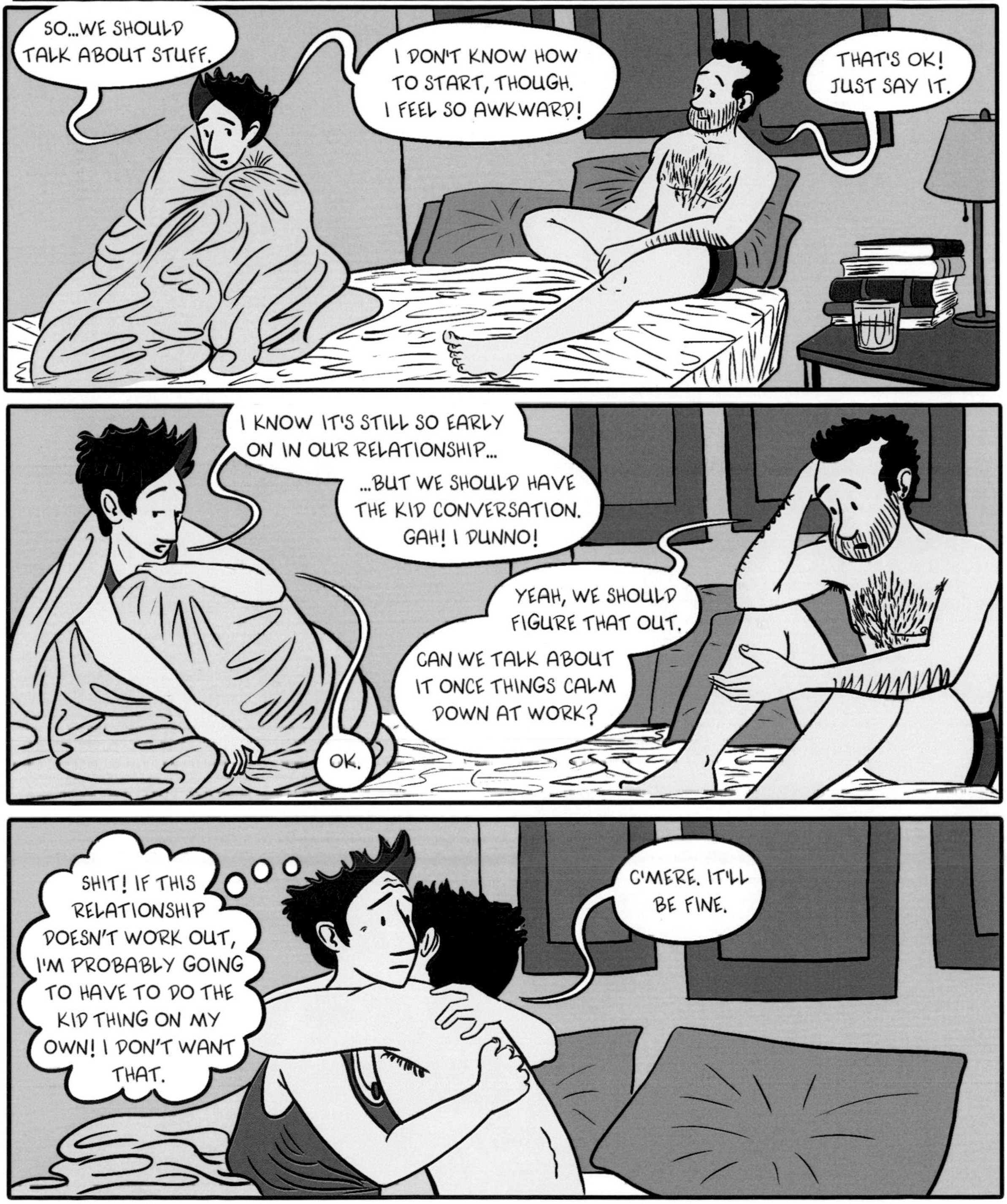
SO...WE SHOULD TALK ABOUT STUFF.
I DON'T KNOW HOW TO START, THOUGH. I FEEL SO AWKWARD!
THAT'S OK! JUST SAY IT.
I KNOW IT'S STILL SO EARLY ON IN OUR RELATIONSHIP...
...BUT WE SHOULD HAVE THE KID CONVERSATION. GAH! I DUNNO!
YEAH, WE SHOULD FIGURE THAT OUT.
CAN WE TALK ABOUT IT ONCE THINGS CALM DOWN AT WORK?
OK.
SHIT! IF THIS RELATIONSHIP DOESN'T WORK OUT, I'M PROBABLY GOING TO HAVE TO DO THE KID THING ON MY OWN! I DON'T WANT THAT.
C'MERE. IT'LL BE FINE.

The conversation was put on hold. That summer turned out to be rife with colossal upheavals. Steve's dad died just as I was seriously considering shutting down my festival. I went into caregiver mode for him and added yet another layer of self-abnegation to the mix. Yet, I still thought everything was fine with the relationship.

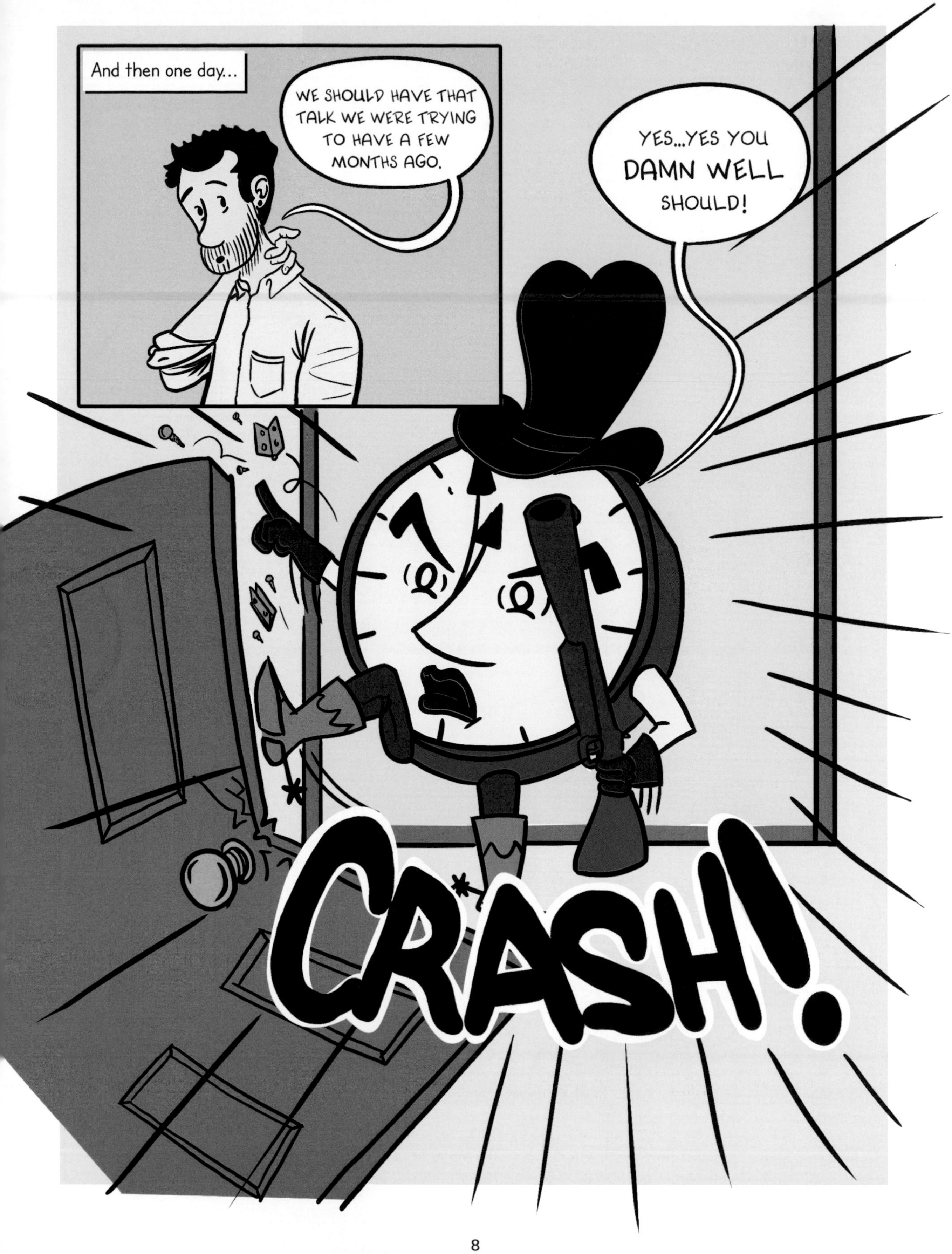
And then one day...
WE SHOULD HAVE THAT TALK WE WERE TRYING TO HAVE A FEW MONTHS AGO.
YES...YES YOU DAMN WELL SHOULD!
CRASH!

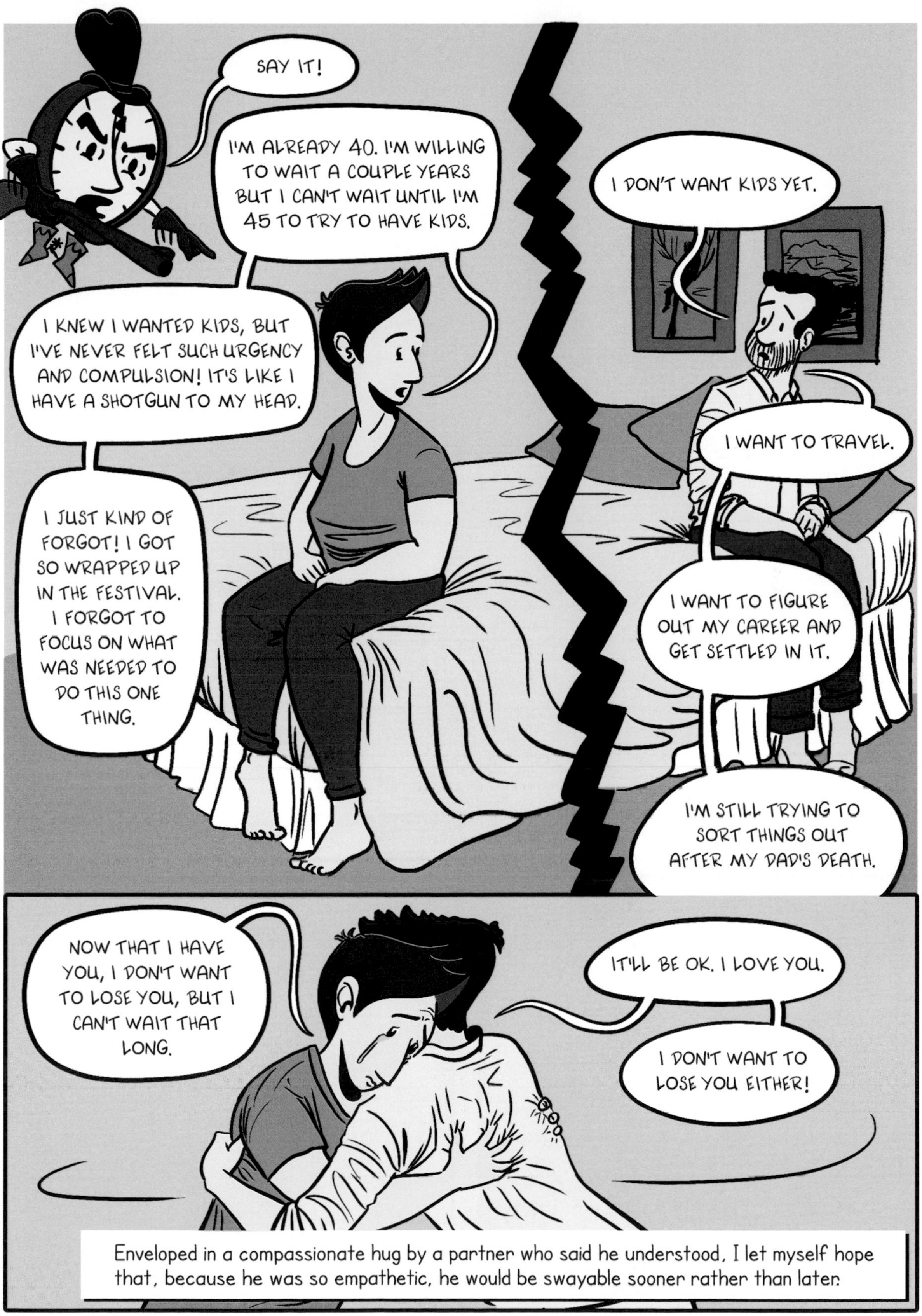
SAY IT!
I'M ALREADY 40. I'M WILLING TO WAIT A COUPLE YEARS BUT I CAN'T WAIT UNTIL I'M 45 TO TRY TO HAVE KIDS.
I KNEW I WANTED KIDS, BUT I'VE NEVER FELT SUCH URGENCY AND COMPULSION! IT'S LIKE I HAVE A SHOTGUN TO MY HEAD.
I JUST KIND OF FORGOT! I GOT SO WRAPPED UP IN THE FESTIVAL. I FORGOT TO FOCUS ON WHAT WAS NEEDED TO DO THIS ONE THING.
I DON'T WANT KIDS YET.
I WANT TO TRAVEL.
I WANT TO FIGURE OUT MY CAREER AND GET SETTLED IN IT.
I'M STILL TRYING TO SORT THINGS OUT AFTER MY DAD'S DEATH.
NOW THAT I HAVE YOU, I DON'T WANT TO LOSE YOU, BUT I CAN'T WAIT THAT LONG.
IT'LL BE OK. I LOVE YOU.
I DON'T WANT TO LOSE YOU EITHER!

Enveloped in a compassionate hug by a partner who said he understood, I let myself hope that, because he was so empathetic, he would be swayable sooner rather than later.

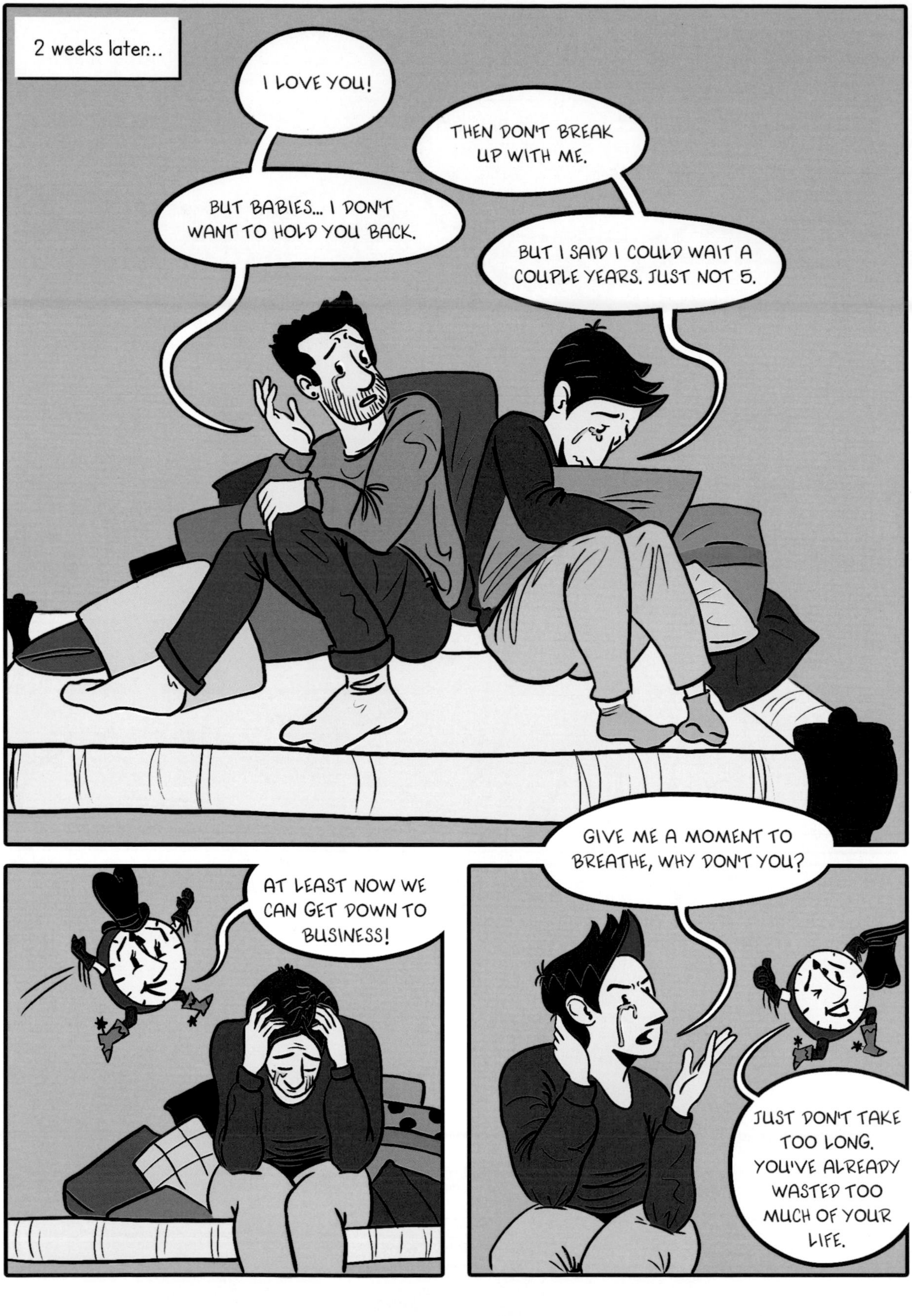
2 weeks later...
I LOVE YOU!
BUT BABIES... I DON'T WANT TO HOLD YOU BACK.
THEN DON'T BREAK UP WITH ME.
BUT I SAID I COULD WAIT A COUPLE YEARS. JUST NOT 5.
AT LEAST NOW WE CAN GET DOWN TO BUSINESS!
GIVE ME A MOMENT TO BREATHE, WHY DON'T YOU?
JUST DON'T TAKE TOO LONG. YOU'VE ALREADY WASTED TOO MUCH OF YOUR LIFE.

Biological Clock was right. In the face of the big 4-0, I finally understood just how much the festival had dominated my life. Time had always seemed like a bottomless resource, and my loneliness was all too often subsumed by the needs of the festival.

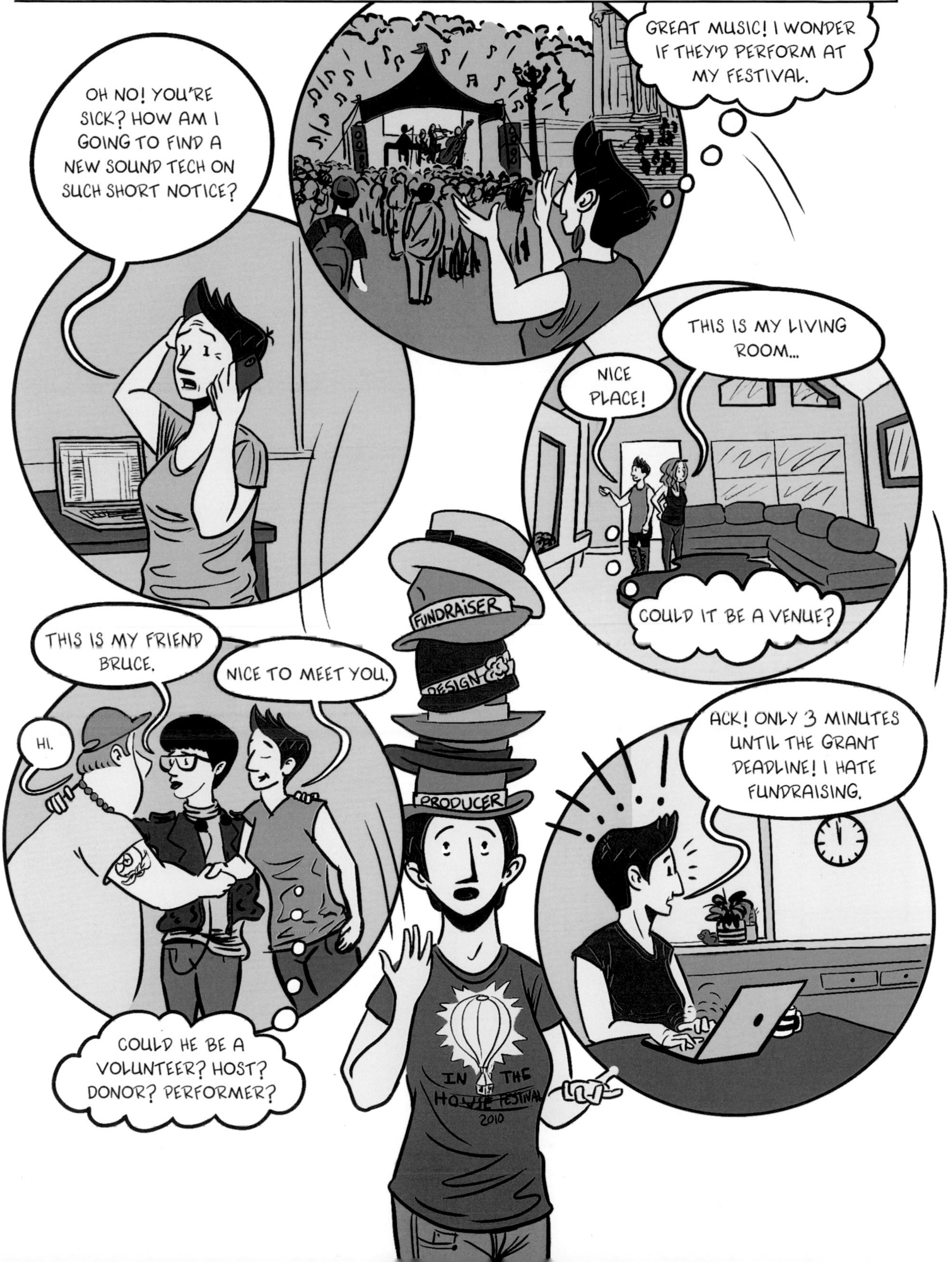
GREAT MUSIC! I WONDER IF THEY'D PERFORM AT MY FESTIVAL.
OH NO! YOU'RE SICK? HOW AM I GOING TO FIND A NEW SOUND TECH ON SUCH SHORT NOTICE?
THIS IS MY LIVING ROOM...
NICE PLACE!
COULD IT BE A VENUE?
FUNDRAISER
DESIGN
PRODUCER
THIS IS MY FRIEND BRUCE.
NICE TO MEET YOU.
HI.
COULD HE BE A VOLUNTEER? HOST? DONOR? PERFORMER?
ACK! ONLY 3 MINUTES UNTIL THE GRANT DEADLINE! I HATE FUNDRAISING.
IN THE HOUSE FESTIVAL 2010

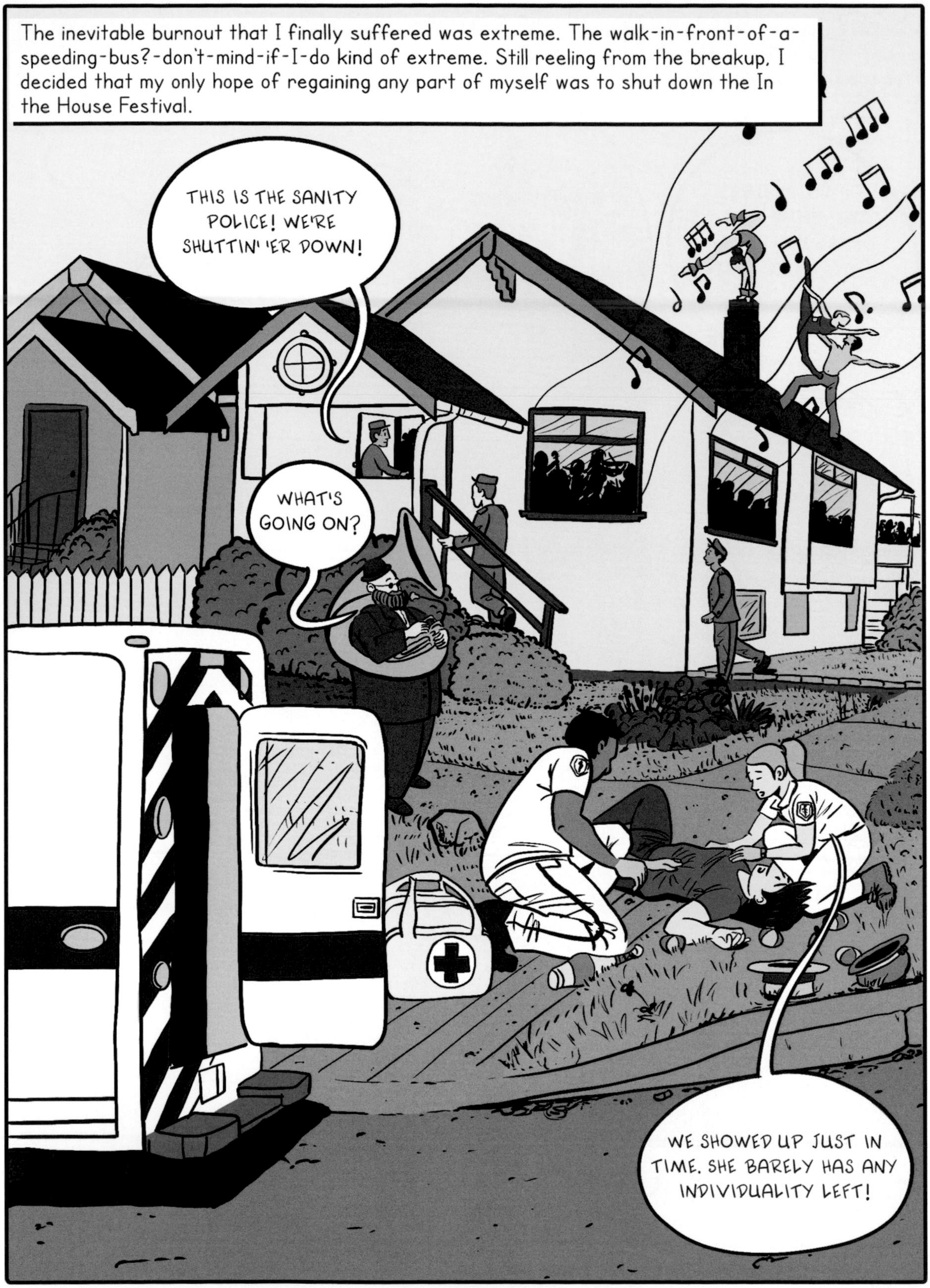
The inevitable burnout that I finally suffered was extreme. The walk-in-front-of-a-speeding-bus?-don't-mind-if-I-do kind of extreme. Still reeling from the breakup, I decided that my only hope of regaining any part of myself was to shut down the In the House Festival.
THIS IS THE SANITY POLICE! WE'RE SHUTTIN' 'ER DOWN!
WHAT'S GOING ON?
WE SHOWED UP JUST IN TIME. SHE BARELY HAS ANY INDIVIDUALITY LEFT!

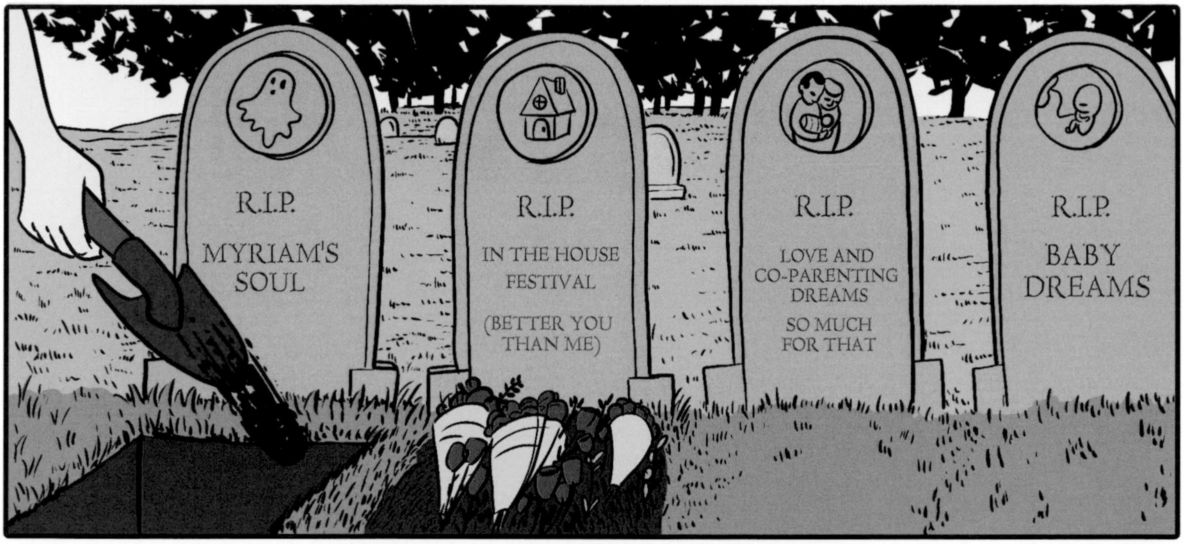
R.I.P.
MYRIAM'S SOUL
R.I.P.
IN THE HOUSE FESTIVAL
(BETTER YOU THAN ME)
R.I.P.
LOVE AND CO-PARENTING DREAMS
SO MUCH FOR THAT
R.I.P.
BABY DREAMS

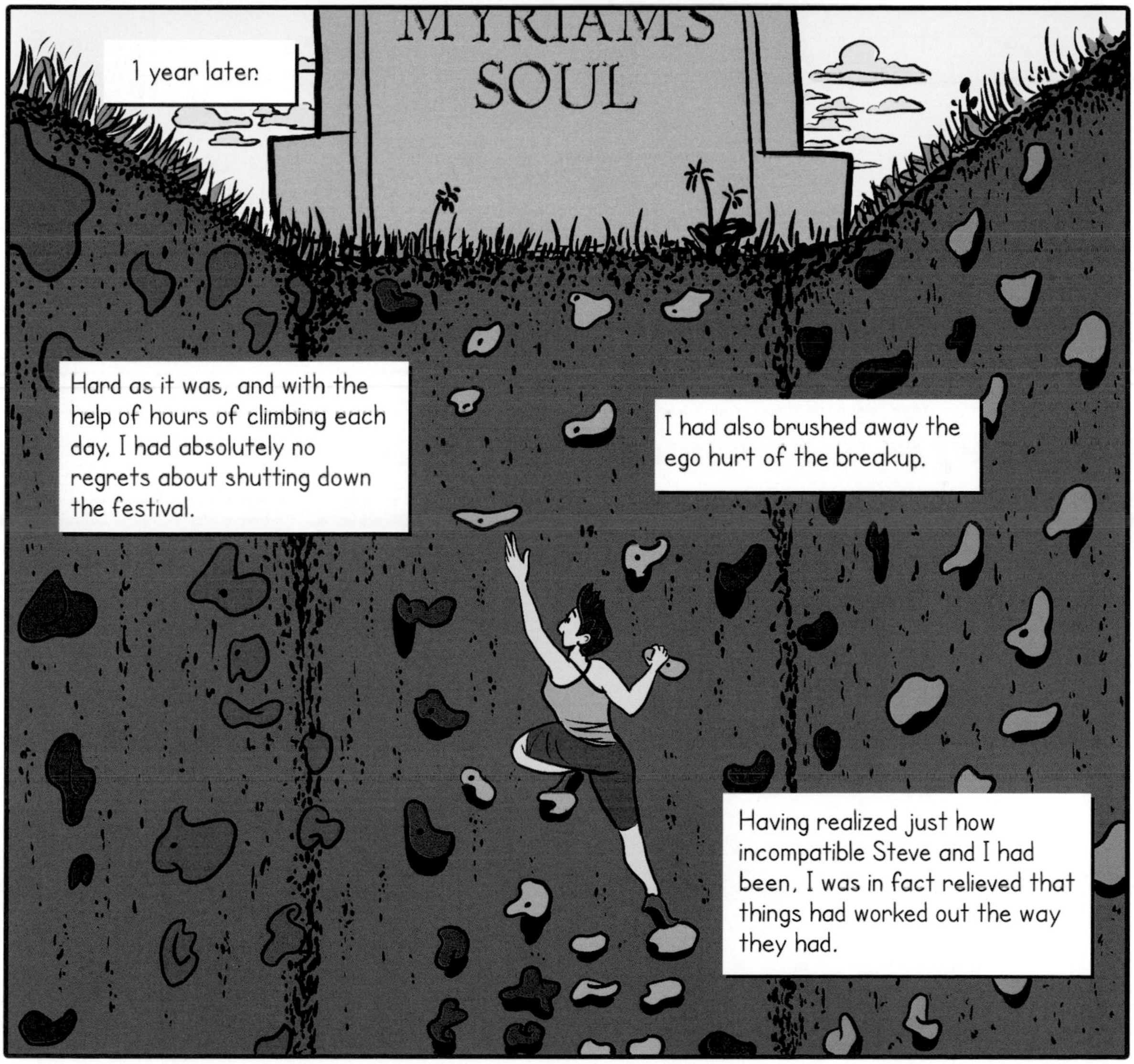
1 year later.
MYRIAM'S SOUL
Hard as it was, and with the help of hours of climbing each day, I had absolutely no regrets about shutting down the festival.
I had also brushed away the ego hurt of the breakup.
Having realized just how incompatible Steve and I had been, I was in fact relieved that things had worked out the way they had.

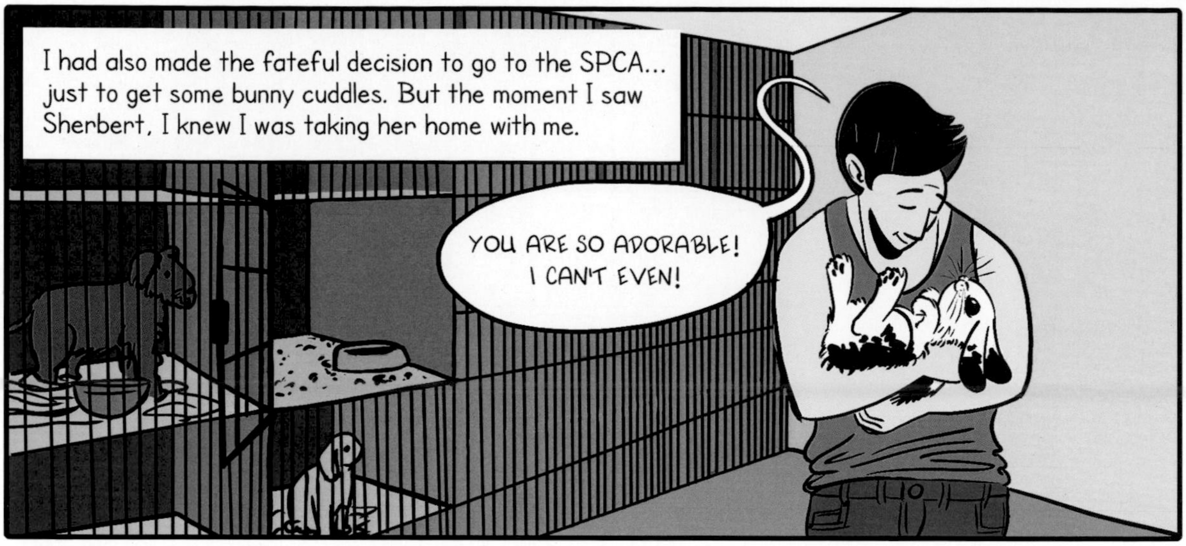
I had also made the fateful decision to go to the SPCA... just to get some bunny cuddles. But the moment I saw Sherbert, I knew I was taking her home with me.
YOU ARE SO ADORABLE! I CAN'T EVEN!

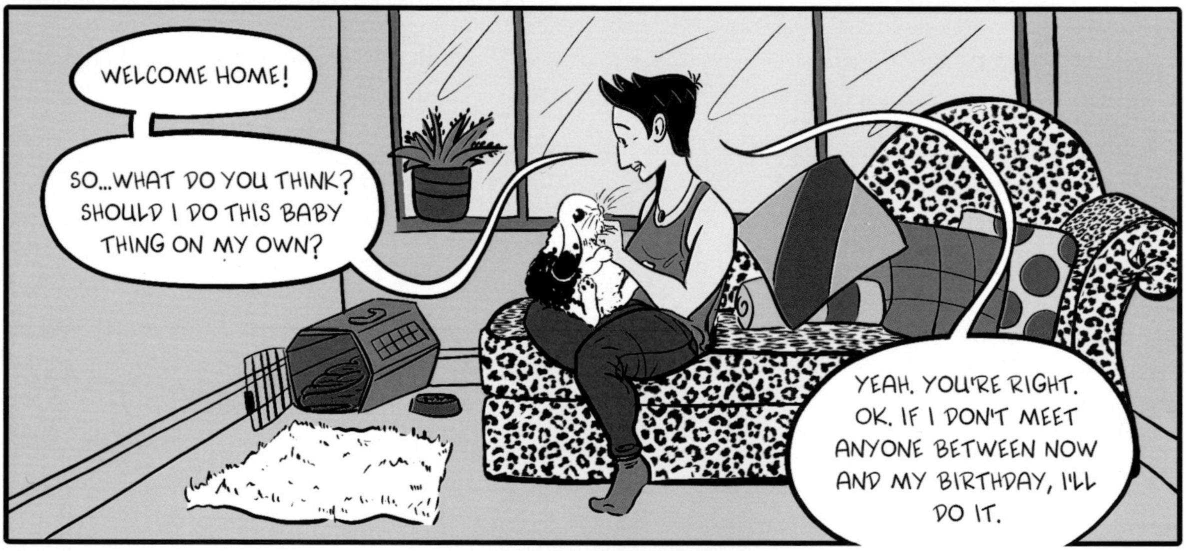
WELCOME HOME!
SO...WHAT DO YOU THINK? SHOULD I DO THIS BABY THING ON MY OWN?
YEAH. YOU'RE RIGHT. OK. IF I DON'T MEET ANYONE BETWEEN NOW AND MY BIRTHDAY, I'LL DO IT.

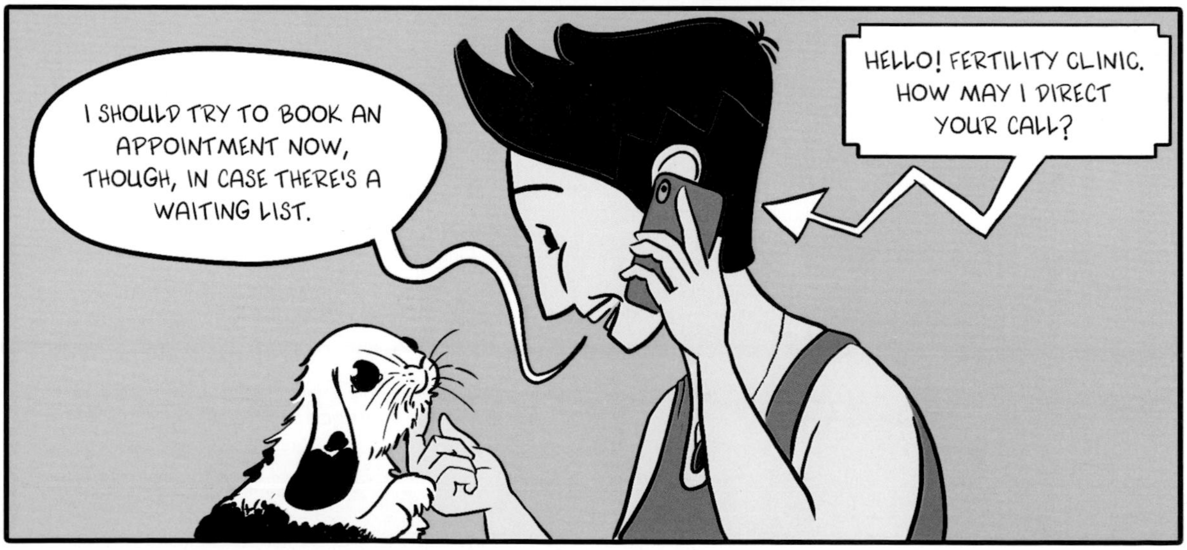
I SHOULD TRY TO BOOK AN APPOINTMENT NOW, THOUGH, IN CASE THERE'S A WAITING LIST.
HELLO! FERTILITY CLINIC. HOW MAY I DIRECT YOUR CALL?

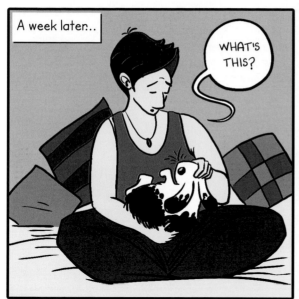

A week later...

WHAT'S THIS?

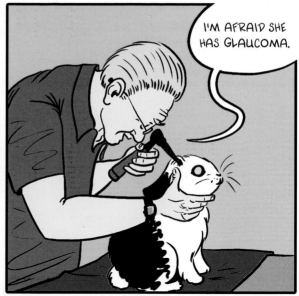

I'M AFRAID SHE HAS GLAUCOMA.

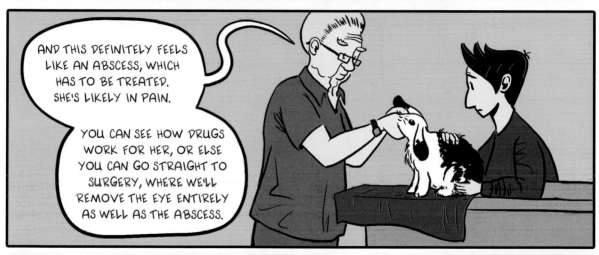

AND THIS DEFINITELY FEELS LIKE AN ABSCESS, WHICH HAS TO BE TREATED. SHE'S LIKELY IN PAIN.

YOU CAN SEE HOW DRUGS WORK FOR HER, OR ELSE YOU CAN GO STRAIGHT TO SURGERY, WHERE WE'LL REMOVE THE EYE ENTIRELY AS WELL AS THE ABSCESS.

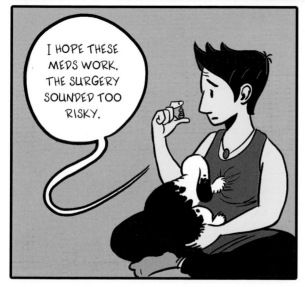

I HOPE THESE MEDS WORK. THE SURGERY SOUNDED TOO RISKY.

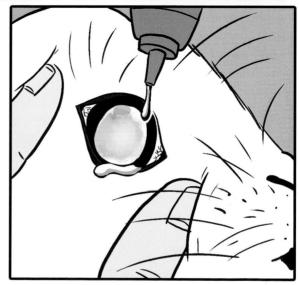

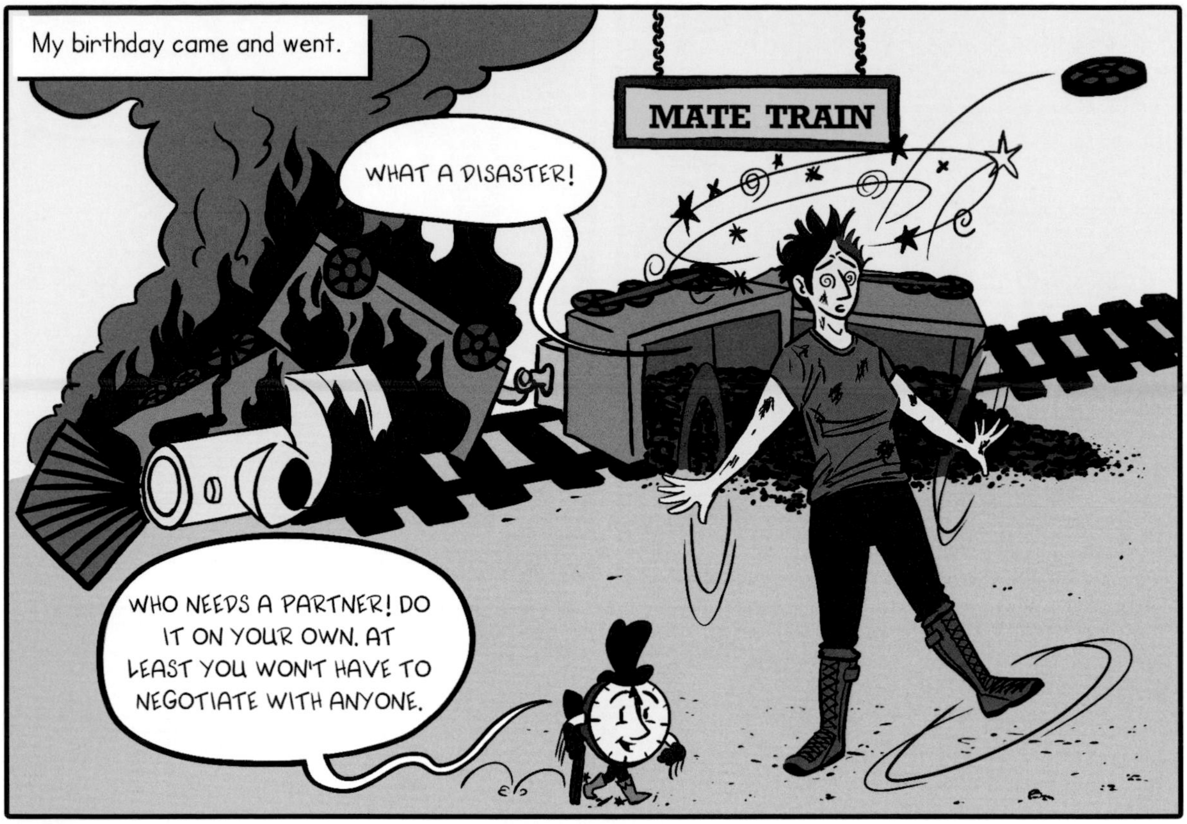
My birthday came and went.
MATE TRAIN
WHAT A DISASTER!
WHO NEEDS A PARTNER! DO IT ON YOUR OWN. AT LEAST YOU WON'T HAVE TO NEGOTIATE WITH ANYONE.

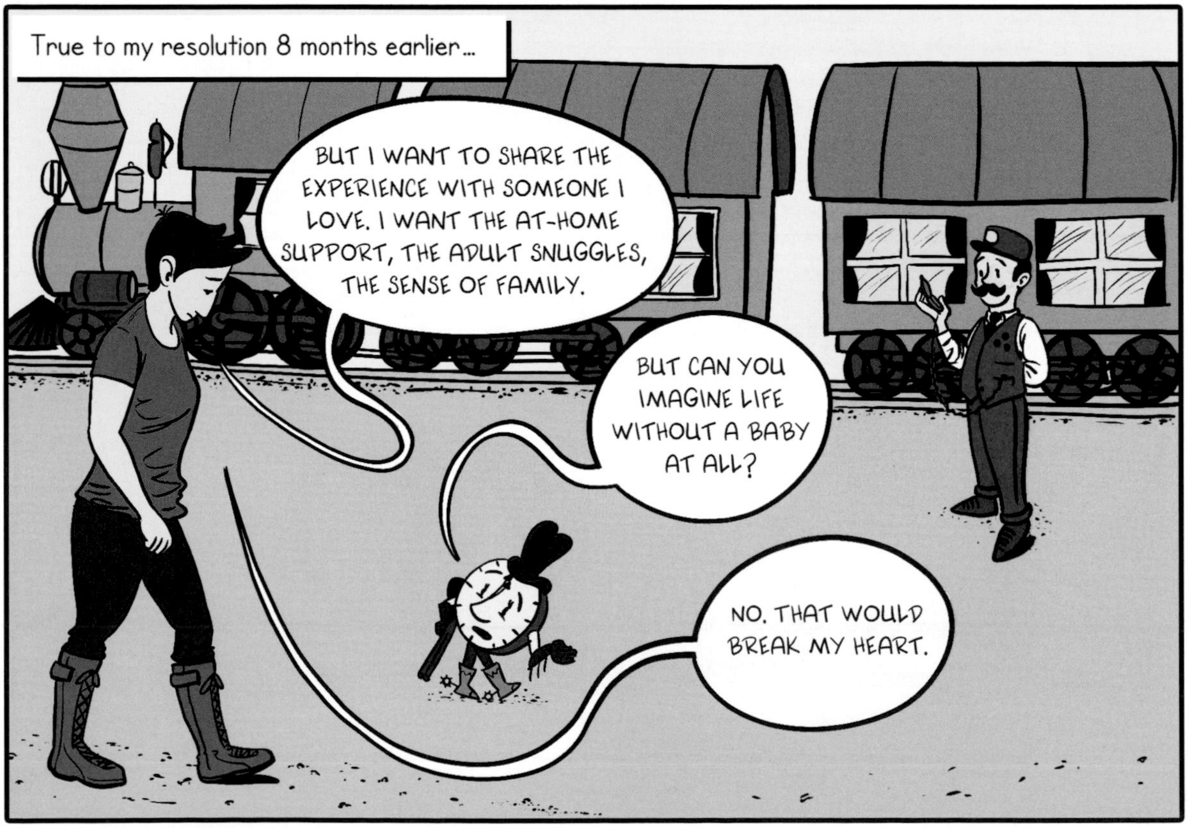
True to my resolution 8 months earlier...
BUT I WANT TO SHARE THE EXPERIENCE WITH SOMEONE I LOVE. I WANT THE AT-HOME SUPPORT, THE ADULT SNUGGLES, THE SENSE OF FAMILY.
BUT CAN YOU IMAGINE LIFE WITHOUT A BABY AT ALL?
NO. THAT WOULD BREAK MY HEART.

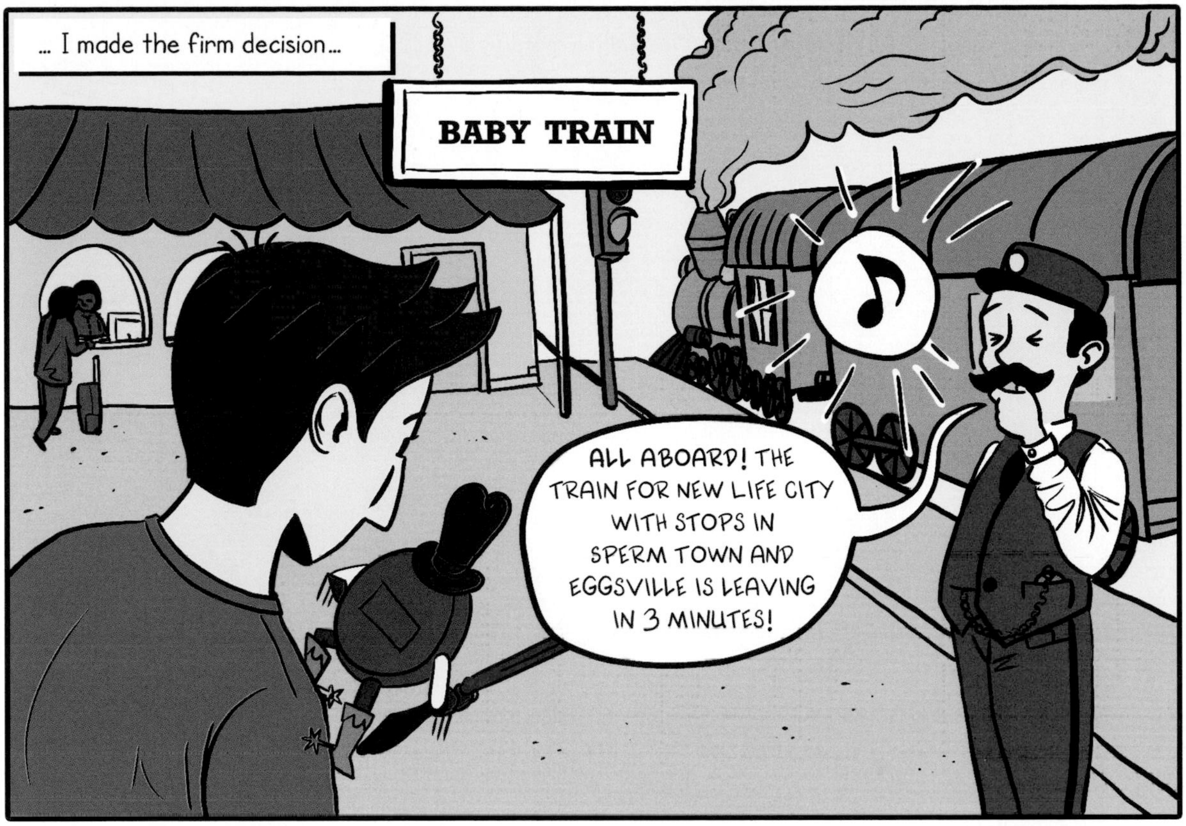
... I made the firm decision...
BABY TRAIN
ALL ABOARD! THE TRAIN FOR NEW LIFE CITY WITH STOPS IN SPERM TOWN AND EGGSVILLE IS LEAVING IN 3 MINUTES!

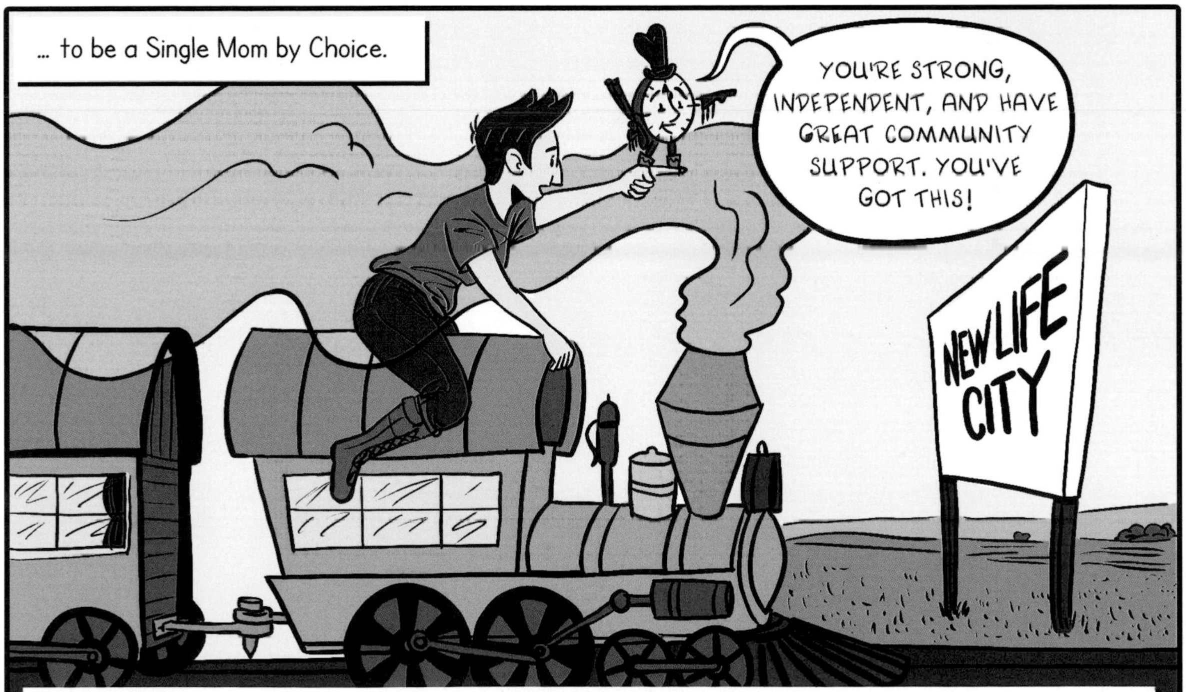
... to be a Single Mom by Choice.
YOU'RE STRONG, INDEPENDENT, AND HAVE GREAT COMMUNITY SUPPORT. YOU'VE GOT THIS!
NEW LIFE CITY
I was sad that my family life would be so vastly different from my fantasy of it, but I was also relieved to be proactive about the one life-changing event that had a rapidly approaching expiration date.

YEAR TWO

MAY 2O15–JULY 2O16

Turkey Basting

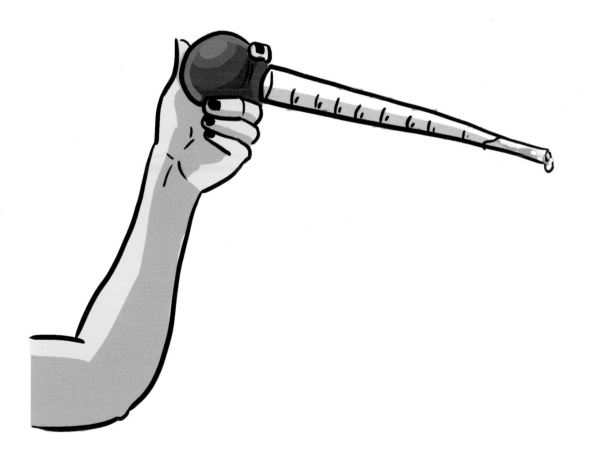

Chapter 1

Dahlia

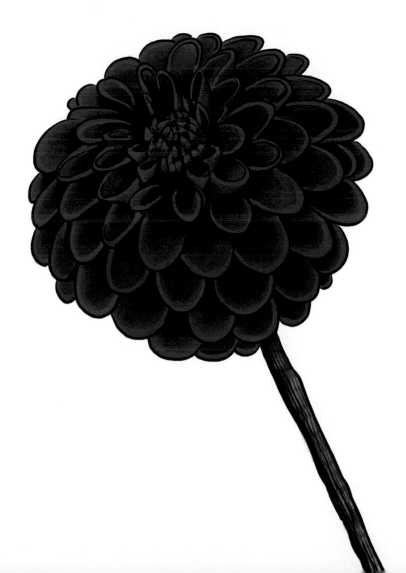

Once set in my decision, I saw no reason to keep it a secret.

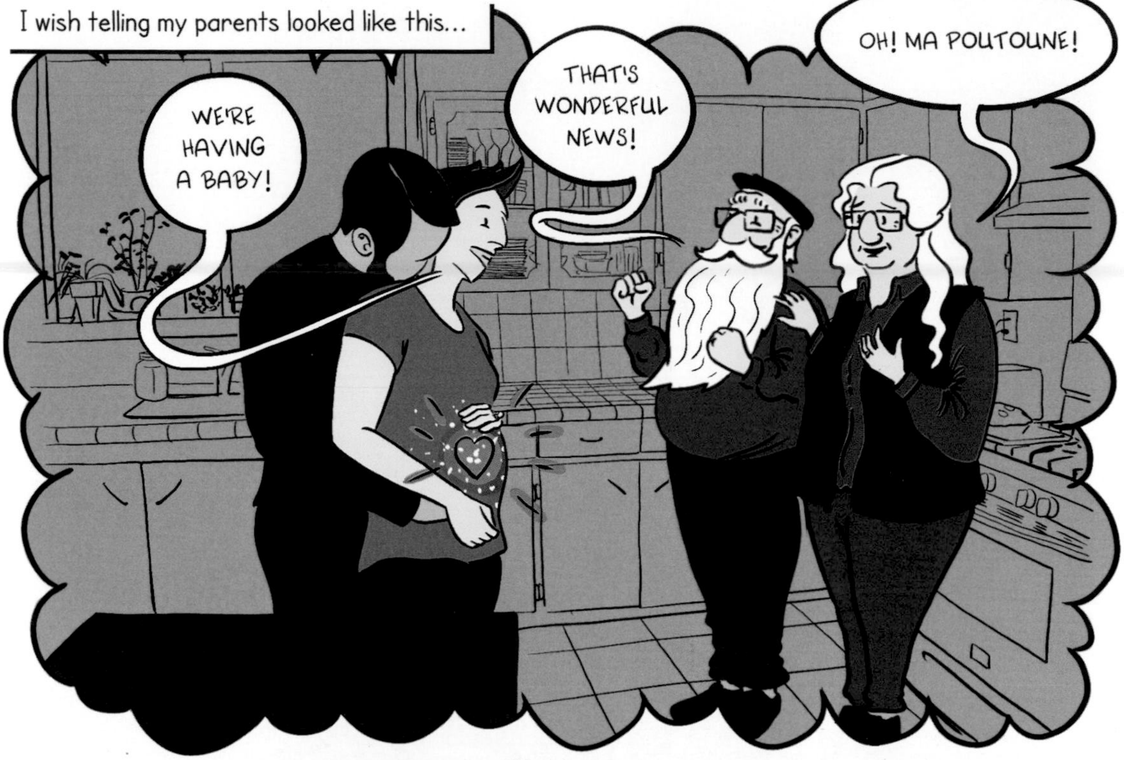
I wish telling my parents looked like this...
WE'RE HAVING A BABY!
THAT'S WONDERFUL NEWS!
OH! MA POUTOUNE!

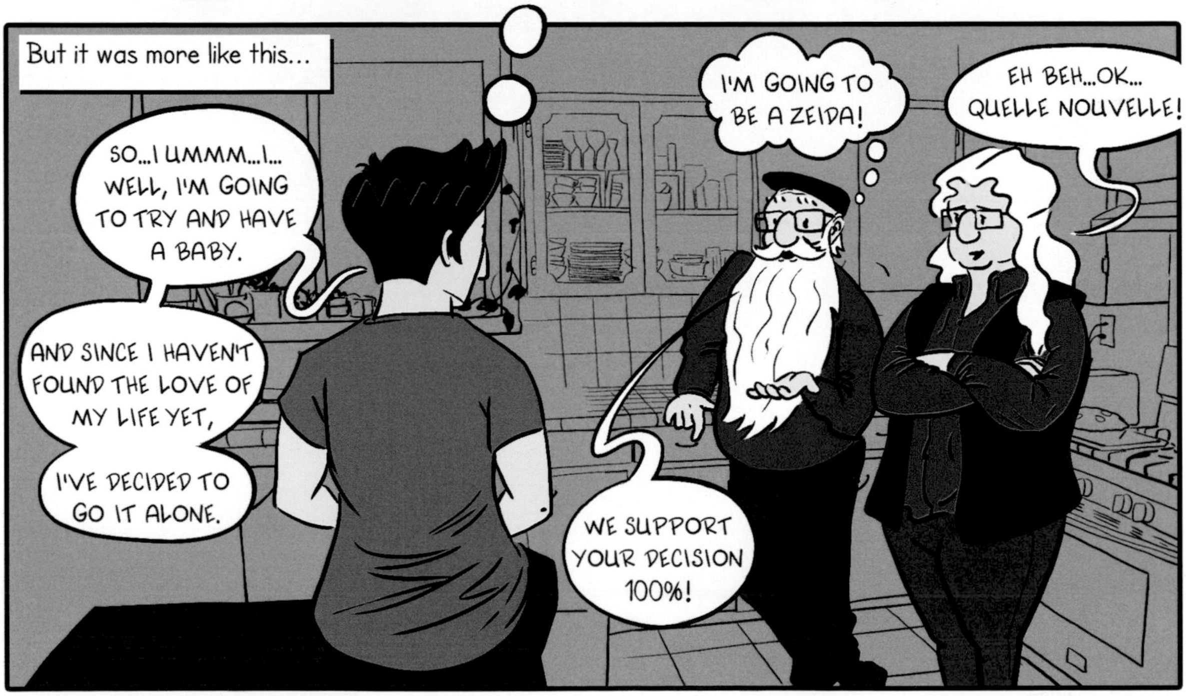
But it was more like this...
SO...I UMMM...I... WELL, I'M GOING TO TRY AND HAVE A BABY.
AND SINCE I HAVEN'T FOUND THE LOVE OF MY LIFE YET,
I'VE DECIDED TO GO IT ALONE.
I'M GOING TO BE A ZEIDA!
EH BEH...OK... QUELLE NOUVELLE!
WE SUPPORT YOUR DECISION 100%!

Knowing that I had the backing of the people close to me made everything a smidge less daunting.

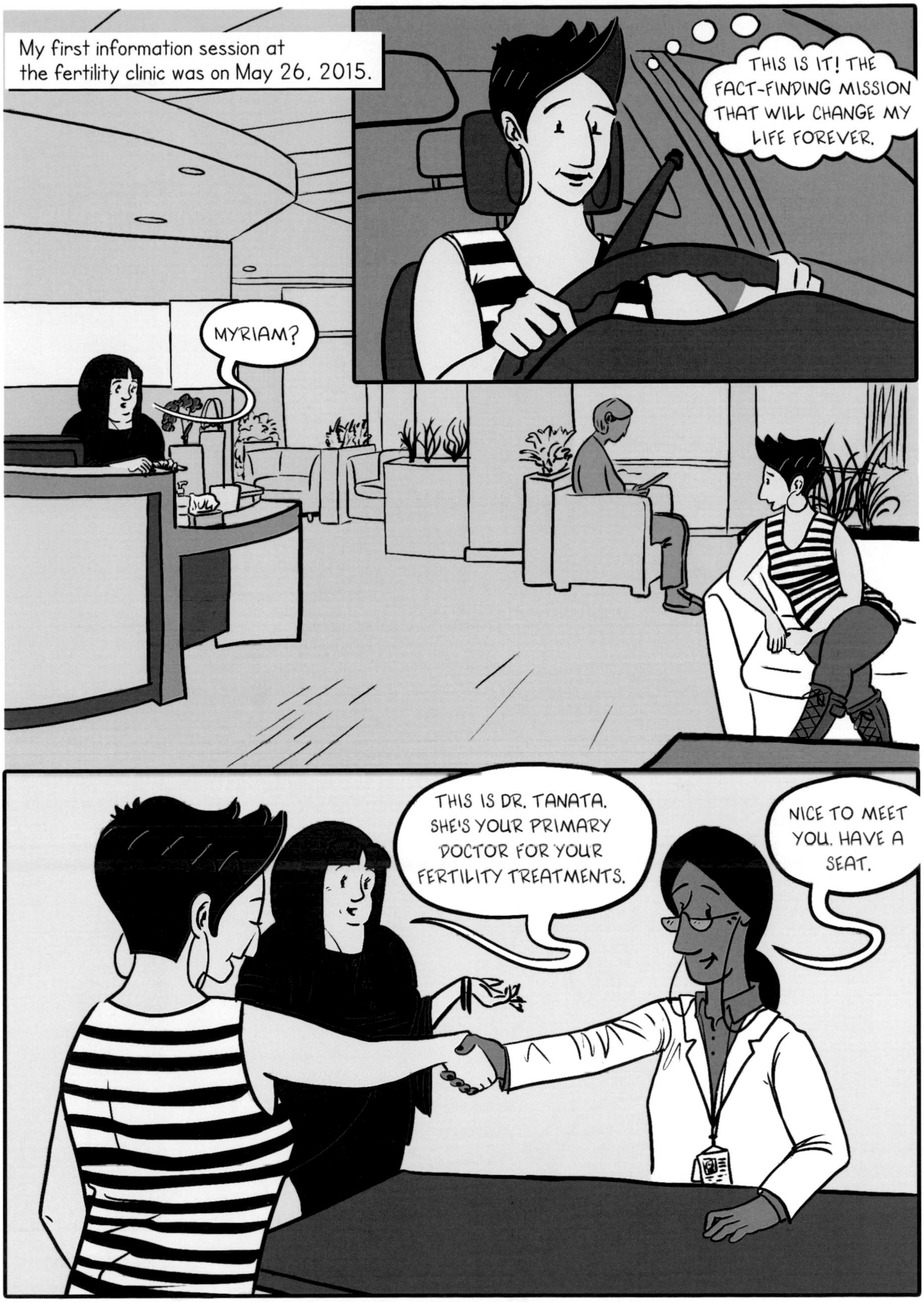
My first information session at the fertility clinic was on May 26, 2015.
THIS IS IT! THE FACT-FINDING MISSION THAT WILL CHANGE MY LIFE FOREVER.
MYRIAM?
THIS IS DR. TANATA. SHE'S YOUR PRIMARY DOCTOR FOR YOUR FERTILITY TREATMENTS.
NICE TO MEET YOU. HAVE A SEAT.

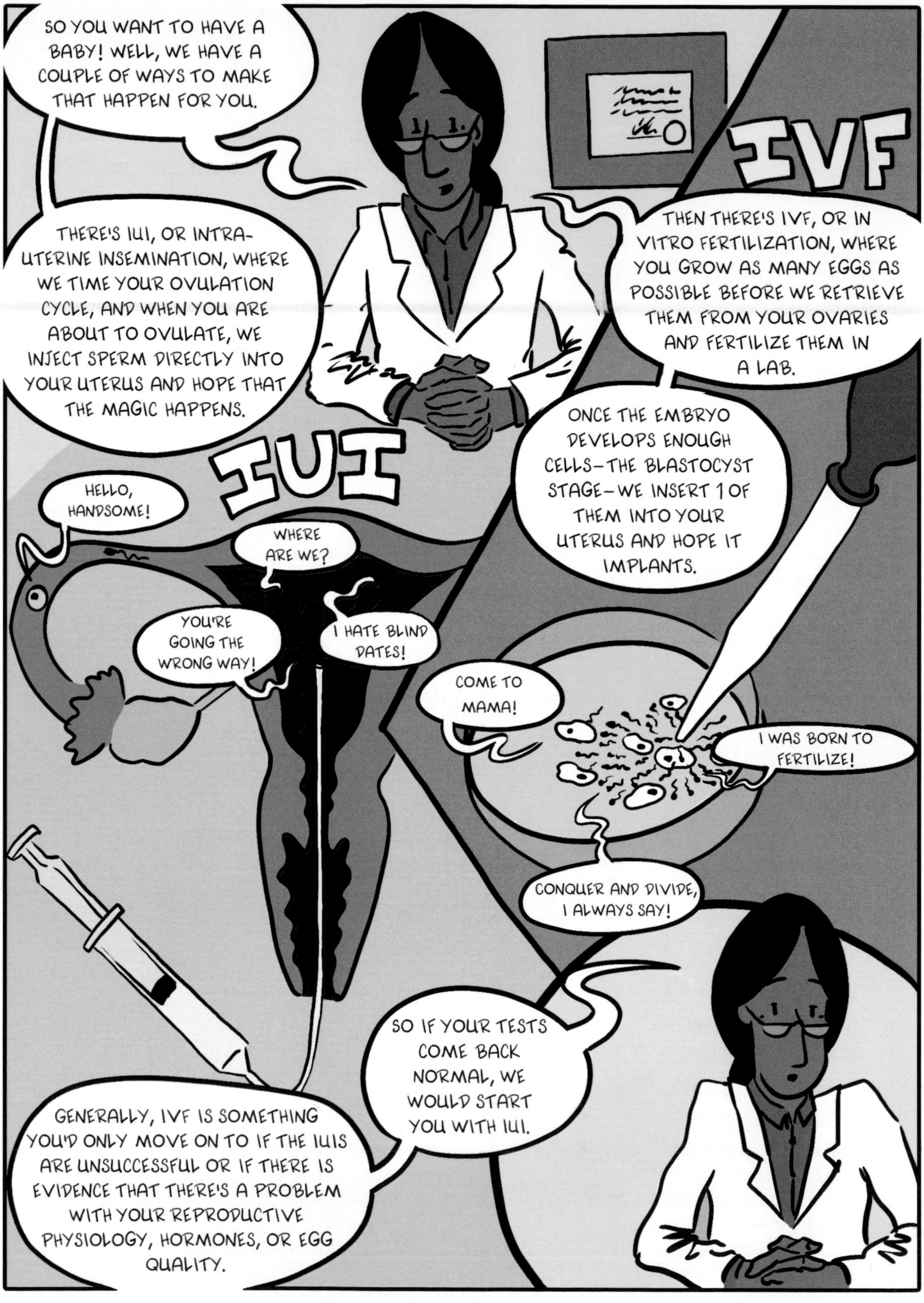

SO YOU WANT TO HAVE A BABY! WELL, WE HAVE A COUPLE OF WAYS TO MAKE THAT HAPPEN FOR YOU.
THERE'S IUI, OR INTRA-UTERINE INSEMINATION, WHERE WE TIME YOUR OVULATION CYCLE, AND WHEN YOU ARE ABOUT TO OVULATE, WE INJECT SPERM DIRECTLY INTO YOUR UTERUS AND HOPE THAT THE MAGIC HAPPENS.
IUI
HELLO, HANDSOME!
WHERE ARE WE?
YOU'RE GOING THE WRONG WAY!
I HATE BLIND DATES!
IVF
THEN THERE'S IVF, OR IN VITRO FERTILIZATION, WHERE YOU GROW AS MANY EGGS AS POSSIBLE BEFORE WE RETRIEVE THEM FROM YOUR OVARIES AND FERTILIZE THEM IN A LAB.
ONCE THE EMBRYO DEVELOPS ENOUGH CELLS—THE BLASTOCYST STAGE—WE INSERT 1 OF THEM INTO YOUR UTERUS AND HOPE IT IMPLANTS.
COME TO MAMA!
I WAS BORN TO FERTILIZE!
CONQUER AND DIVIDE, I ALWAYS SAY!
SO IF YOUR TESTS COME BACK NORMAL, WE WOULD START YOU WITH IUI.
GENERALLY, IVF IS SOMETHING YOU'D ONLY MOVE ON TO IF THE IUIS ARE UNSUCCESSFUL OR IF THERE IS EVIDENCE THAT THERE'S A PROBLEM WITH YOUR REPRODUCTIVE PHYSIOLOGY, HORMONES, OR EGG QUALITY.

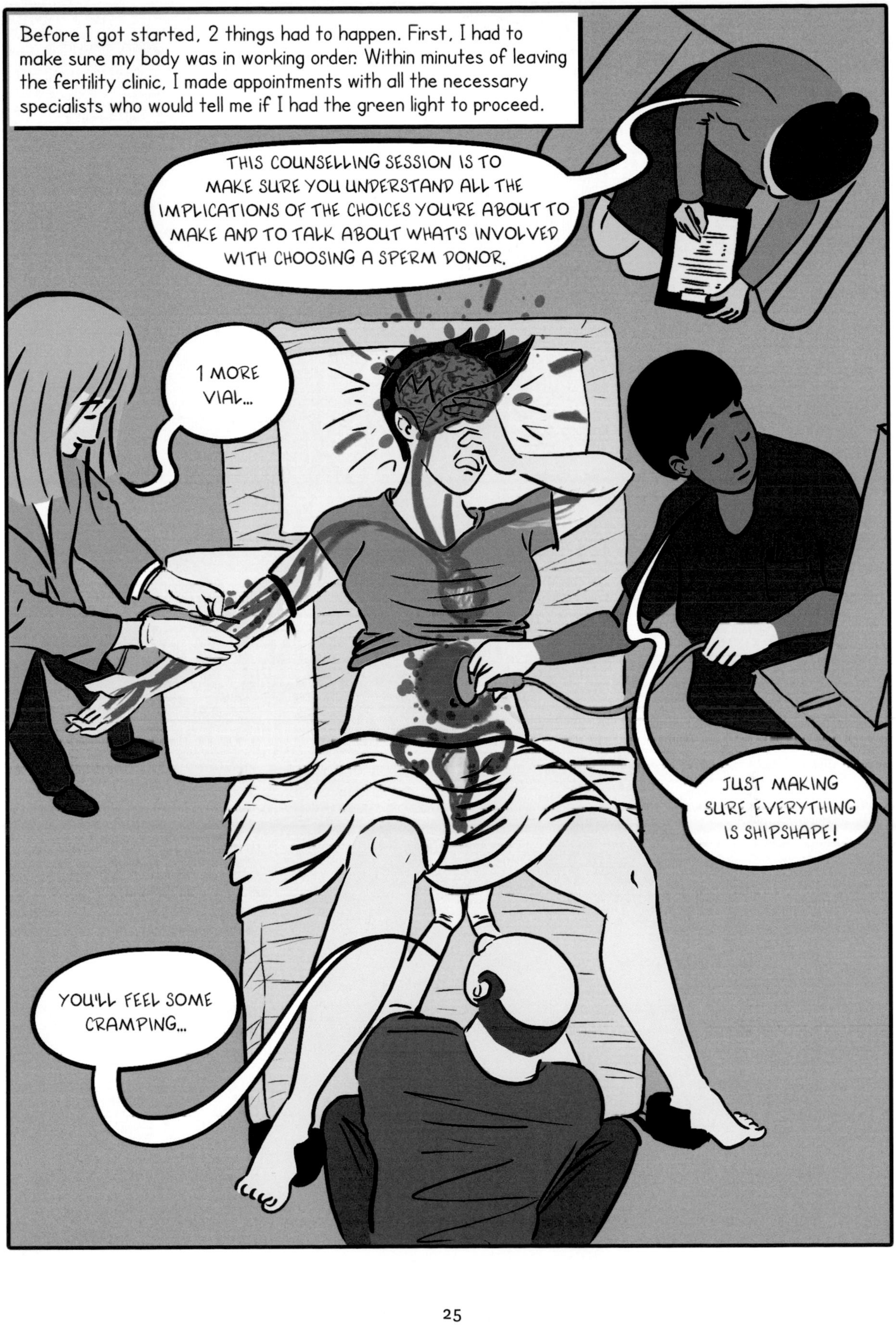
Before I got started, 2 things had to happen. First, I had to make sure my body was in working order. Within minutes of leaving the fertility clinic, I made appointments with all the necessary specialists who would tell me if I had the green light to proceed.
THIS COUNSELLING SESSION IS TO MAKE SURE YOU UNDERSTAND ALL THE IMPLICATIONS OF THE CHOICES YOU'RE ABOUT TO MAKE AND TO TALK ABOUT WHAT'S INVOLVED WITH CHOOSING A SPERM DONOR.
1 MORE VIAL...
JUST MAKING SURE EVERYTHING IS SHIPSHAPE!
YOU'LL FEEL SOME CRAMPING...

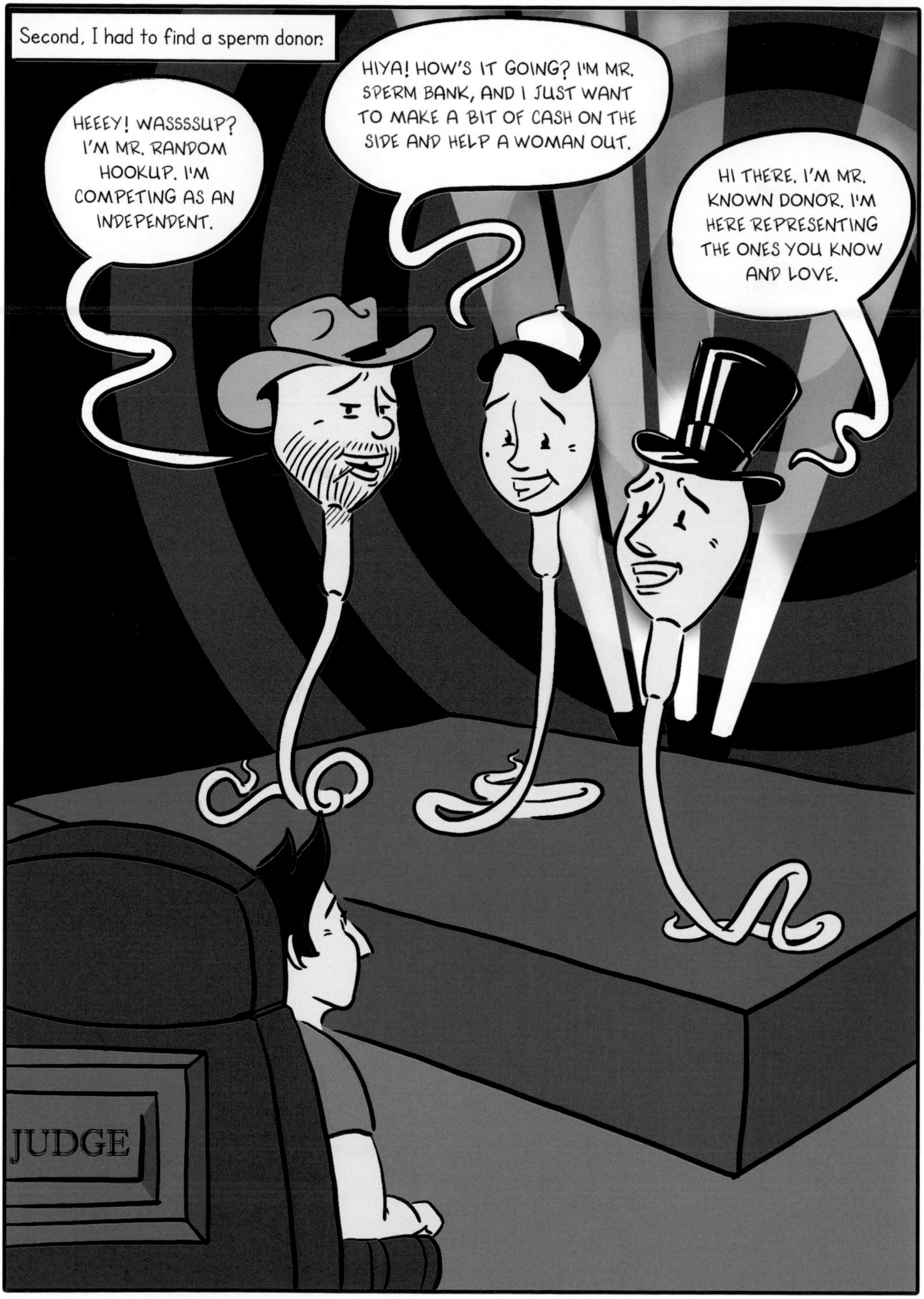
Second, I had to find a sperm donor.
HEEEY! WASSSSUP? I'M MR. RANDOM HOOKUP. I'M COMPETING AS AN INDEPENDENT.
HIYA! HOW'S IT GOING? I'M MR. SPERM BANK, AND I JUST WANT TO MAKE A BIT OF CASH ON THE SIDE AND HELP A WOMAN OUT.
HI THERE. I'M MR. KNOWN DONOR. I'M HERE REPRESENTING THE ONES YOU KNOW AND LOVE.
JUDGE

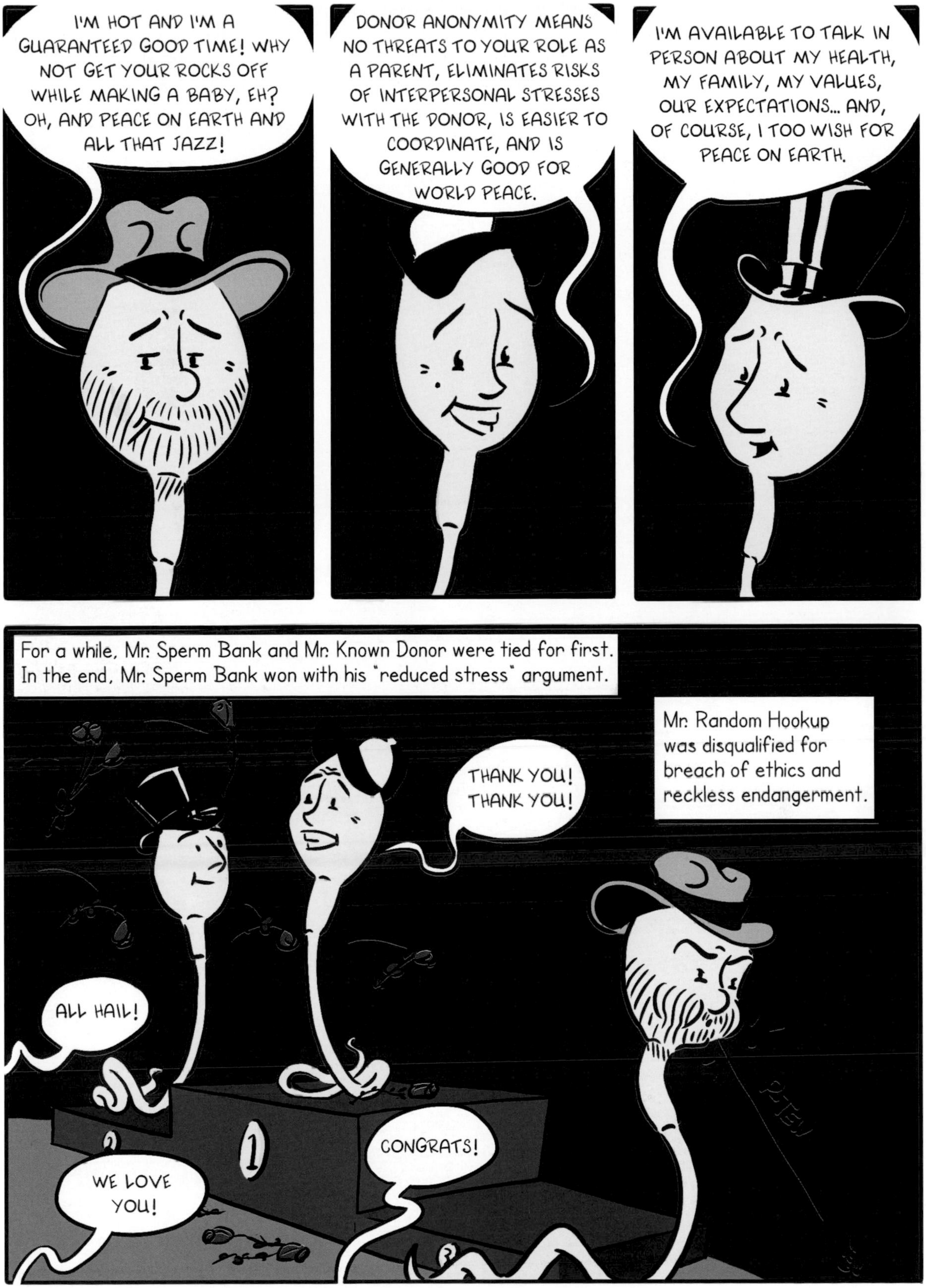

I'M HOT AND I'M A GUARANTEED GOOD TIME! WHY NOT GET YOUR ROCKS OFF WHILE MAKING A BABY, EH? OH, AND PEACE ON EARTH AND ALL THAT JAZZ!
DONOR ANONYMITY MEANS NO THREATS TO YOUR ROLE AS A PARENT, ELIMINATES RISKS OF INTERPERSONAL STRESSES WITH THE DONOR, IS EASIER TO COORDINATE, AND IS GENERALLY GOOD FOR WORLD PEACE.
I'M AVAILABLE TO TALK IN PERSON ABOUT MY HEALTH, MY FAMILY, MY VALUES, OUR EXPECTATIONS... AND, OF COURSE, I TOO WISH FOR PEACE ON EARTH.
For a while, Mr. Sperm Bank and Mr. Known Donor were tied for first. In the end, Mr. Sperm Bank won with his "reduced stress" argument.
Mr. Random Hookup was disqualified for breach of ethics and reckless endangerment.
THANK YOU! THANK YOU!
ALL HAIL!
CONGRATS!
WE LOVE YOU!

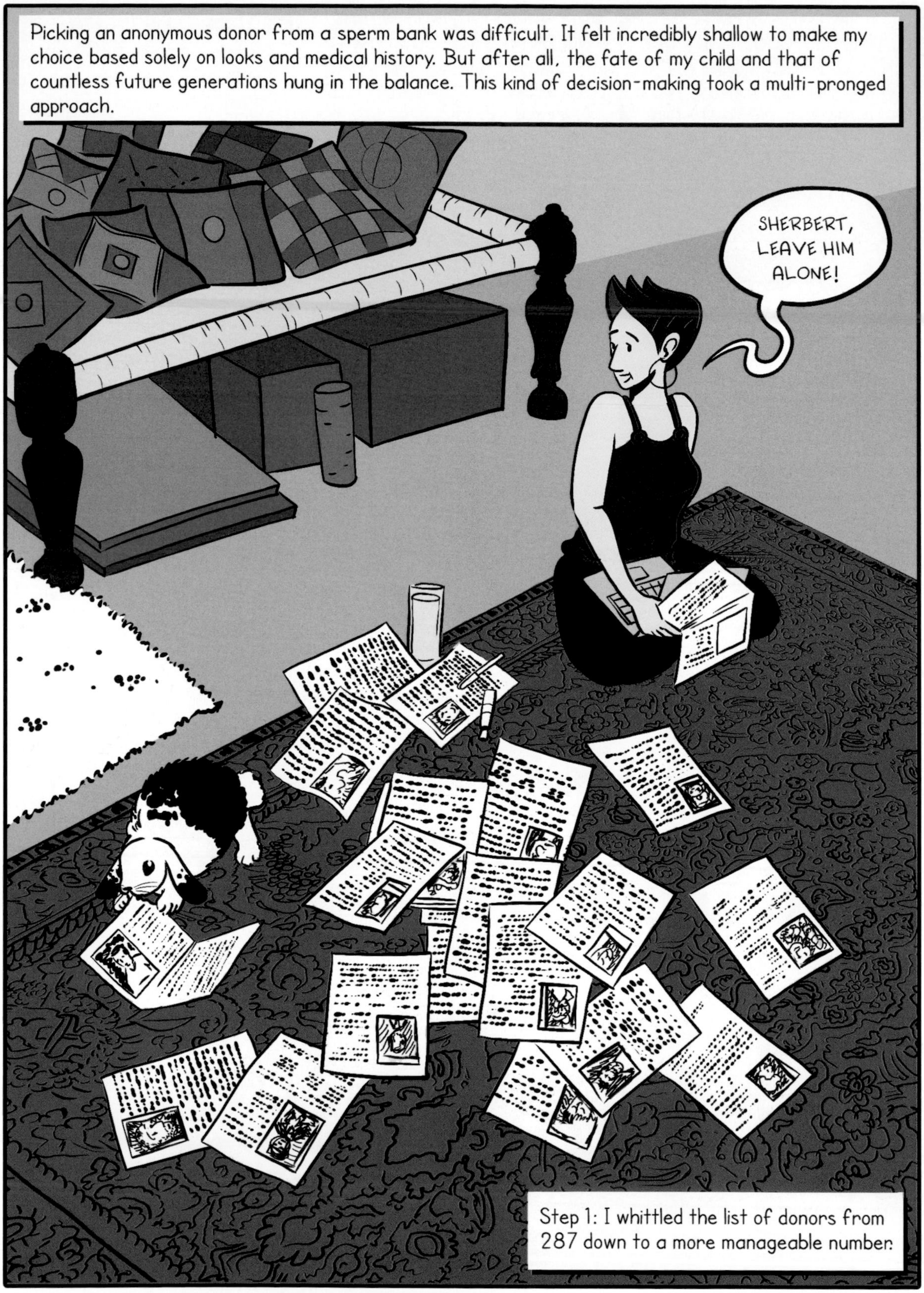
Picking an anonymous donor from a sperm bank was difficult. It felt incredibly shallow to make my choice based solely on looks and medical history. But after all, the fate of my child and that of countless future generations hung in the balance. This kind of decision-making took a multi-pronged approach.
SHERBERT, LEAVE HIM ALONE!
Step 1: I whittled the list of donors from 287 down to a more manageable number.

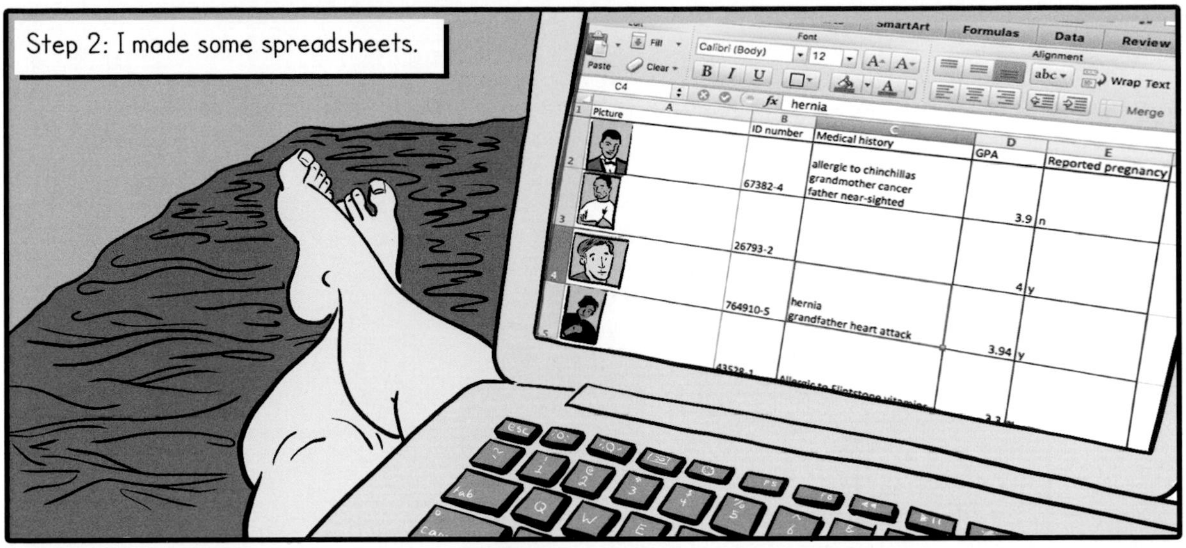
Step 2: I made some spreadsheets.
Formulas
Data
Review
Paste
Fill
Clear
Calibri (Body)
12
Wrap Text
Merge
C4
hernia
Picture
ID number
Medical history
GPA
Reported pregnancy
67382-4
allergic to chinchillas
grandmother cancer
father near-sighted
3.9 n
26793-2
4 y
764910-5
hernia
grandfather heart attack
3.94 y

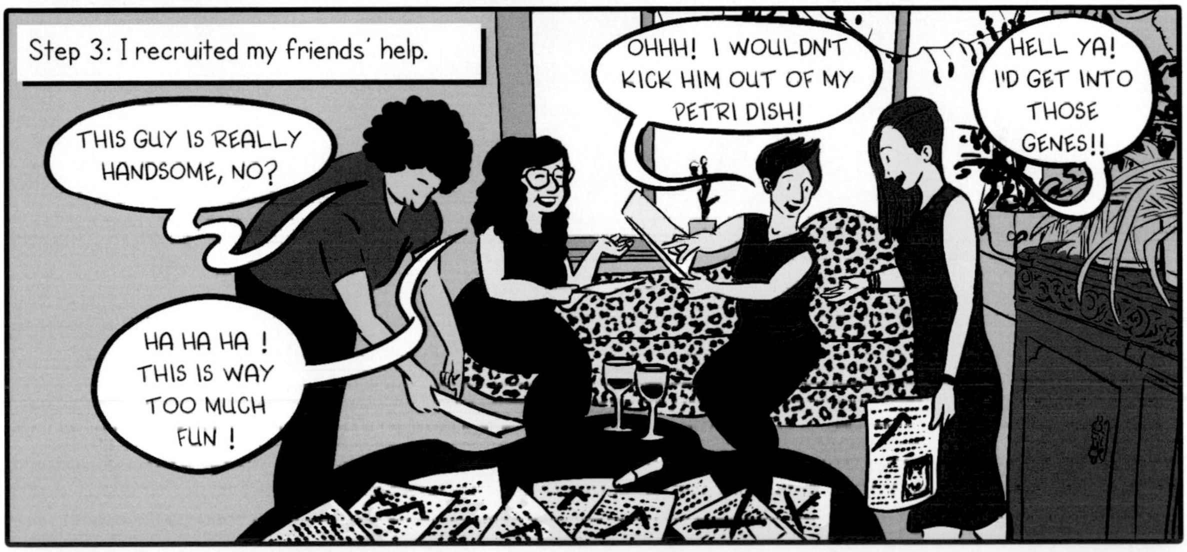
Step 3: I recruited my friends' help.
THIS GUY IS REALLY HANDSOME, NO?
HA HA HA ! THIS IS WAY TOO MUCH FUN !
OHHH! I WOULDN'T KICK HIM OUT OF MY PETRI DISH!
HELL YA! I'D GET INTO THOSE GENES!!

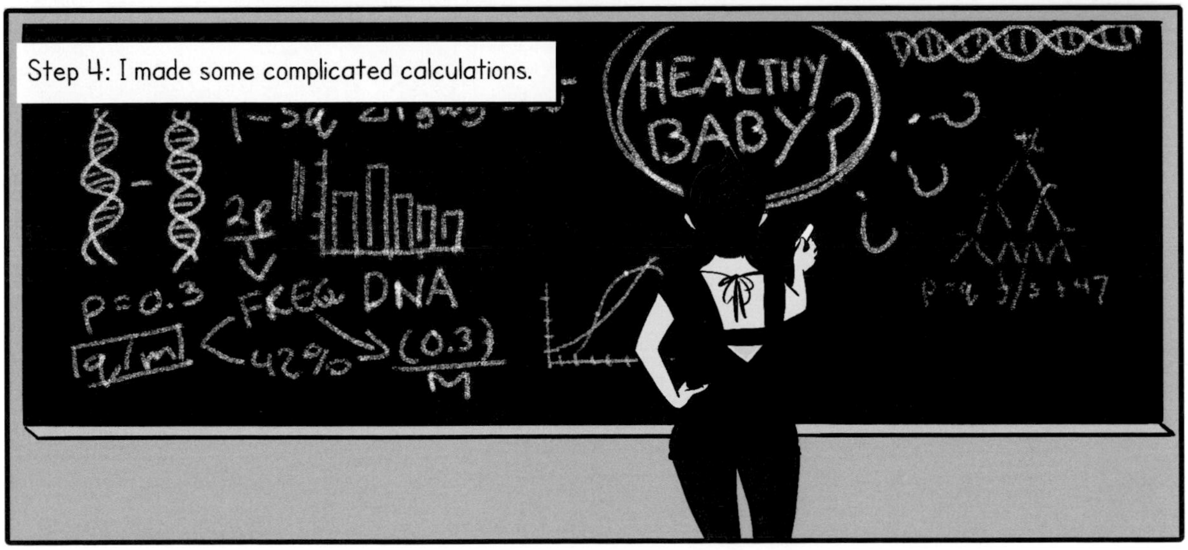
Step 4: I made some complicated calculations.
HEALTHY BABY?
P=0.3
FREQ DNA
42%
(0.3)
M

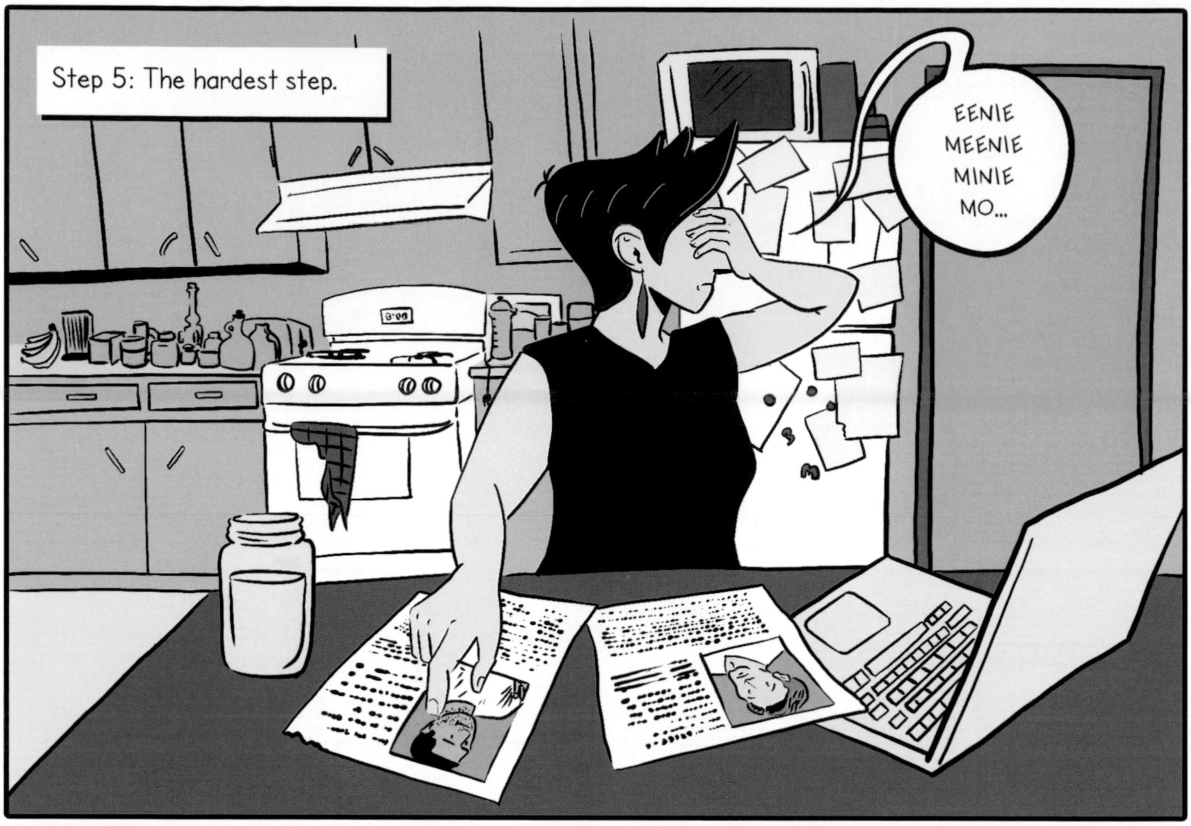
Step 5: The hardest step.
EENIE MEENIE MINIE MO...

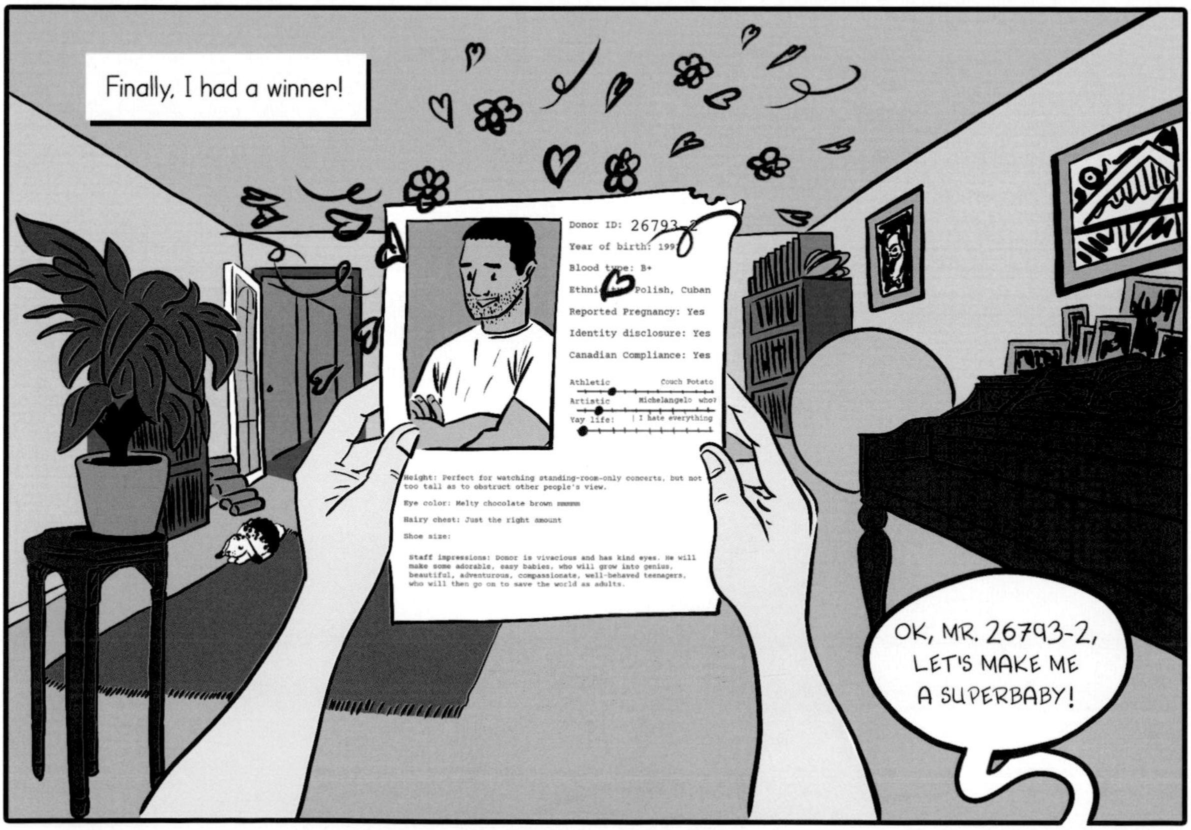
Finally, I had a winner!
Donor ID: 26793
Year of birth: 199
Blood type: B+
Polish, Cuban
Reported Pregnancy: Yes
Identity disclosure: Yes
Canadian Compliance: Yes
Athletic Couch Potato
Artistic Michelangelo who?
Yay life! I hate everything
Height: Perfect for watching standing-room-only concerts, but not too tall as to obstruct other people's view.
Eye color: Melty chocolate brown mmmmm
Hairy chest: Just the right amount
Shoe size:
Staff impressions: Donor is vivacious and has kind eyes. He will make some adorable, easy babies, who will grow into genius, beautiful, adventurous, compassionate, well-behaved teenagers, who will then go on to save the world as adults.
OK, MR. 26793-2, LET'S MAKE ME A SUPERBABY!

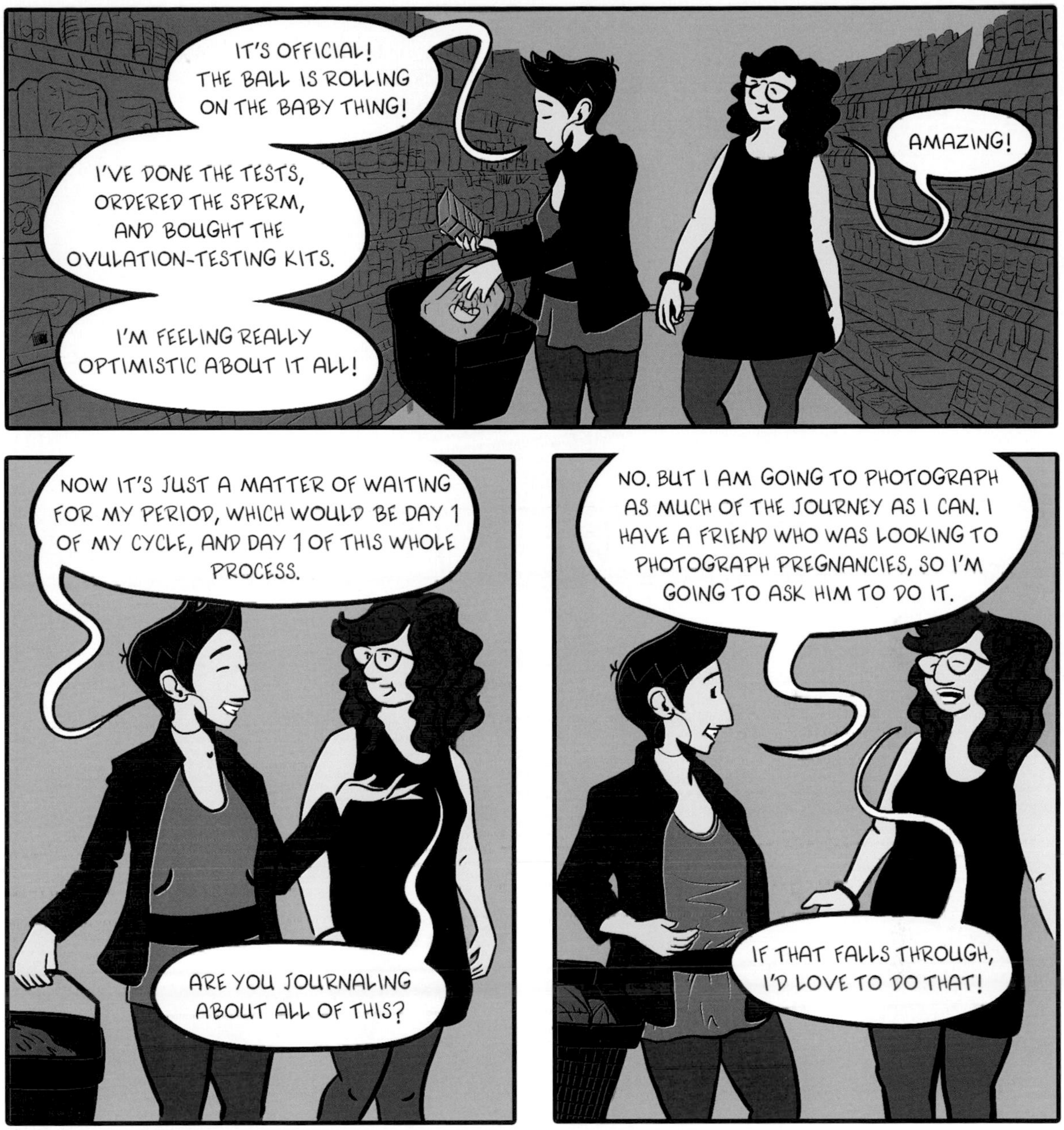
IT'S OFFICIAL! THE BALL IS ROLLING ON THE BABY THING!
I'VE DONE THE TESTS, ORDERED THE SPERM, AND BOUGHT THE OVULATION-TESTING KITS.
I'M FEELING REALLY OPTIMISTIC ABOUT IT ALL!
AMAZING!
NOW IT'S JUST A MATTER OF WAITING FOR MY PERIOD, WHICH WOULD BE DAY 1 OF MY CYCLE, AND DAY 1 OF THIS WHOLE PROCESS.
ARE YOU JOURNALING ABOUT ALL OF THIS?
NO. BUT I AM GOING TO PHOTOGRAPH AS MUCH OF THE JOURNEY AS I CAN. I HAVE A FRIEND WHO WAS LOOKING TO PHOTOGRAPH PREGNANCIES, SO I'M GOING TO ASK HIM TO DO IT.
IF THAT FALLS THROUGH, I'D LOVE TO DO THAT!

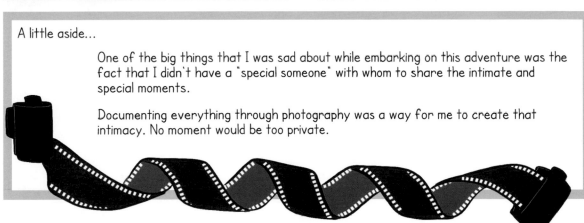

A little aside…

One of the big things that I was sad about while embarking on this adventure was the fact that I didn't have a "special someone" with whom to share the intimate and special moments.

Documenting everything through photography was a way for me to create that intimacy. No moment would be too private.

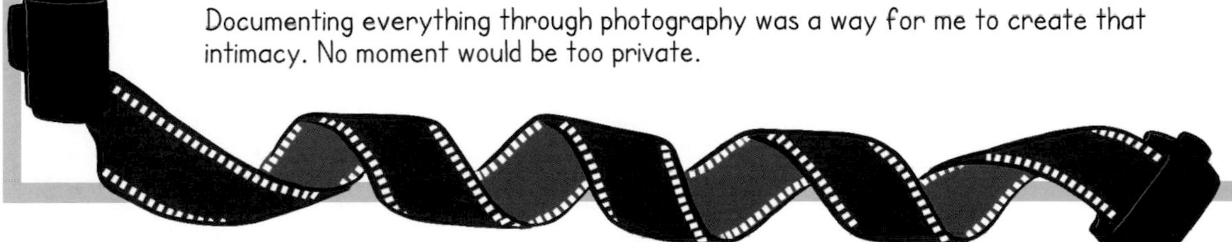

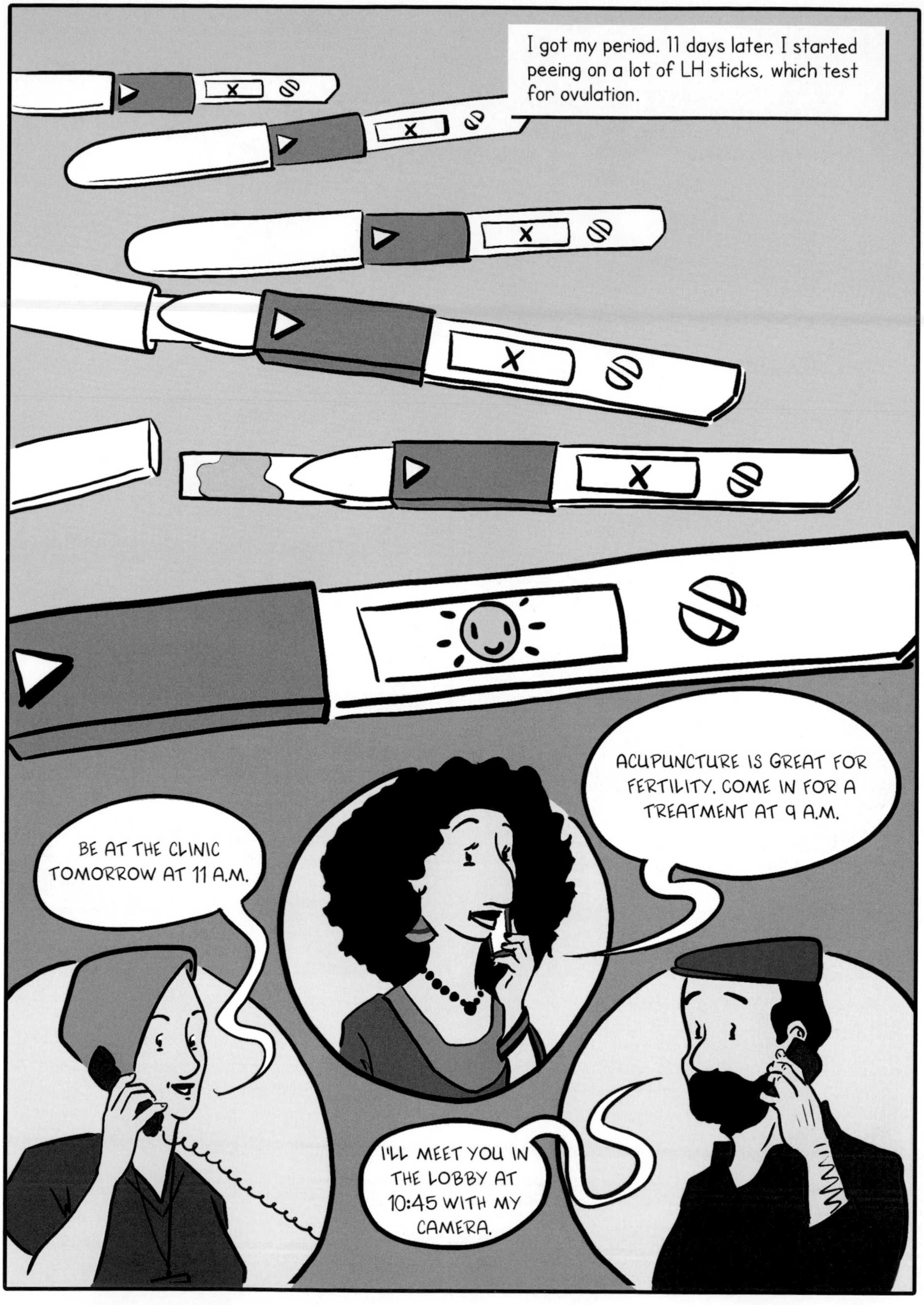
I got my period. 11 days later, I started peeing on a lot of LH sticks, which test for ovulation.
BE AT THE CLINIC TOMORROW AT 11 A.M.
ACUPUNCTURE IS GREAT FOR FERTILITY. COME IN FOR A TREATMENT AT 9 A.M.
I'LL MEET YOU IN THE LOBBY AT 10:45 WITH MY CAMERA.

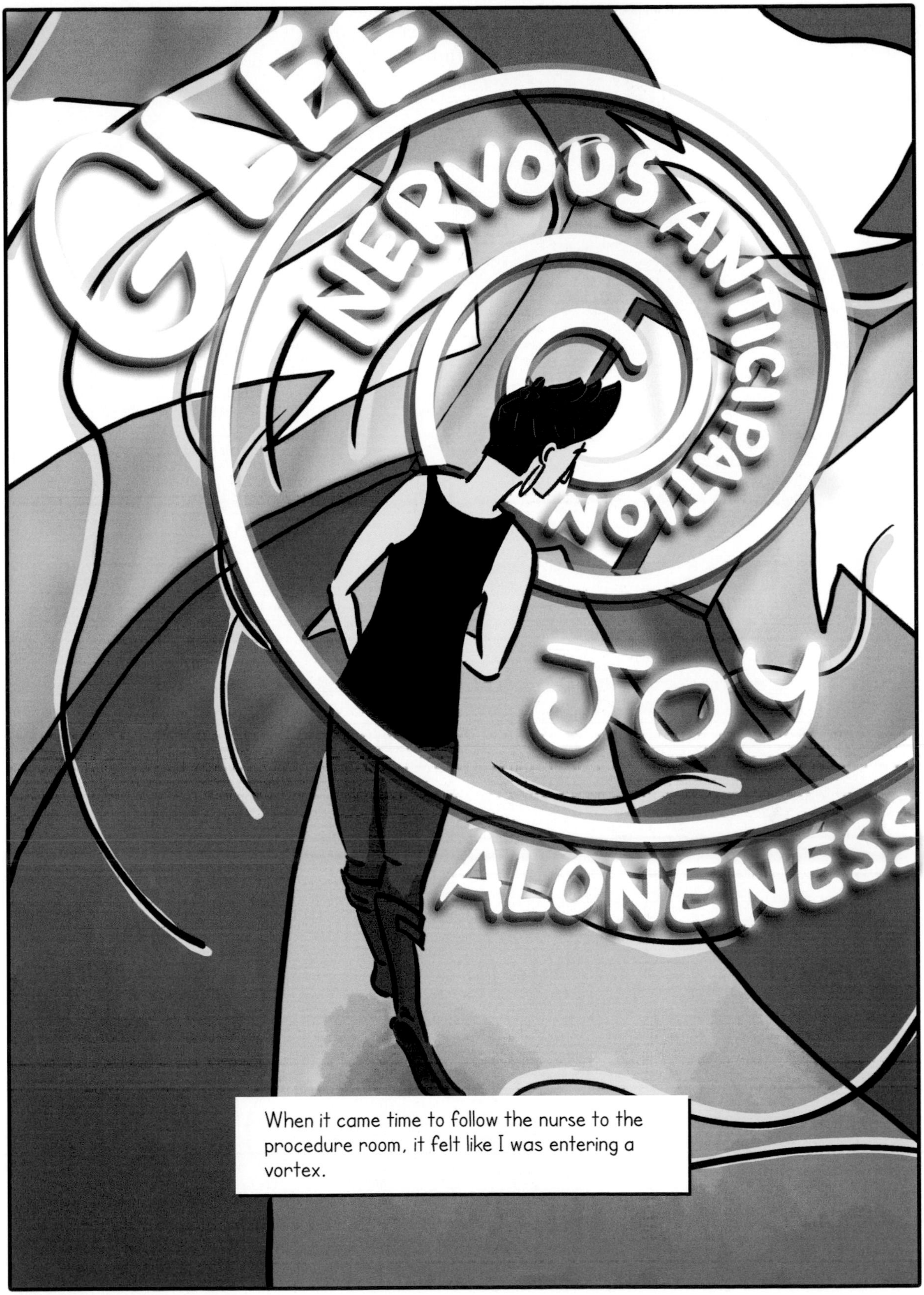
GLEE
NERVOUS ANTICIPATION
JOY
ALONENESS
When it came time to follow the nurse to the procedure room, it felt like I was entering a vortex.

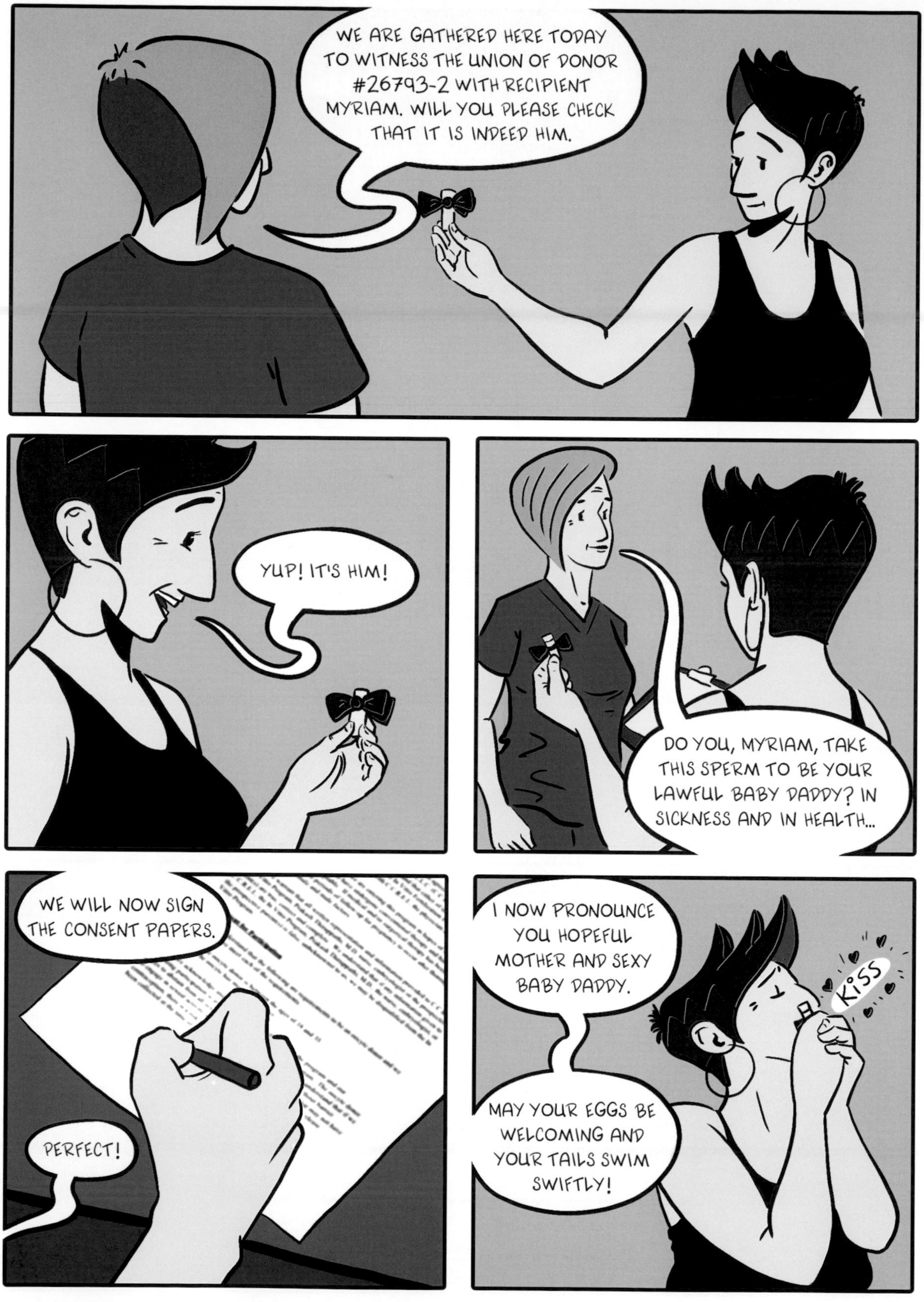
WE ARE GATHERED HERE TODAY TO WITNESS THE UNION OF DONOR #26793-2 WITH RECIPIENT MYRIAM. WILL YOU PLEASE CHECK THAT IT IS INDEED HIM.
YUP! IT'S HIM!
DO YOU, MYRIAM, TAKE THIS SPERM TO BE YOUR LAWFUL BABY DADDY? IN SICKNESS AND IN HEALTH...
WE WILL NOW SIGN THE CONSENT PAPERS.
PERFECT!
I NOW PRONOUNCE YOU HOPEFUL MOTHER AND SEXY BABY DADDY.
KISS
MAY YOUR EGGS BE WELCOMING AND YOUR TAILS SWIM SWIFTLY!

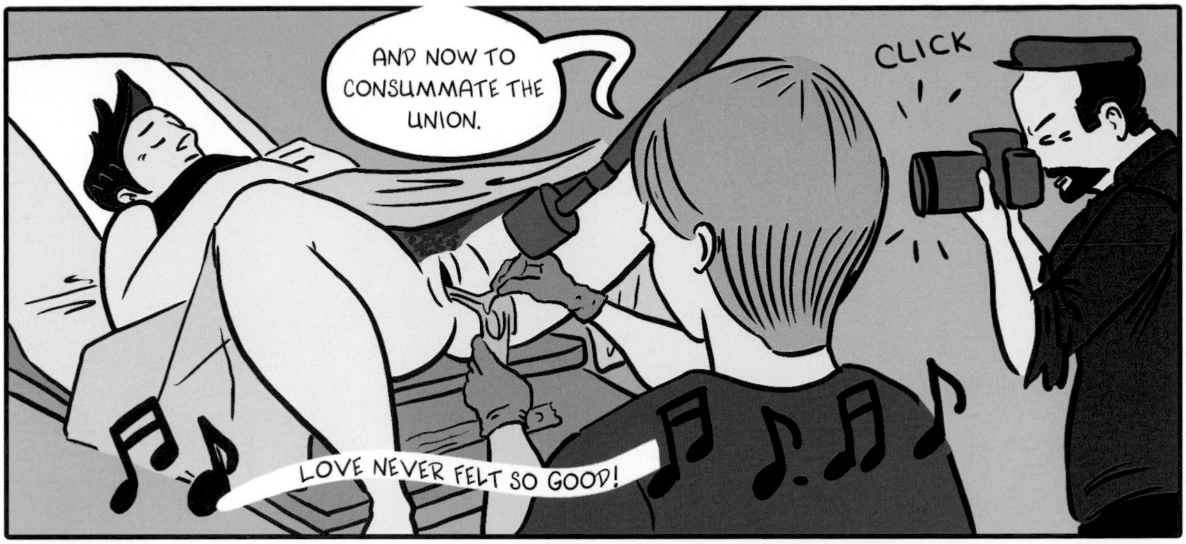
AND NOW TO CONSUMMATE THE UNION.
CLICK
LOVE NEVER FELT SO GOOD!

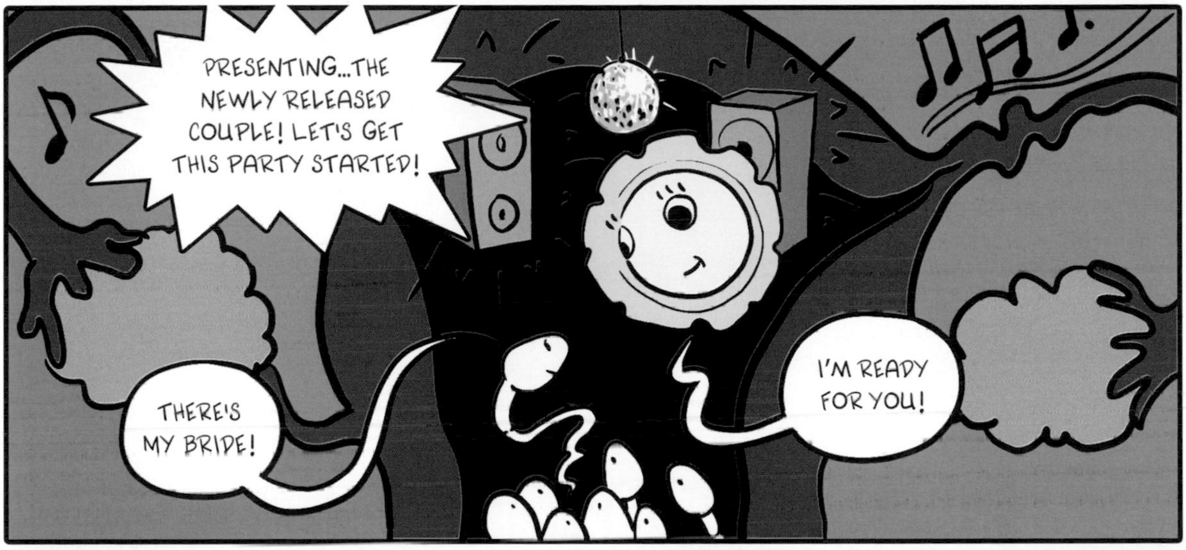
PRESENTING...THE NEWLY RELEASED COUPLE! LET'S GET THIS PARTY STARTED!
THERE'S MY BRIDE!
I'M READY FOR YOU!

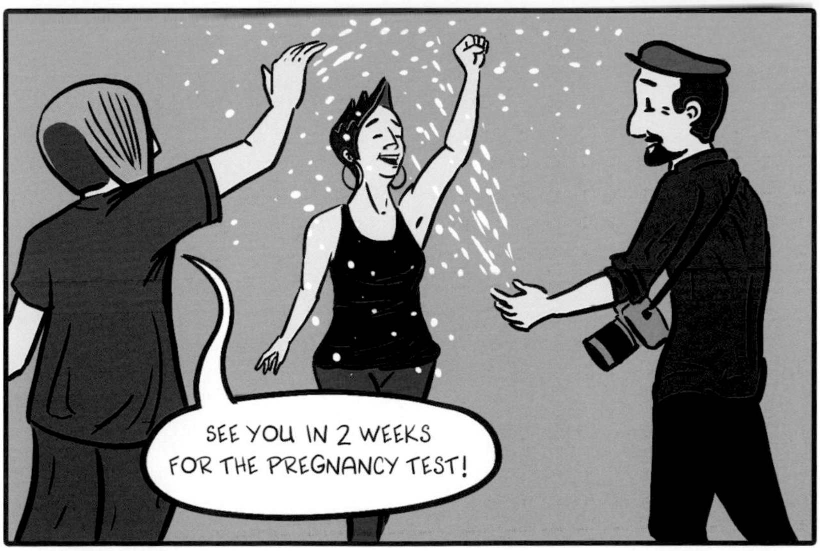
SEE YOU IN 2 WEEKS FOR THE PREGNANCY TEST!

That was it. Either I was going to be pregnant or I wasn't.

All that prep, one big (yet short) party...

and then life went on "as usual."

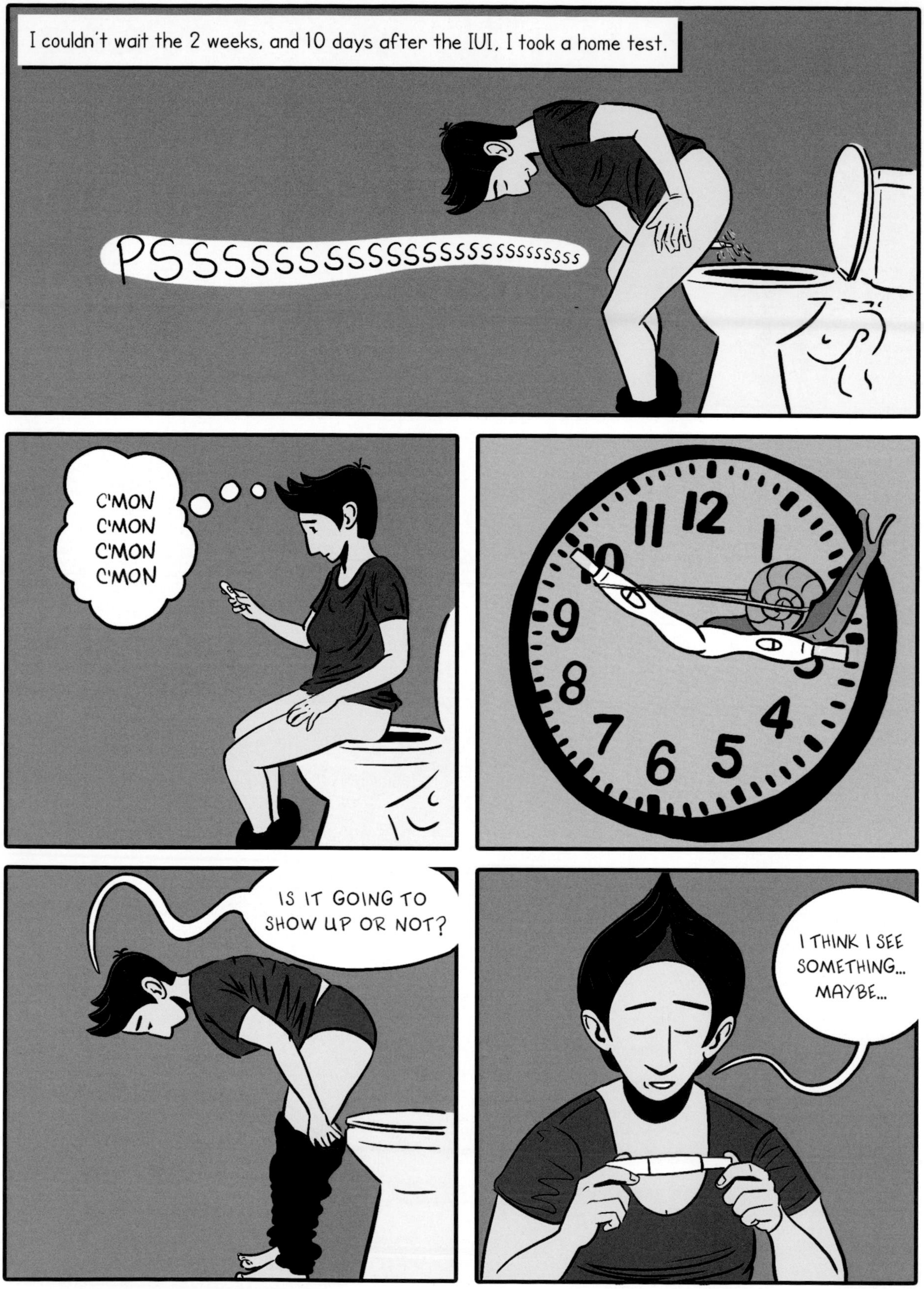
I couldn't wait the 2 weeks, and 10 days after the IUI, I took a home test.
PSSSSSSSSSSSSSSSSSSSSSSSSS
C'MON C'MON C'MON C'MON
IS IT GOING TO SHOW UP OR NOT?
I THINK I SEE SOMETHING... MAYBE...

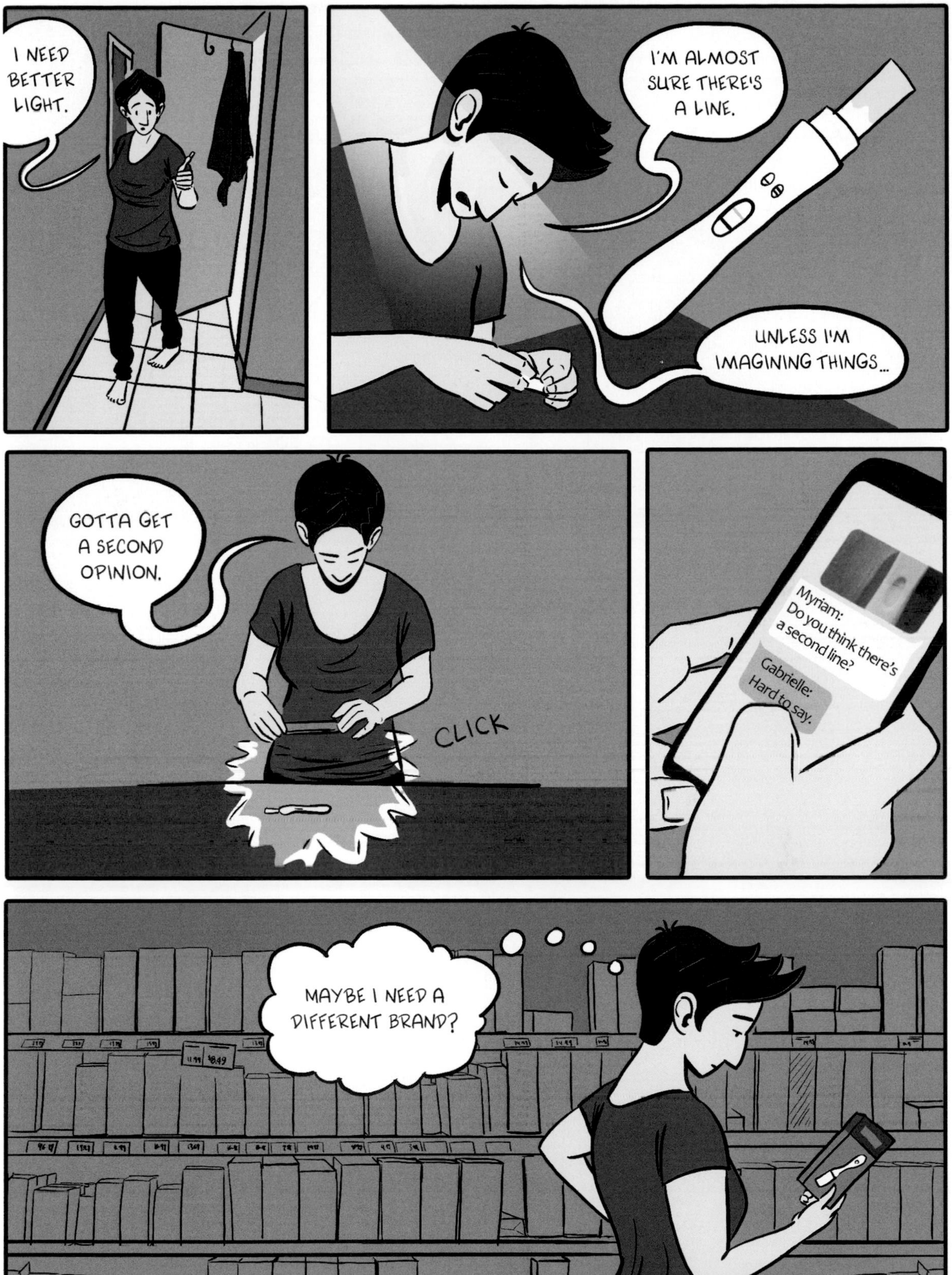
I NEED BETTER LIGHT.
I'M ALMOST SURE THERE'S A LINE.
UNLESS I'M IMAGINING THINGS...
GOTTA GET A SECOND OPINION.
CLICK
Myriam: Do you think there's a second line?
Gabrielle: Hard to say.
MAYBE I NEED A DIFFERENT BRAND?

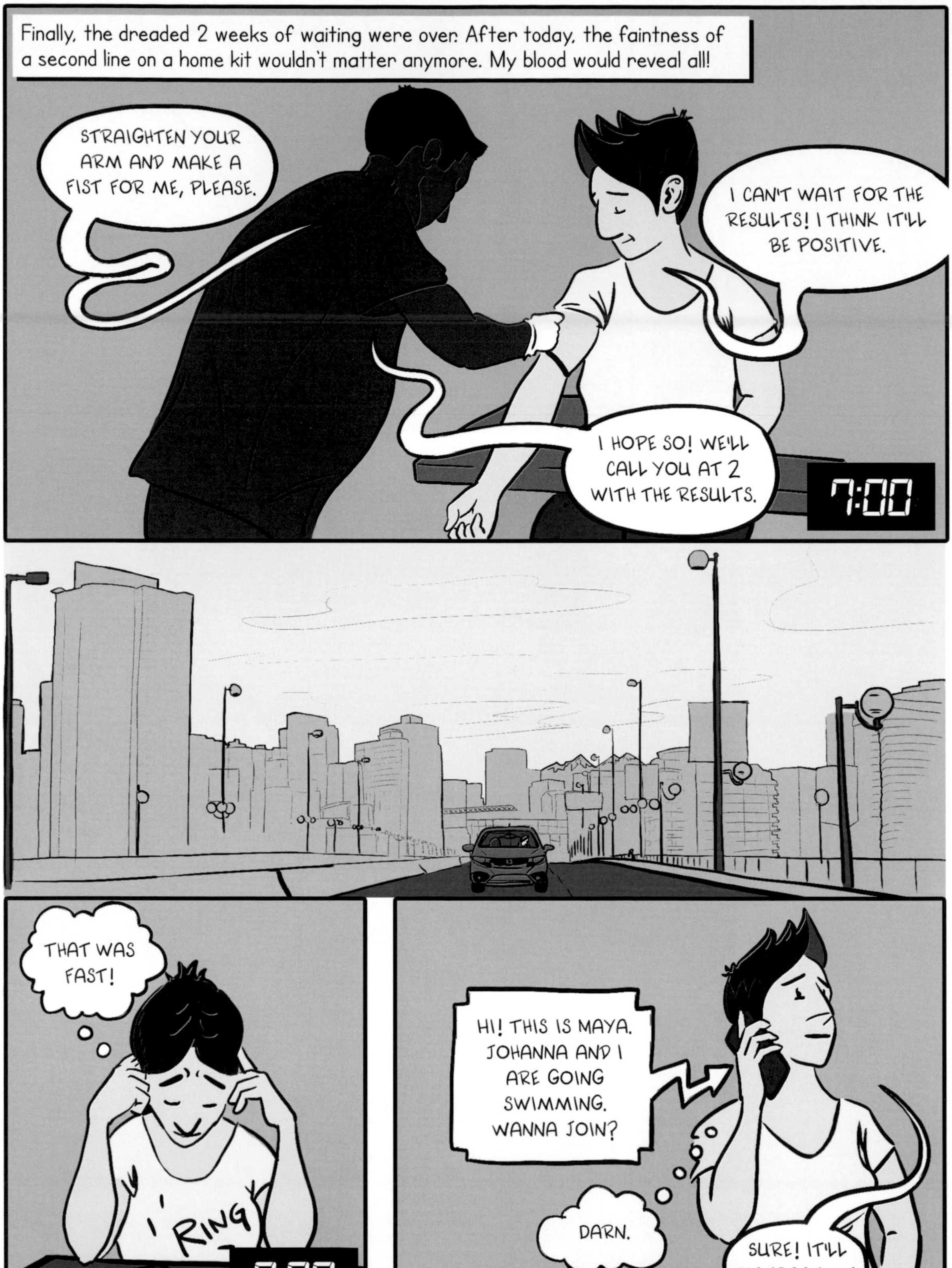

Finally, the dreaded 2 weeks of waiting were over. After today, the faintness of a second line on a home kit wouldn't matter anymore. My blood would reveal all!
STRAIGHTEN YOUR ARM AND MAKE A FIST FOR ME, PLEASE.
I CAN'T WAIT FOR THE RESULTS! I THINK IT'LL BE POSITIVE.
I HOPE SO! WE'LL CALL YOU AT 2 WITH THE RESULTS.
7:00
THAT WAS FAST!
RING
9:00
HI! THIS IS MAYA. JOHANNA AND I ARE GOING SWIMMING. WANNA JOIN?
DARN.
SURE! IT'LL DISTRACT ME.

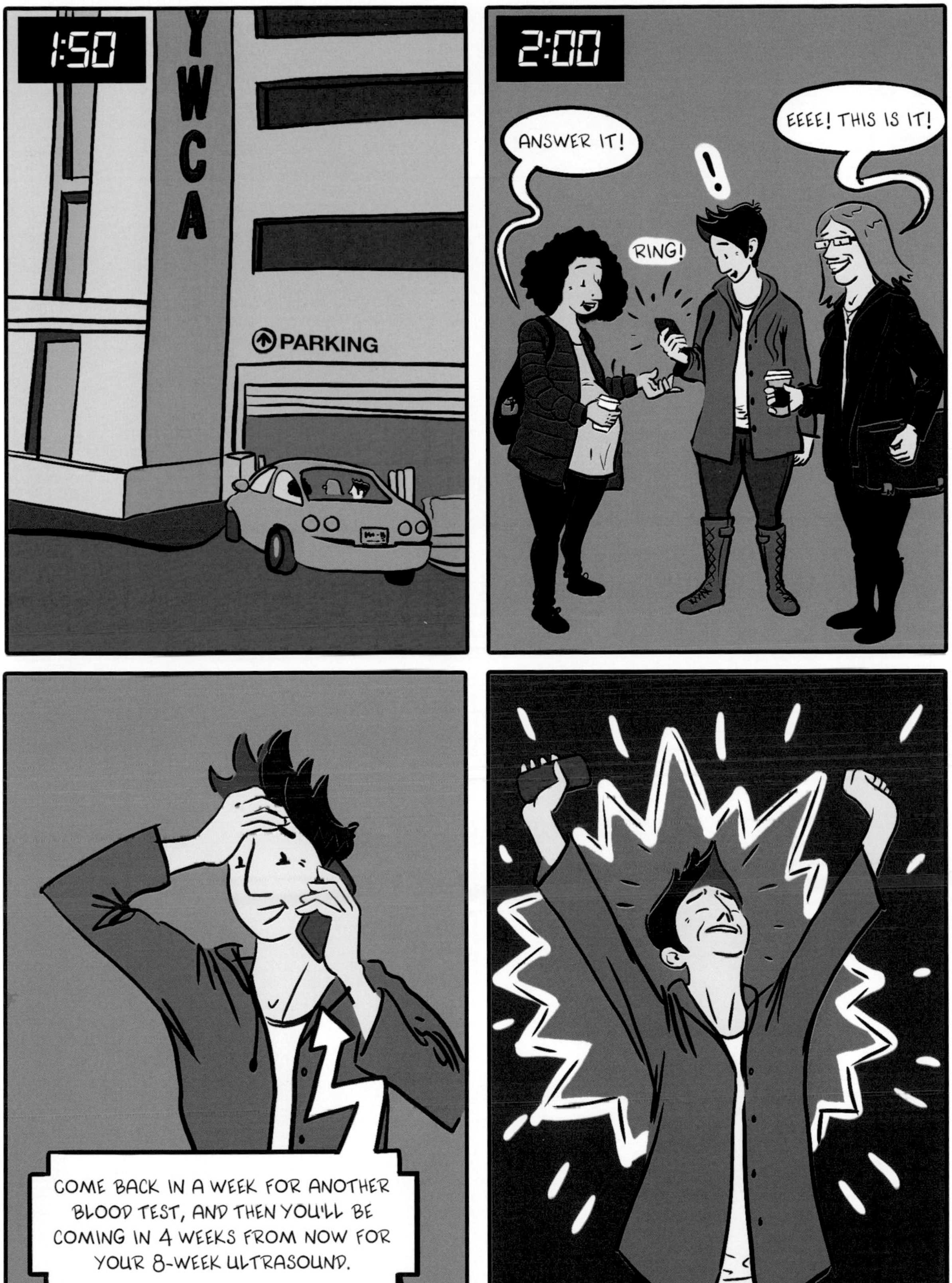
1:50
YWCA
PARKING
2:00
ANSWER IT!
!
RING!
EEEE! THIS IS IT!
COME BACK IN A WEEK FOR ANOTHER BLOOD TEST, AND THEN YOU'LL BE COMING IN 4 WEEKS FROM NOW FOR YOUR 8-WEEK ULTRASOUND.

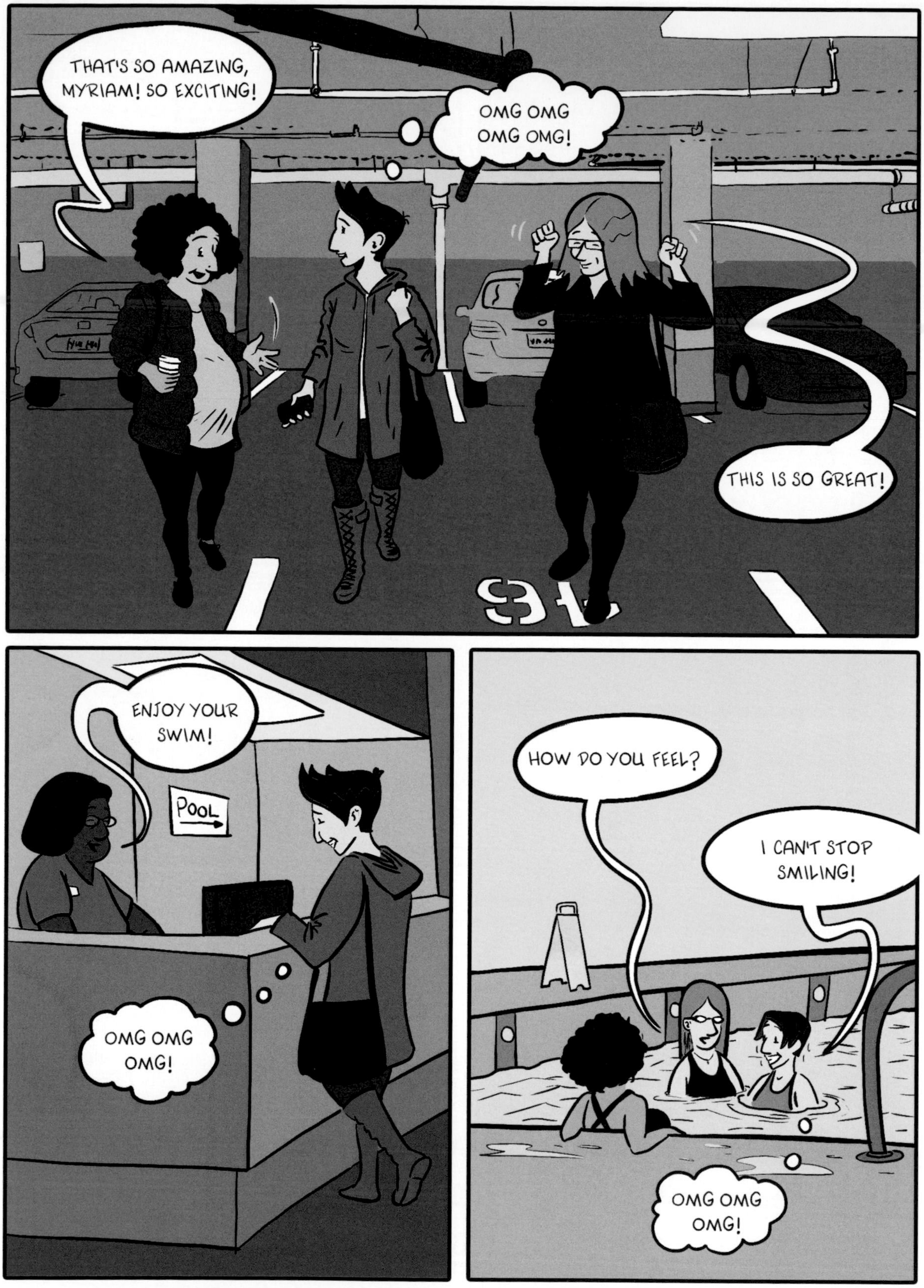
THAT'S SO AMAZING, MYRIAM! SO EXCITING!
OMG OMG OMG OMG!
THIS IS SO GREAT!
ENJOY YOUR SWIM!
POOL
OMG OMG OMG!
HOW DO YOU FEEL?
I CAN'T STOP SMILING!
OMG OMG OMG!

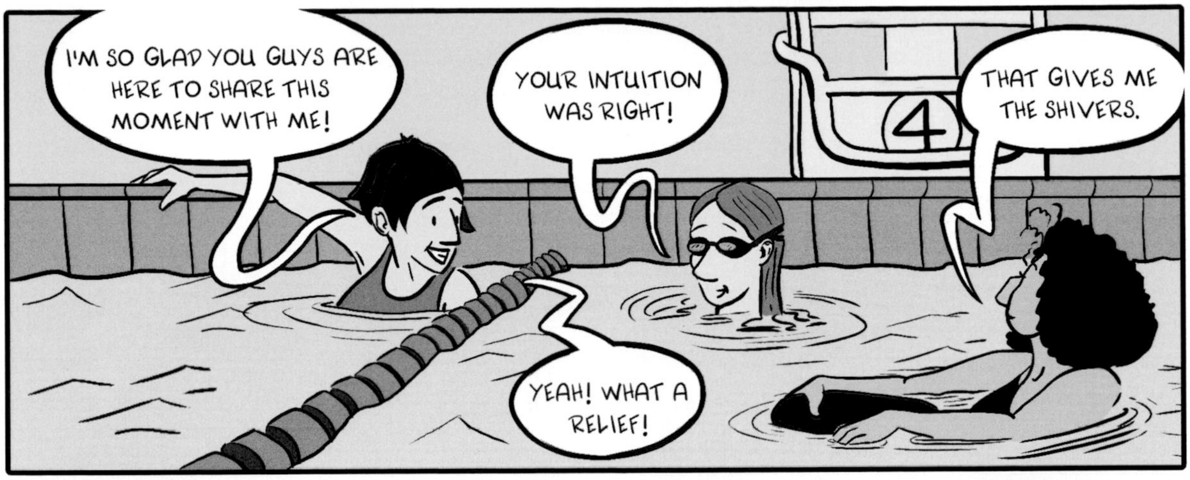
I'M SO GLAD YOU GUYS ARE HERE TO SHARE THIS MOMENT WITH ME!
YOUR INTUITION WAS RIGHT!
THAT GIVES ME THE SHIVERS.
YEAH! WHAT A RELIEF!
4

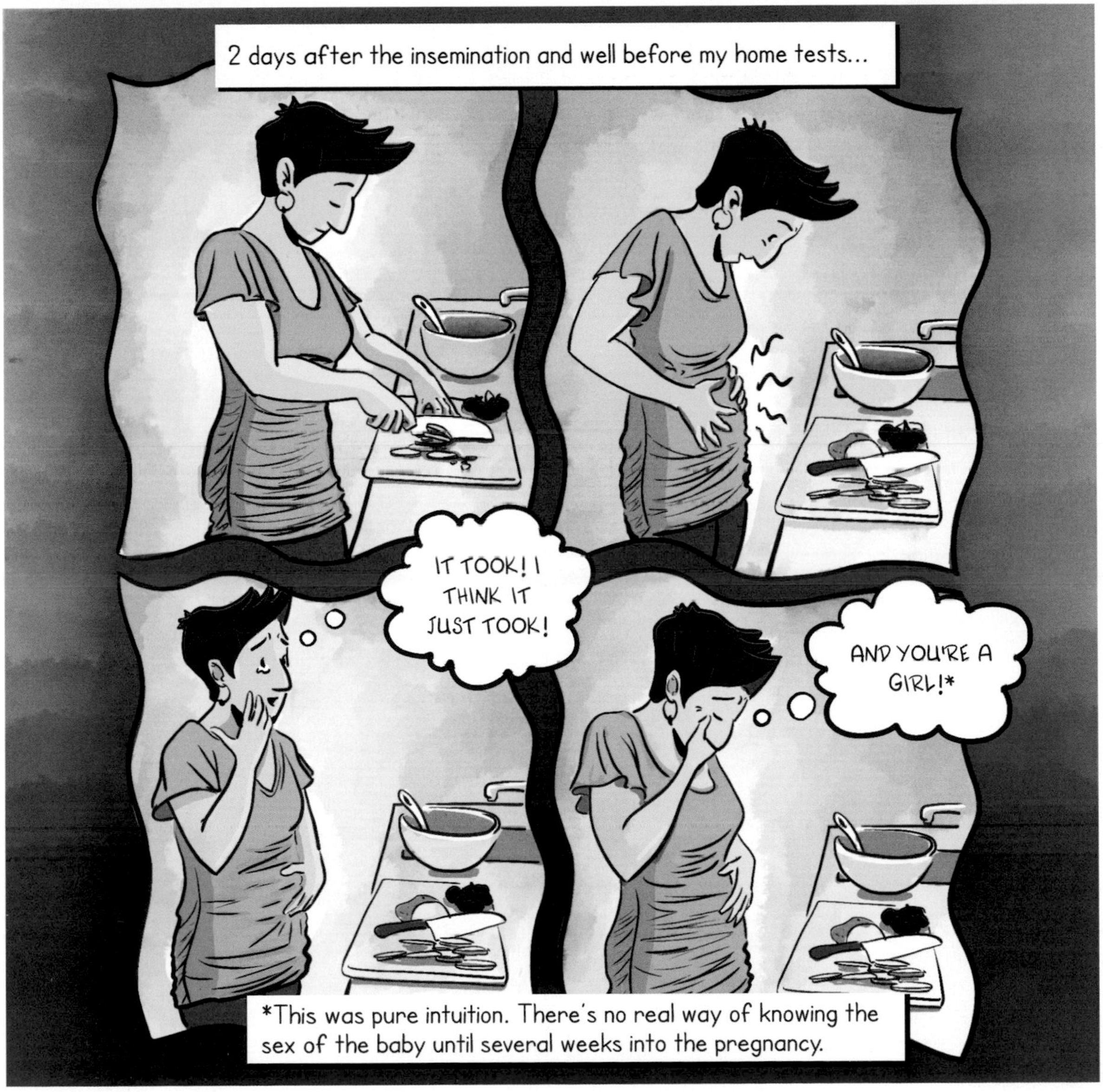
2 days after the insemination and well before my home tests...
IT TOOK! I THINK IT JUST TOOK!
AND YOU'RE A GIRL!*
*This was pure intuition. There's no real way of knowing the sex of the baby until several weeks into the pregnancy.

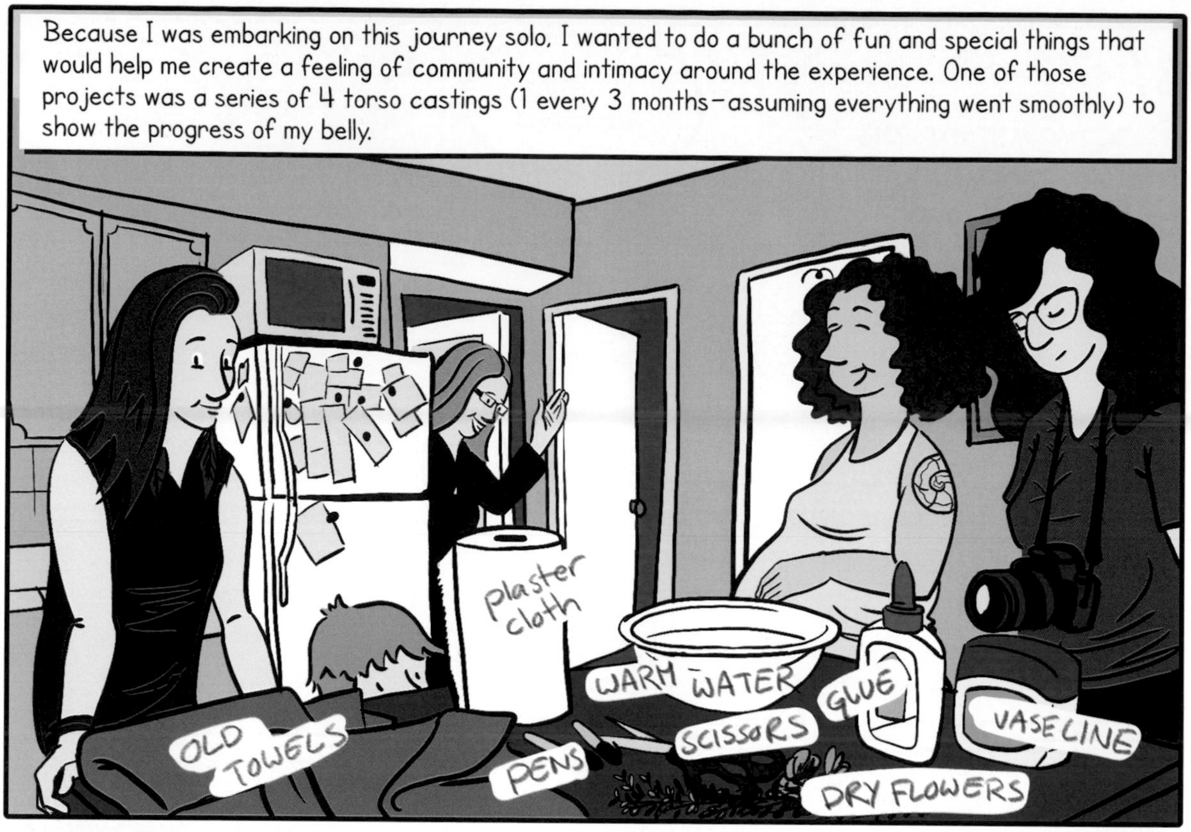
Because I was embarking on this journey solo, I wanted to do a bunch of fun and special things that would help me create a feeling of community and intimacy around the experience. One of those projects was a series of 4 torso castings (1 every 3 months–assuming everything went smoothly) to show the progress of my belly.
plaster cloth
WARM WATER
GLUE
OLD TOWELS
PENS
SCISSORS
VASELINE
DRY FLOWERS

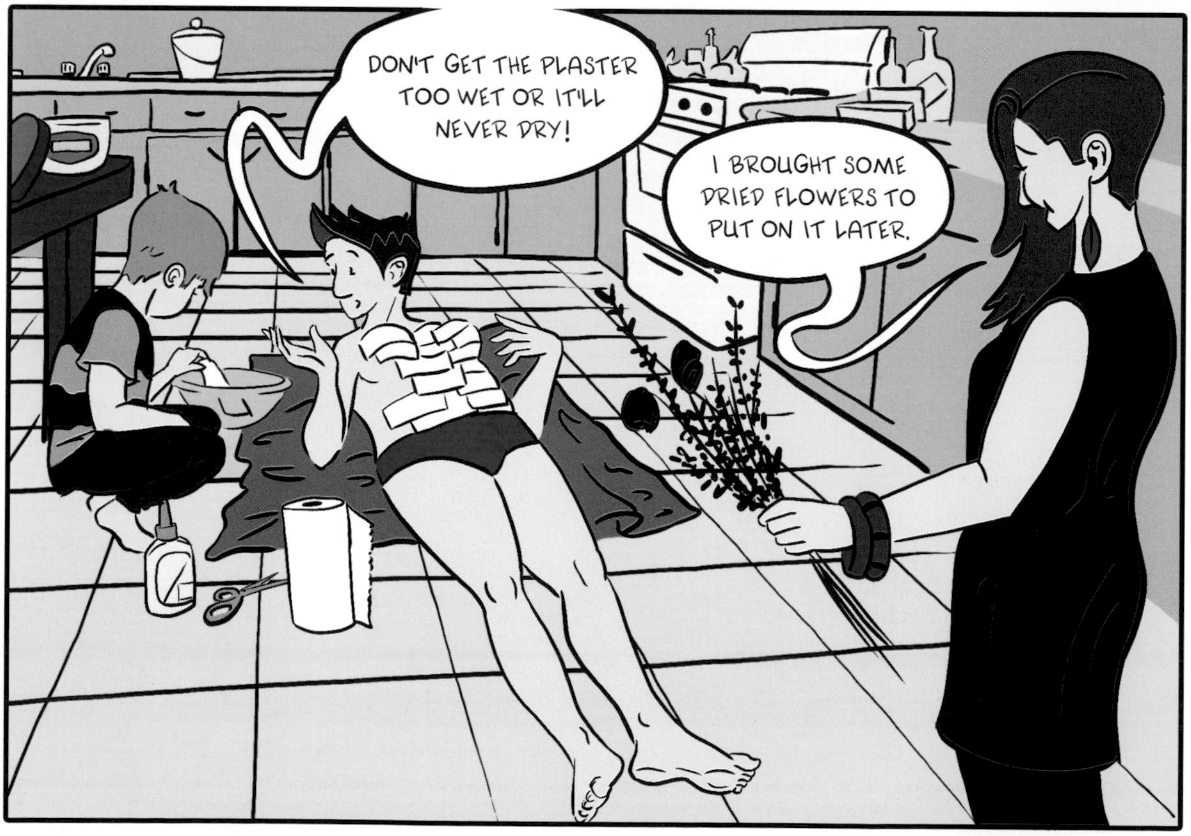
DON'T GET THE PLASTER TOO WET OR IT'LL NEVER DRY!
I BROUGHT SOME DRIED FLOWERS TO PUT ON IT LATER.

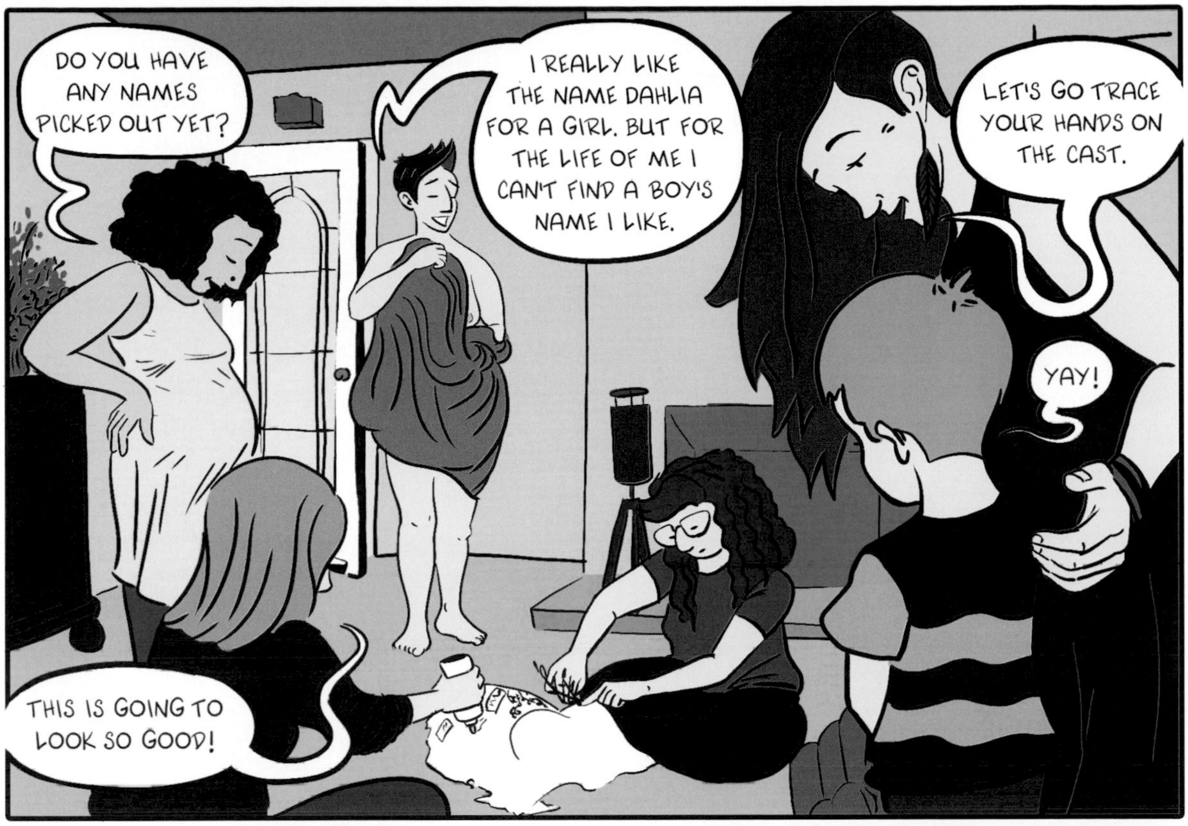
DO YOU HAVE ANY NAMES PICKED OUT YET?
I REALLY LIKE THE NAME DAHLIA FOR A GIRL. BUT FOR THE LIFE OF ME I CAN'T FIND A BOY'S NAME I LIKE.
LET'S GO TRACE YOUR HANDS ON THE CAST.
YAY!
THIS IS GOING TO LOOK SO GOOD!

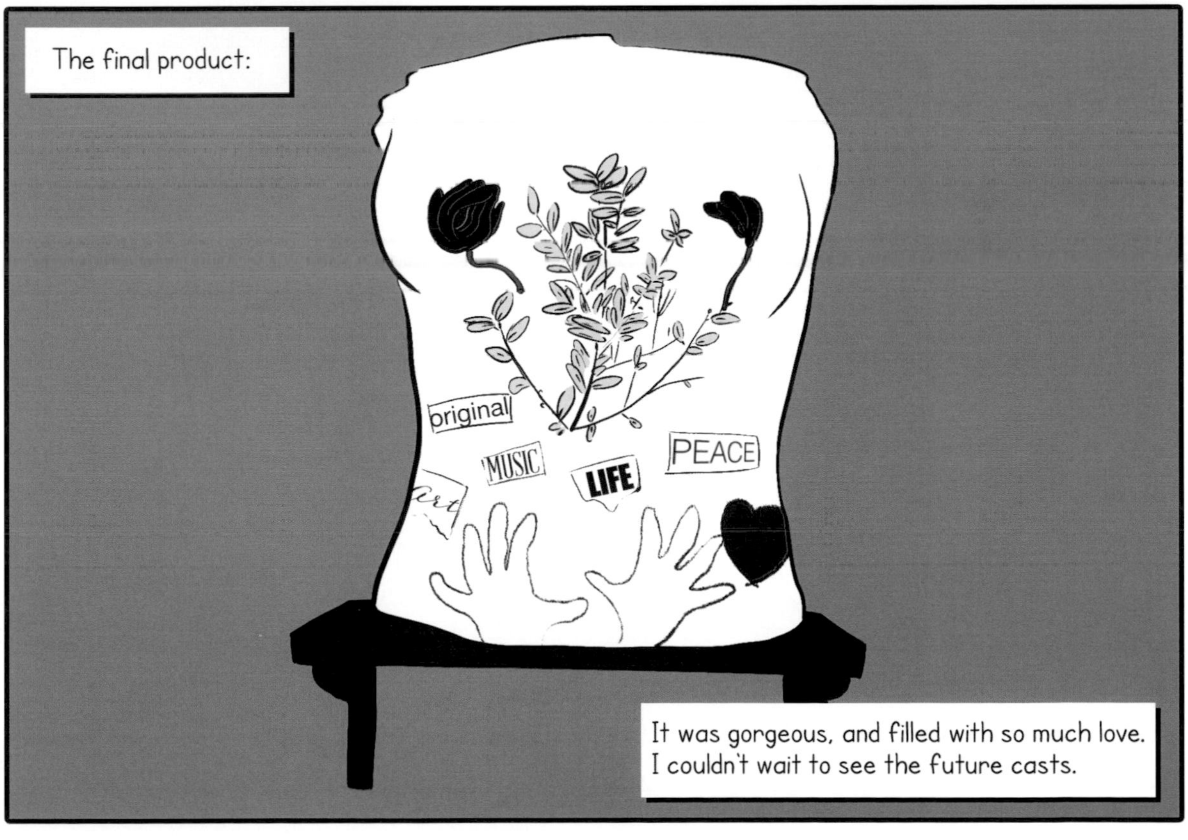
The final product:
original
MUSIC
LIFE
PEACE
It was gorgeous, and filled with so much love. I couldn't wait to see the future casts.

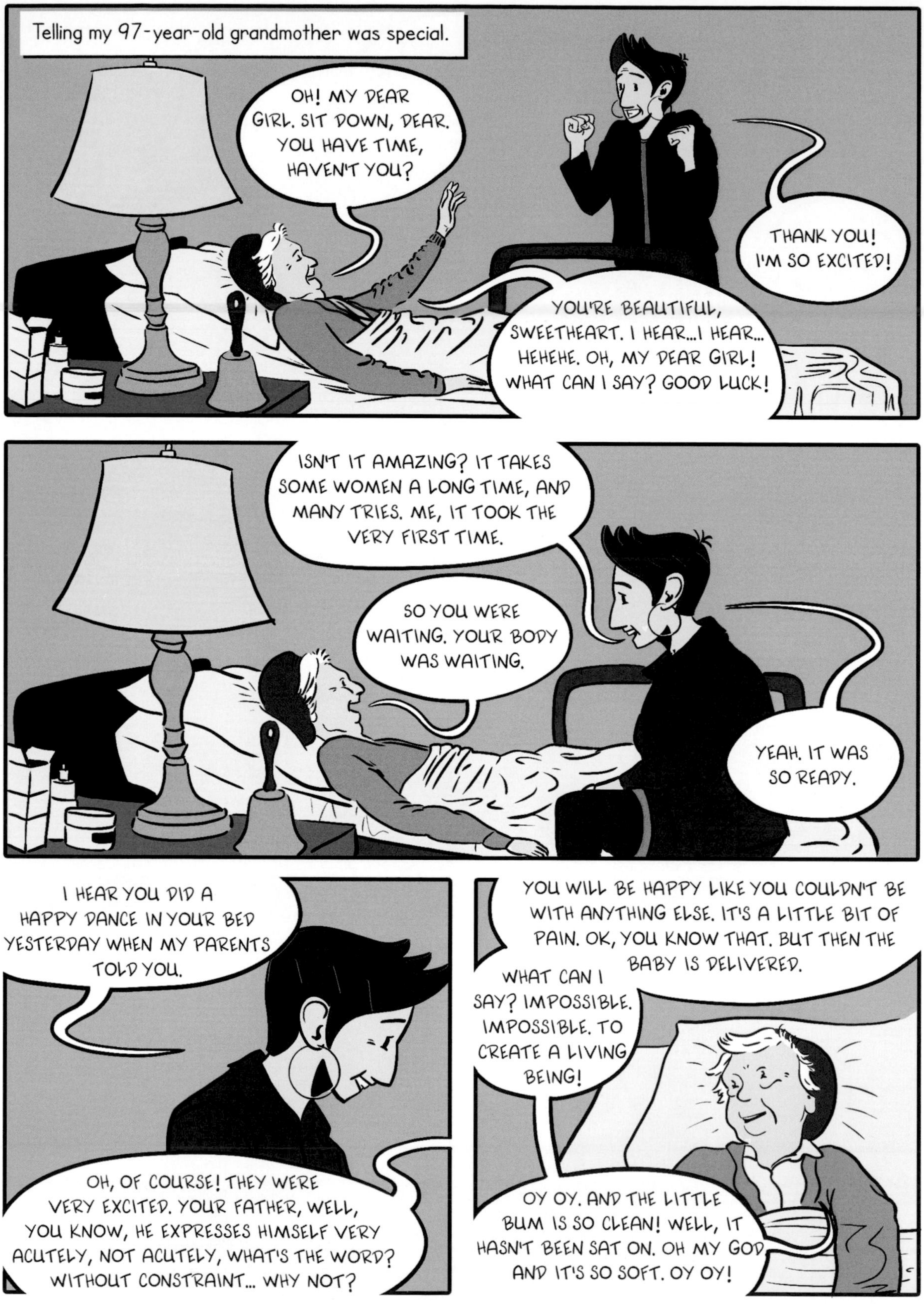

Telling my 97-year-old grandmother was special.
OH! MY DEAR GIRL. SIT DOWN, DEAR. YOU HAVE TIME, HAVEN'T YOU?
THANK YOU! I'M SO EXCITED!
YOU'RE BEAUTIFUL, SWEETHEART. I HEAR...I HEAR... HEHEHE. OH, MY DEAR GIRL! WHAT CAN I SAY? GOOD LUCK!
ISN'T IT AMAZING? IT TAKES SOME WOMEN A LONG TIME, AND MANY TRIES. ME, IT TOOK THE VERY FIRST TIME.
SO YOU WERE WAITING. YOUR BODY WAS WAITING.
YEAH. IT WAS SO READY.
I HEAR YOU DID A HAPPY DANCE IN YOUR BED YESTERDAY WHEN MY PARENTS TOLD YOU.
OH, OF COURSE! THEY WERE VERY EXCITED. YOUR FATHER, WELL, YOU KNOW, HE EXPRESSES HIMSELF VERY ACUTELY, NOT ACUTELY, WHAT'S THE WORD? WITHOUT CONSTRAINT... WHY NOT?
YOU WILL BE HAPPY LIKE YOU COULDN'T BE WITH ANYTHING ELSE. IT'S A LITTLE BIT OF PAIN. OK, YOU KNOW THAT. BUT THEN THE BABY IS DELIVERED.
WHAT CAN I SAY? IMPOSSIBLE. IMPOSSIBLE. TO CREATE A LIVING BEING!
OY OY. AND THE LITTLE BUM IS SO CLEAN! WELL, IT HASN'T BEEN SAT ON. OH MY GOD AND IT'S SO SOFT. OY OY!

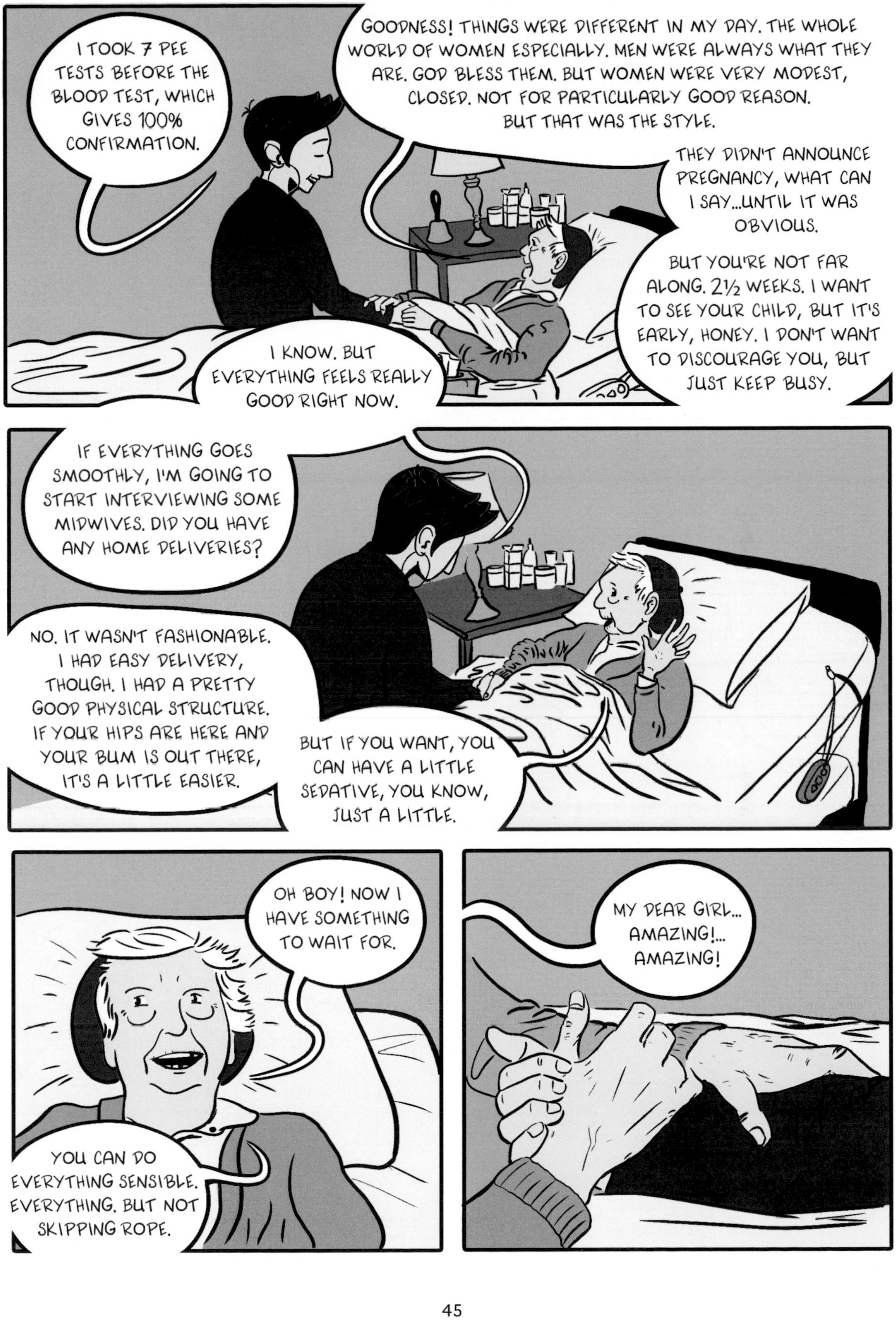
I TOOK 7 PEE TESTS BEFORE THE BLOOD TEST, WHICH GIVES 100% CONFIRMATION.
GOODNESS! THINGS WERE DIFFERENT IN MY DAY. THE WHOLE WORLD OF WOMEN ESPECIALLY. MEN WERE ALWAYS WHAT THEY ARE. GOD BLESS THEM. BUT WOMEN WERE VERY MODEST, CLOSED. NOT FOR PARTICULARLY GOOD REASON. BUT THAT WAS THE STYLE.
THEY DIDN'T ANNOUNCE PREGNANCY, WHAT CAN I SAY...UNTIL IT WAS OBVIOUS.
BUT YOU'RE NOT FAR ALONG. 2½ WEEKS. I WANT TO SEE YOUR CHILD, BUT IT'S EARLY, HONEY. I DON'T WANT TO DISCOURAGE YOU, BUT JUST KEEP BUSY.
I KNOW. BUT EVERYTHING FEELS REALLY GOOD RIGHT NOW.
IF EVERYTHING GOES SMOOTHLY, I'M GOING TO START INTERVIEWING SOME MIDWIVES. DID YOU HAVE ANY HOME DELIVERIES?
NO. IT WASN'T FASHIONABLE. I HAD EASY DELIVERY, THOUGH. I HAD A PRETTY GOOD PHYSICAL STRUCTURE. IF YOUR HIPS ARE HERE AND YOUR BUM IS OUT THERE, IT'S A LITTLE EASIER.
BUT IF YOU WANT, YOU CAN HAVE A LITTLE SEDATIVE, YOU KNOW, JUST A LITTLE.
OH BOY! NOW I HAVE SOMETHING TO WAIT FOR.
YOU CAN DO EVERYTHING SENSIBLE. EVERYTHING. BUT NOT SKIPPING ROPE.
MY DEAR GIRL... AMAZING!... AMAZING!

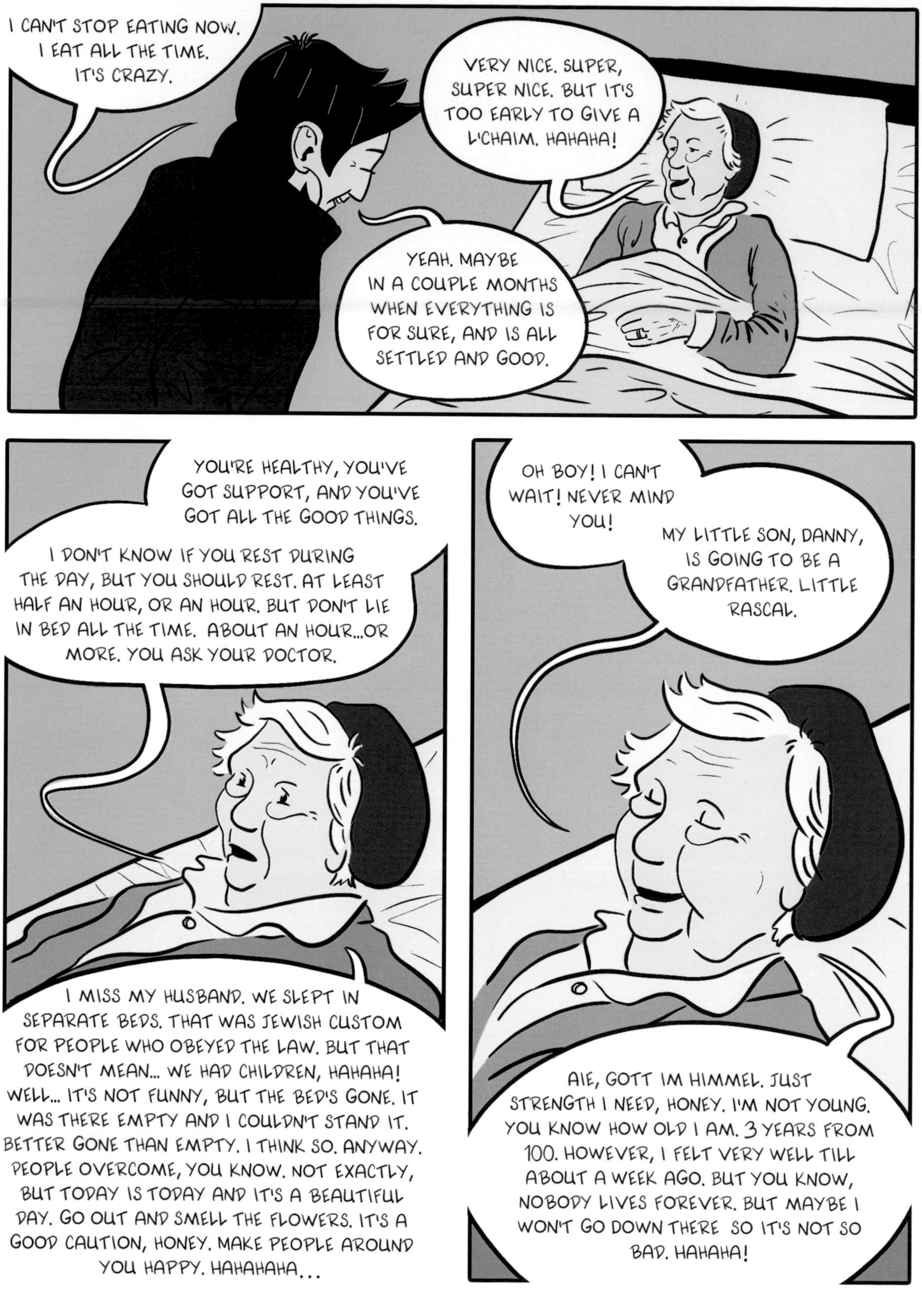
I CAN'T STOP EATING NOW. I EAT ALL THE TIME. IT'S CRAZY.
VERY NICE. SUPER, SUPER NICE. BUT IT'S TOO EARLY TO GIVE A L'CHAIM. HAHAHA!
YEAH. MAYBE IN A COUPLE MONTHS WHEN EVERYTHING IS FOR SURE, AND IS ALL SETTLED AND GOOD.
YOU'RE HEALTHY, YOU'VE GOT SUPPORT, AND YOU'VE GOT ALL THE GOOD THINGS.
I DON'T KNOW IF YOU REST DURING THE DAY, BUT YOU SHOULD REST. AT LEAST HALF AN HOUR, OR AN HOUR. BUT DON'T LIE IN BED ALL THE TIME. ABOUT AN HOUR...OR MORE. YOU ASK YOUR DOCTOR.
I MISS MY HUSBAND. WE SLEPT IN SEPARATE BEDS. THAT WAS JEWISH CUSTOM FOR PEOPLE WHO OBEYED THE LAW. BUT THAT DOESN'T MEAN... WE HAD CHILDREN, HAHAHA! WELL... IT'S NOT FUNNY, BUT THE BED'S GONE. IT WAS THERE EMPTY AND I COULDN'T STAND IT. BETTER GONE THAN EMPTY. I THINK SO. ANYWAY. PEOPLE OVERCOME, YOU KNOW. NOT EXACTLY, BUT TODAY IS TODAY AND IT'S A BEAUTIFUL DAY. GO OUT AND SMELL THE FLOWERS. IT'S A GOOD CAUTION, HONEY. MAKE PEOPLE AROUND YOU HAPPY. HAHAHAHA...
OH BOY! I CAN'T WAIT! NEVER MIND YOU!
MY LITTLE SON, DANNY, IS GOING TO BE A GRANDFATHER. LITTLE RASCAL.
AIE, GOTT IM HIMMEL. JUST STRENGTH I NEED, HONEY. I'M NOT YOUNG. YOU KNOW HOW OLD I AM. 3 YEARS FROM 100. HOWEVER, I FELT VERY WELL TILL ABOUT A WEEK AGO. BUT YOU KNOW, NOBODY LIVES FOREVER. BUT MAYBE I WON'T GO DOWN THERE SO IT'S NOT SO BAD. HAHAHA!

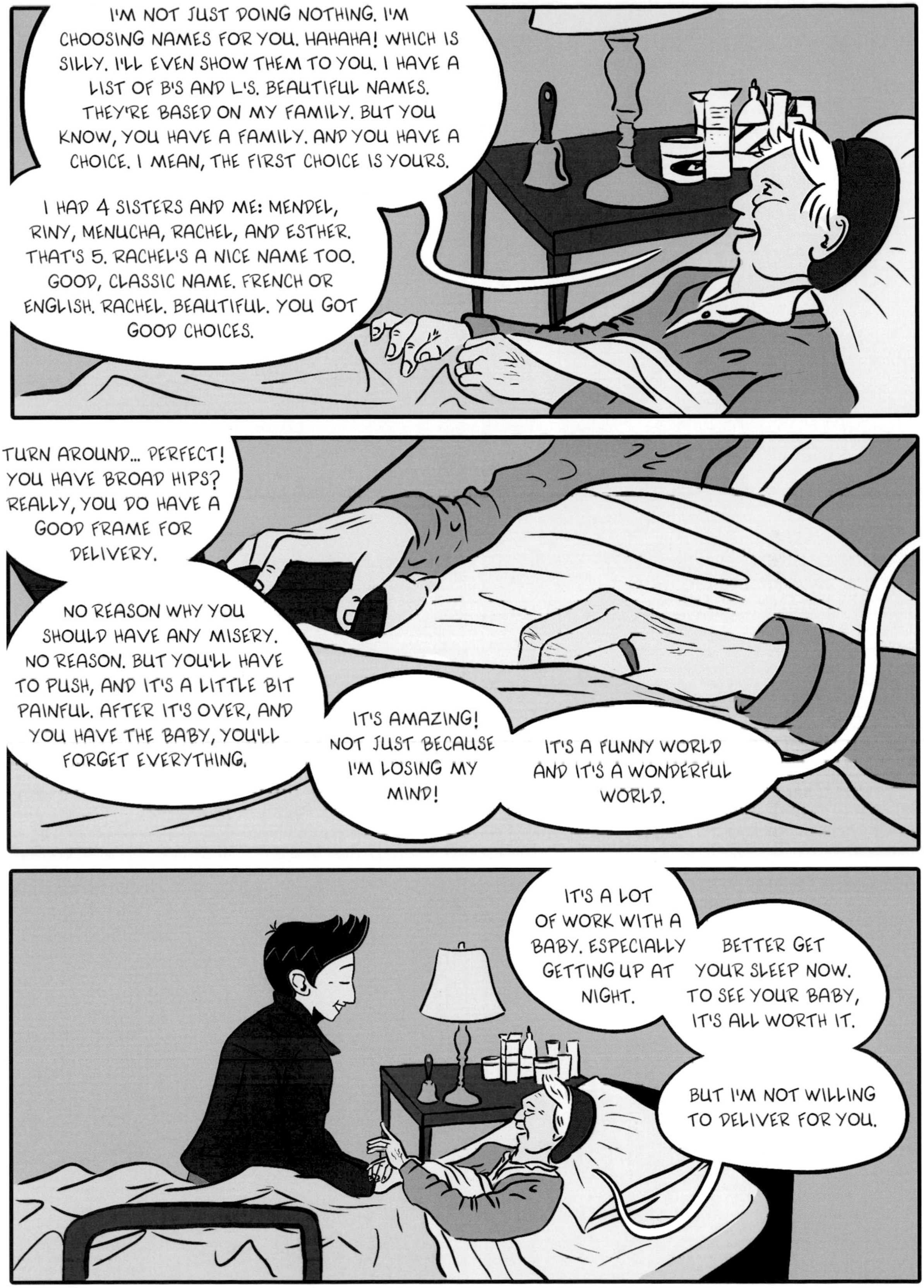
I'M NOT JUST DOING NOTHING. I'M CHOOSING NAMES FOR YOU. HAHAHA! WHICH IS SILLY. I'LL EVEN SHOW THEM TO YOU. I HAVE A LIST OF B'S AND L'S. BEAUTIFUL NAMES. THEY'RE BASED ON MY FAMILY. BUT YOU KNOW, YOU HAVE A FAMILY. AND YOU HAVE A CHOICE. I MEAN, THE FIRST CHOICE IS YOURS.
I HAD 4 SISTERS AND ME: MENDEL, RINY, MENUCHA, RACHEL, AND ESTHER. THAT'S 5. RACHEL'S A NICE NAME TOO. GOOD, CLASSIC NAME. FRENCH OR ENGLISH. RACHEL. BEAUTIFUL. YOU GOT GOOD CHOICES.
TURN AROUND... PERFECT! YOU HAVE BROAD HIPS? REALLY, YOU DO HAVE A GOOD FRAME FOR DELIVERY.
NO REASON WHY YOU SHOULD HAVE ANY MISERY. NO REASON. BUT YOU'LL HAVE TO PUSH, AND IT'S A LITTLE BIT PAINFUL. AFTER IT'S OVER, AND YOU HAVE THE BABY, YOU'LL FORGET EVERYTHING.
IT'S AMAZING! NOT JUST BECAUSE I'M LOSING MY MIND!
IT'S A FUNNY WORLD AND IT'S A WONDERFUL WORLD.
IT'S A LOT OF WORK WITH A BABY. ESPECIALLY GETTING UP AT NIGHT.
BETTER GET YOUR SLEEP NOW. TO SEE YOUR BABY, IT'S ALL WORTH IT.
BUT I'M NOT WILLING TO DELIVER FOR YOU.

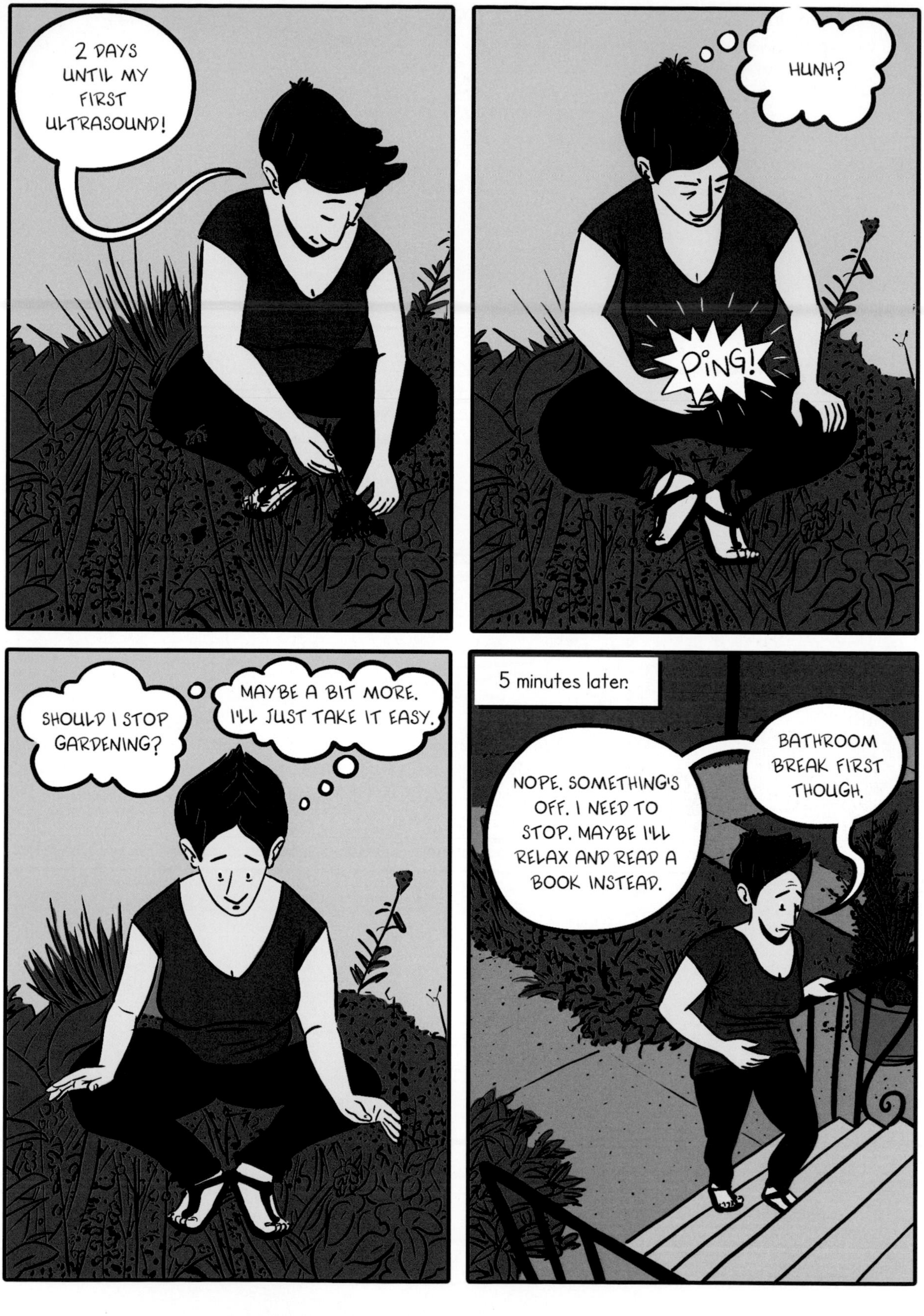

2 DAYS UNTIL MY FIRST ULTRASOUND!
HUNH?
PING!
SHOULD I STOP GARDENING?
MAYBE A BIT MORE. I'LL JUST TAKE IT EASY.
5 minutes later.
NOPE. SOMETHING'S OFF. I NEED TO STOP. MAYBE I'LL RELAX AND READ A BOOK INSTEAD.
BATHROOM BREAK FIRST THOUGH.

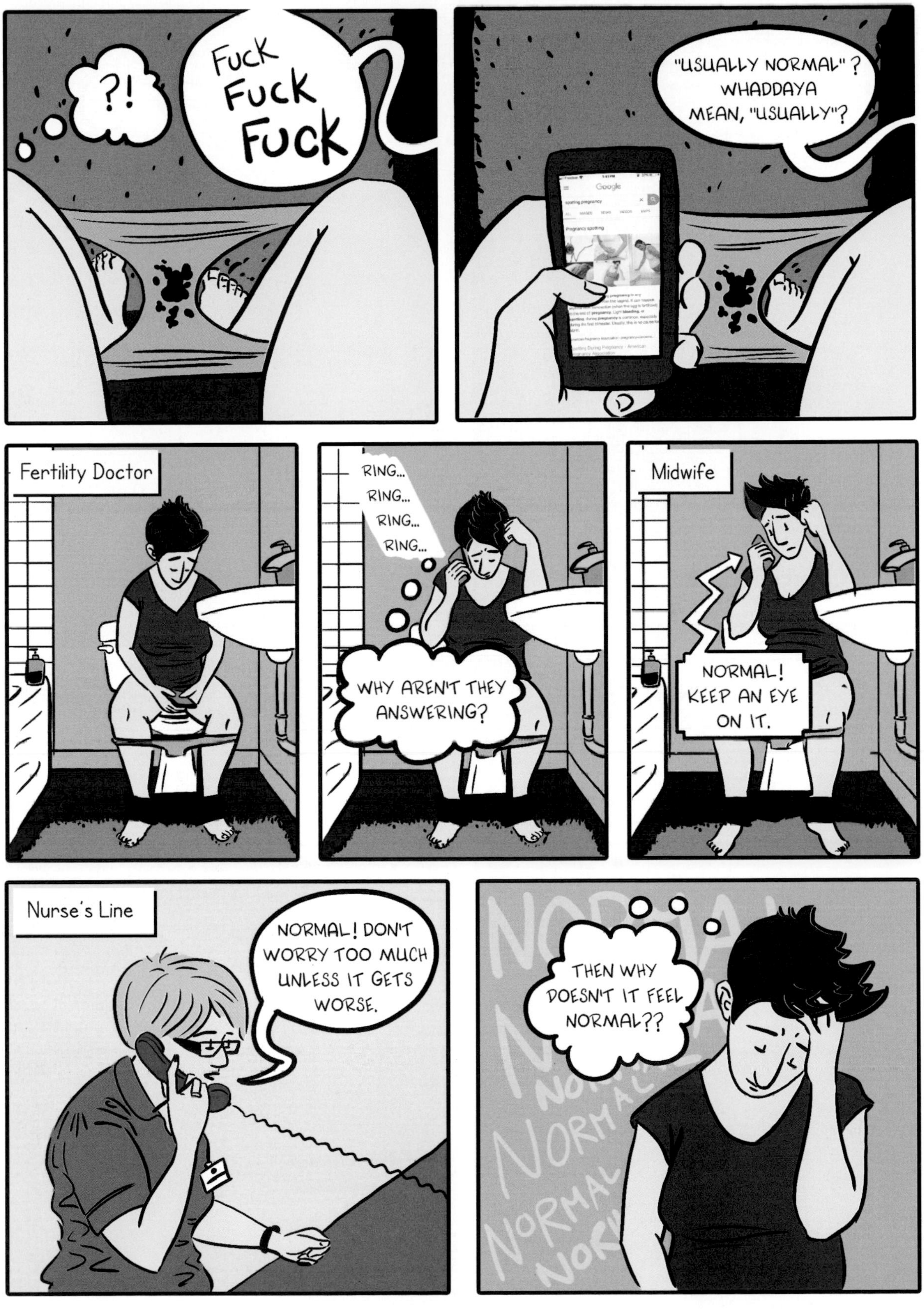
?!
FUCK FUCK FUCK
"USUALLY NORMAL"? WHADDAYA MEAN, "USUALLY"?
Fertility Doctor
RING... RING... RING... RING...
WHY AREN'T THEY ANSWERING?
Midwife
NORMAL! KEEP AN EYE ON IT.
Nurse's Line
NORMAL! DON'T WORRY TOO MUCH UNLESS IT GETS WORSE.
THEN WHY DOESN'T IT FEEL NORMAL??

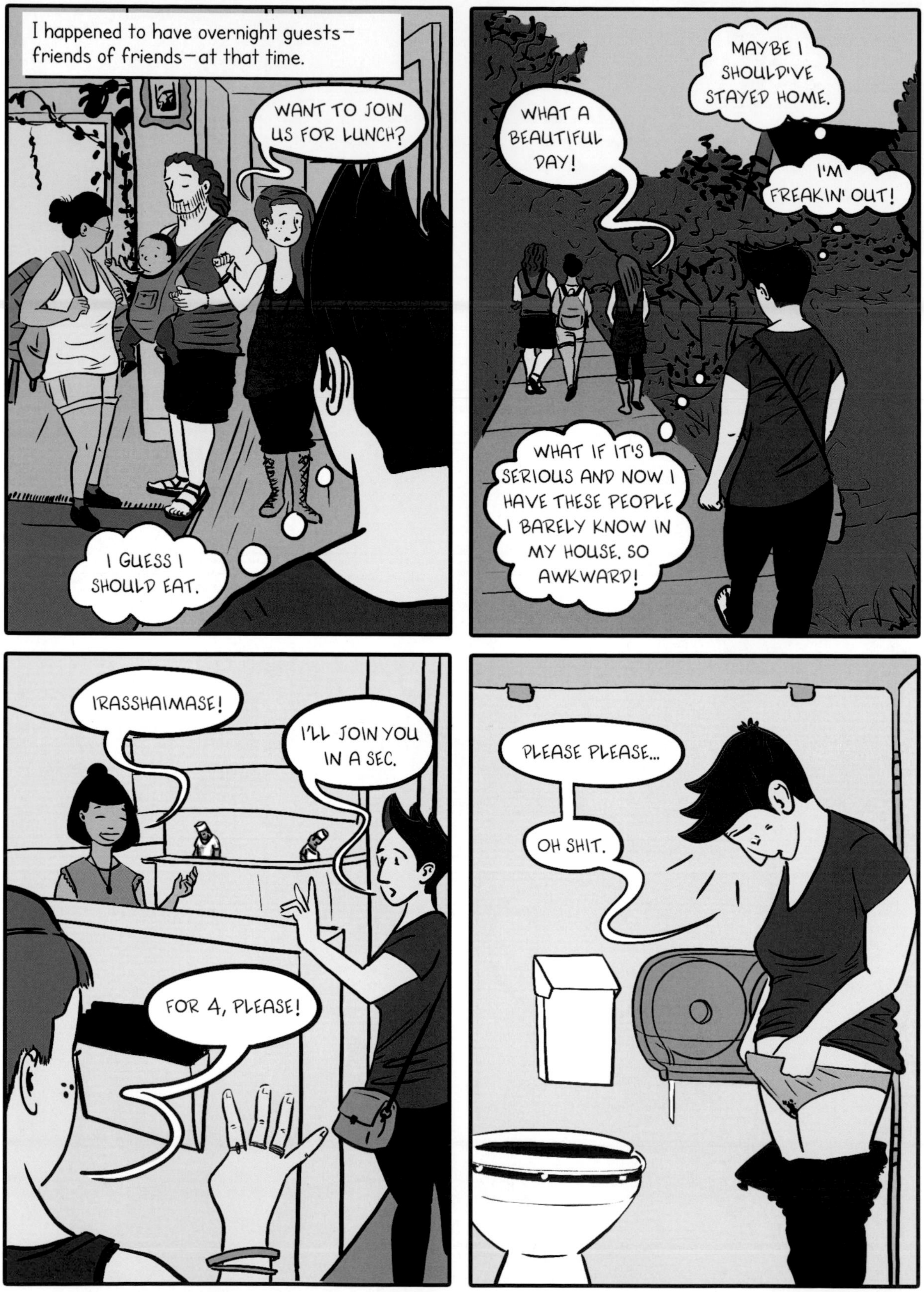
I happened to have overnight guests—friends of friends—at that time.
WANT TO JOIN US FOR LUNCH?
I GUESS I SHOULD EAT.
WHAT A BEAUTIFUL DAY!
MAYBE I SHOULD'VE STAYED HOME.
I'M FREAKIN' OUT!
WHAT IF IT'S SERIOUS AND NOW I HAVE THESE PEOPLE I BARELY KNOW IN MY HOUSE. SO AWKWARD!
IRASSHAIMASE!
I'LL JOIN YOU IN A SEC.
FOR 4, PLEASE!
PLEASE PLEASE...
OH SHIT.

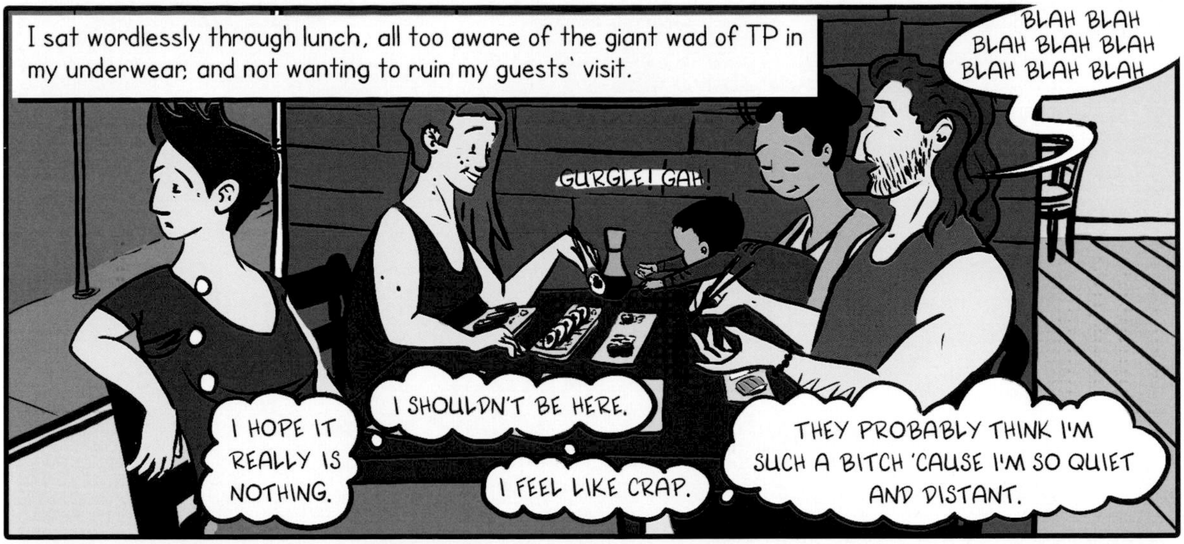
I sat wordlessly through lunch, all too aware of the giant wad of TP in my underwear, and not wanting to ruin my guests' visit.
BLAH BLAH BLAH BLAH BLAH BLAH BLAH BLAH
GURGLE! GAH!
I HOPE IT REALLY IS NOTHING.
I SHOULDN'T BE HERE.
I FEEL LIKE CRAP.
THEY PROBABLY THINK I'M SUCH A BITCH 'CAUSE I'M SO QUIET AND DISTANT.

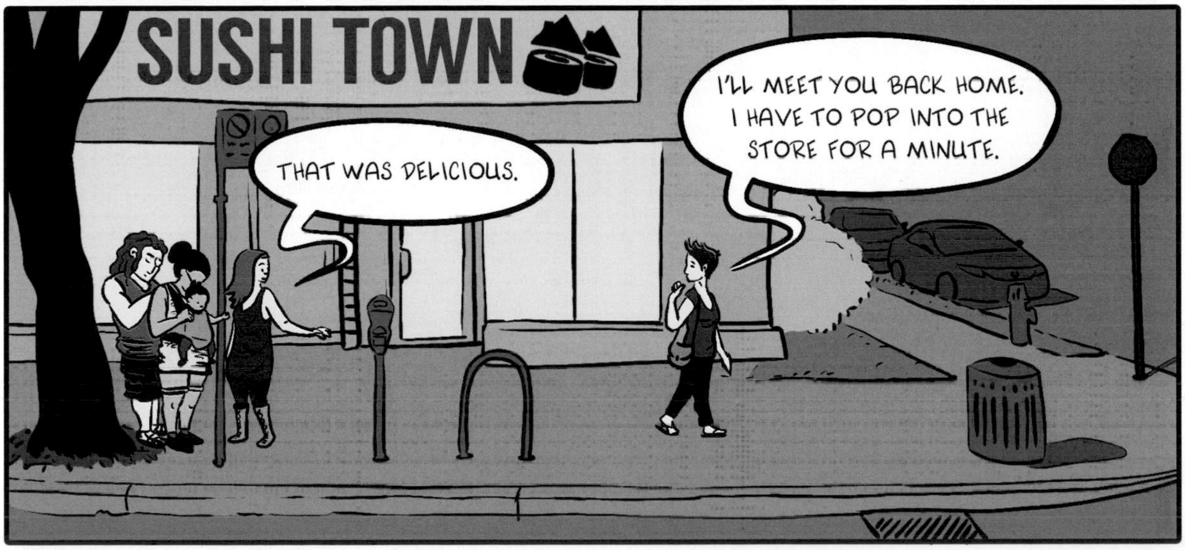
SUSHI TOWN
THAT WAS DELICIOUS.
I'LL MEET YOU BACK HOME. I HAVE TO POP INTO THE STORE FOR A MINUTE.

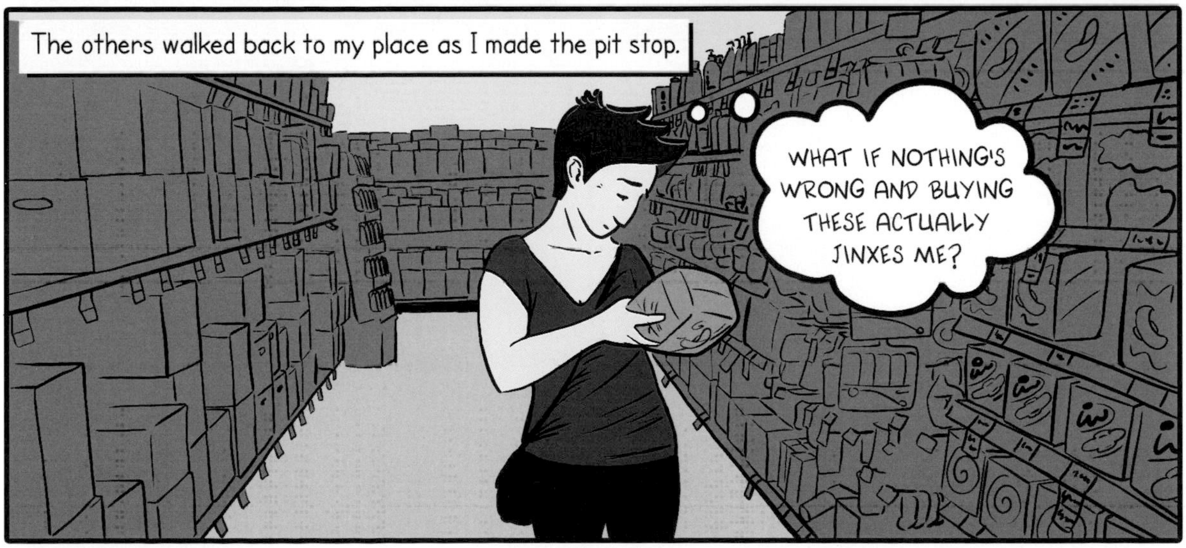
The others walked back to my place as I made the pit stop.
WHAT IF NOTHING'S WRONG AND BUYING THESE ACTUALLY JINXES ME?

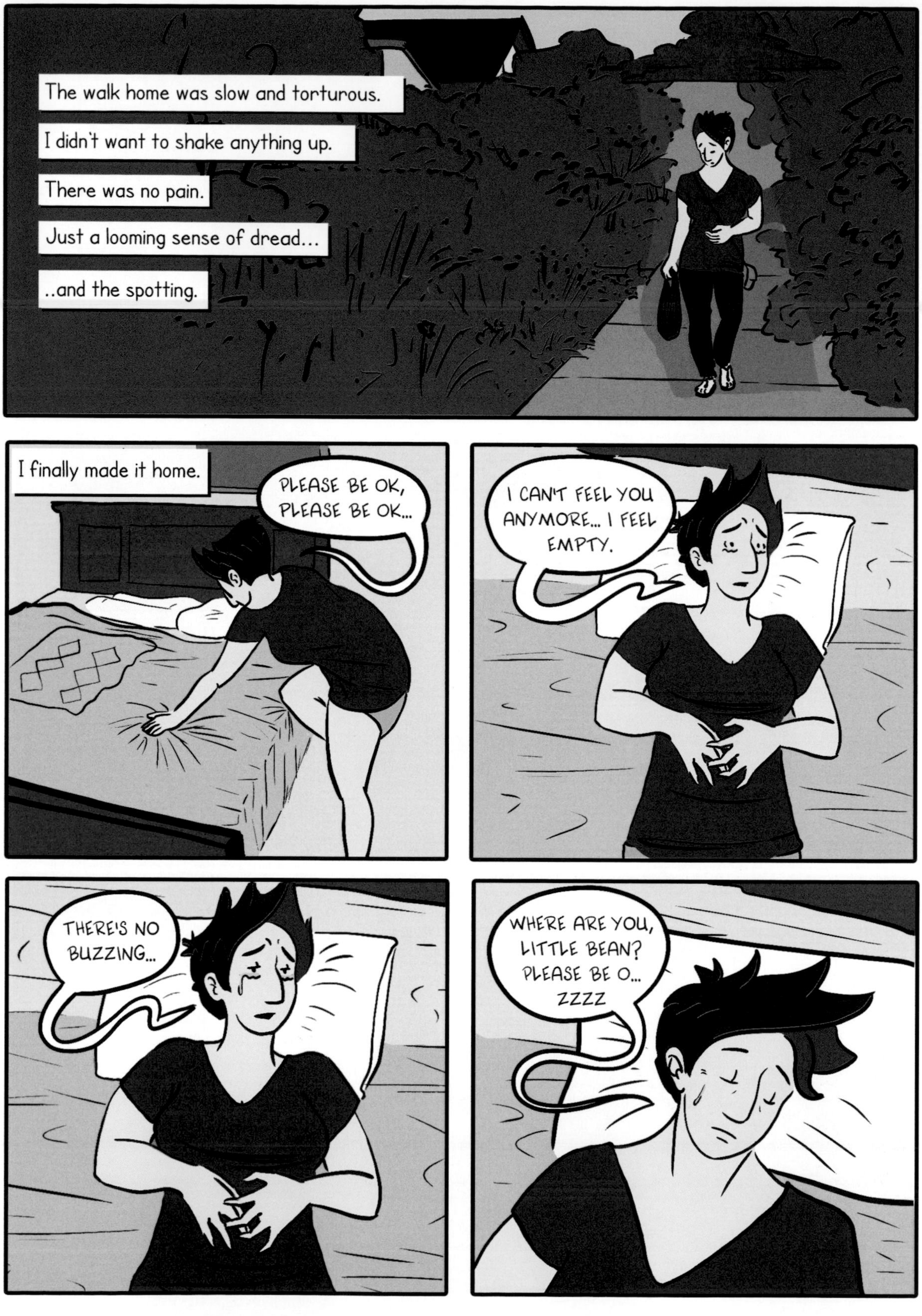
The walk home was slow and torturous.
I didn't want to shake anything up.
There was no pain.
Just a looming sense of dread...
..and the spotting.
I finally made it home.
PLEASE BE OK, PLEASE BE OK...
I CAN'T FEEL YOU ANYMORE... I FEEL EMPTY.
THERE'S NO BUZZING...
WHERE ARE YOU, LITTLE BEAN? PLEASE BE O... ZZZZ

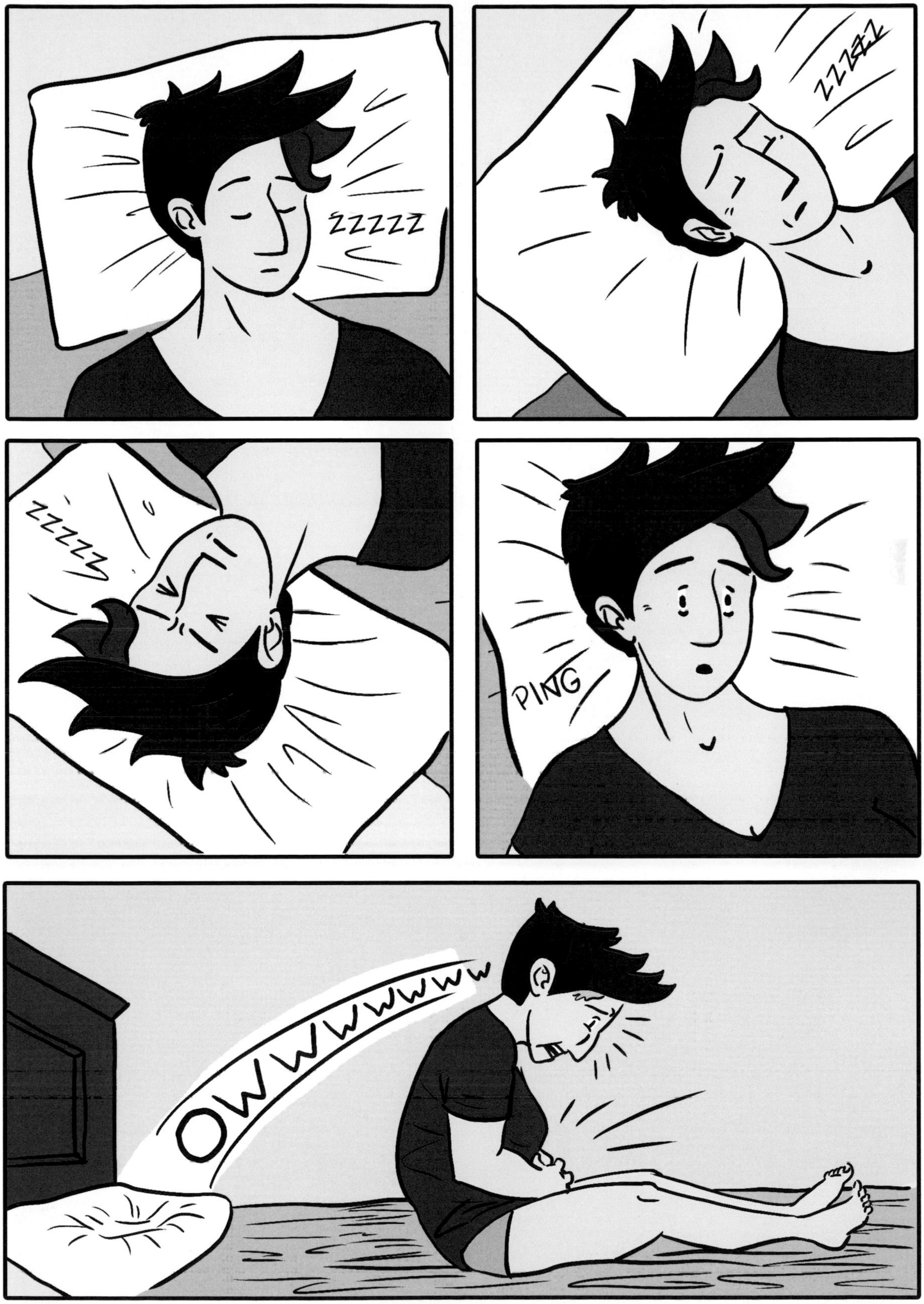
ZZZZZ
ZZZZZ
ZZZZZ
PING
OWWWWWWW

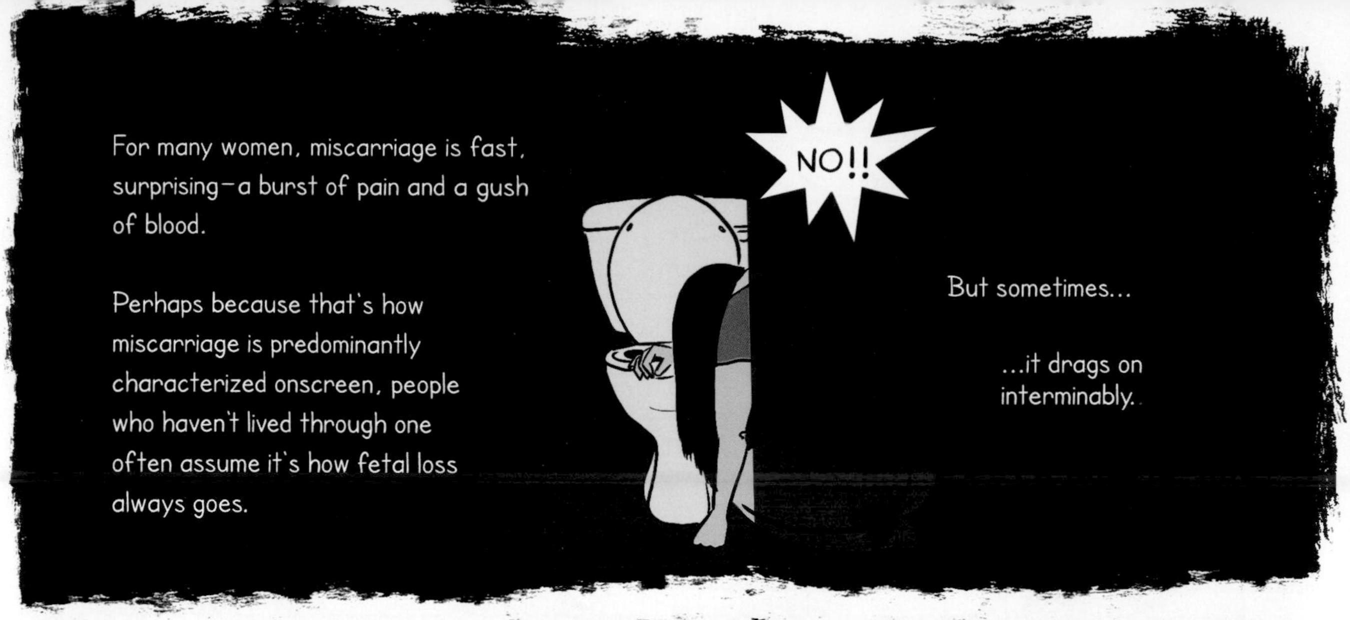
For many women, miscarriage is fast, surprising—a burst of pain and a gush of blood.
Perhaps because that's how miscarriage is predominantly characterized onscreen, people who haven't lived through one often assume it's how fetal loss always goes.
NO!!
But sometimes...
...it drags on interminably.

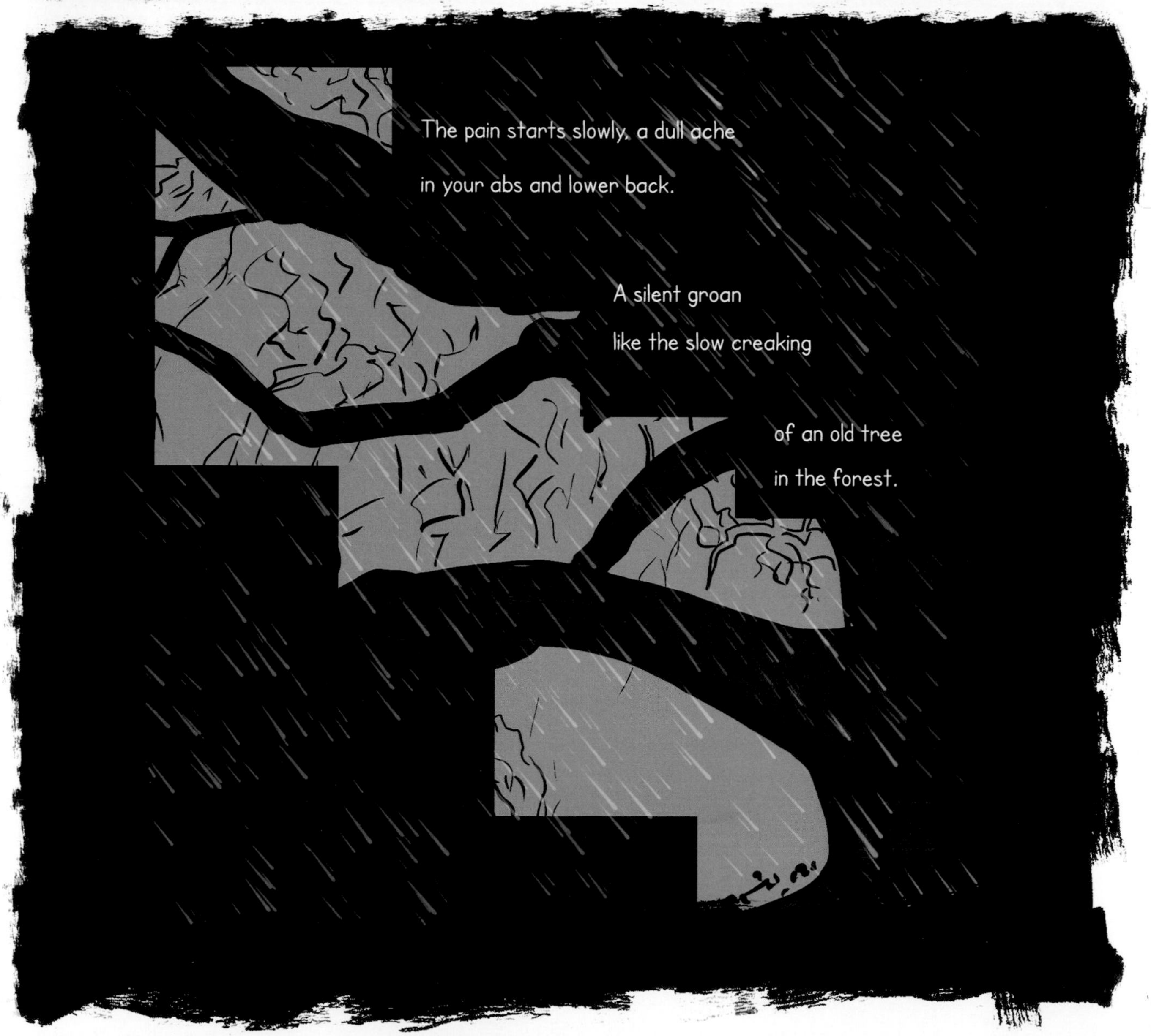
The pain starts slowly, a dull ache
in your abs and lower back.
A silent groan
like the slow creaking
of an old tree
in the forest.

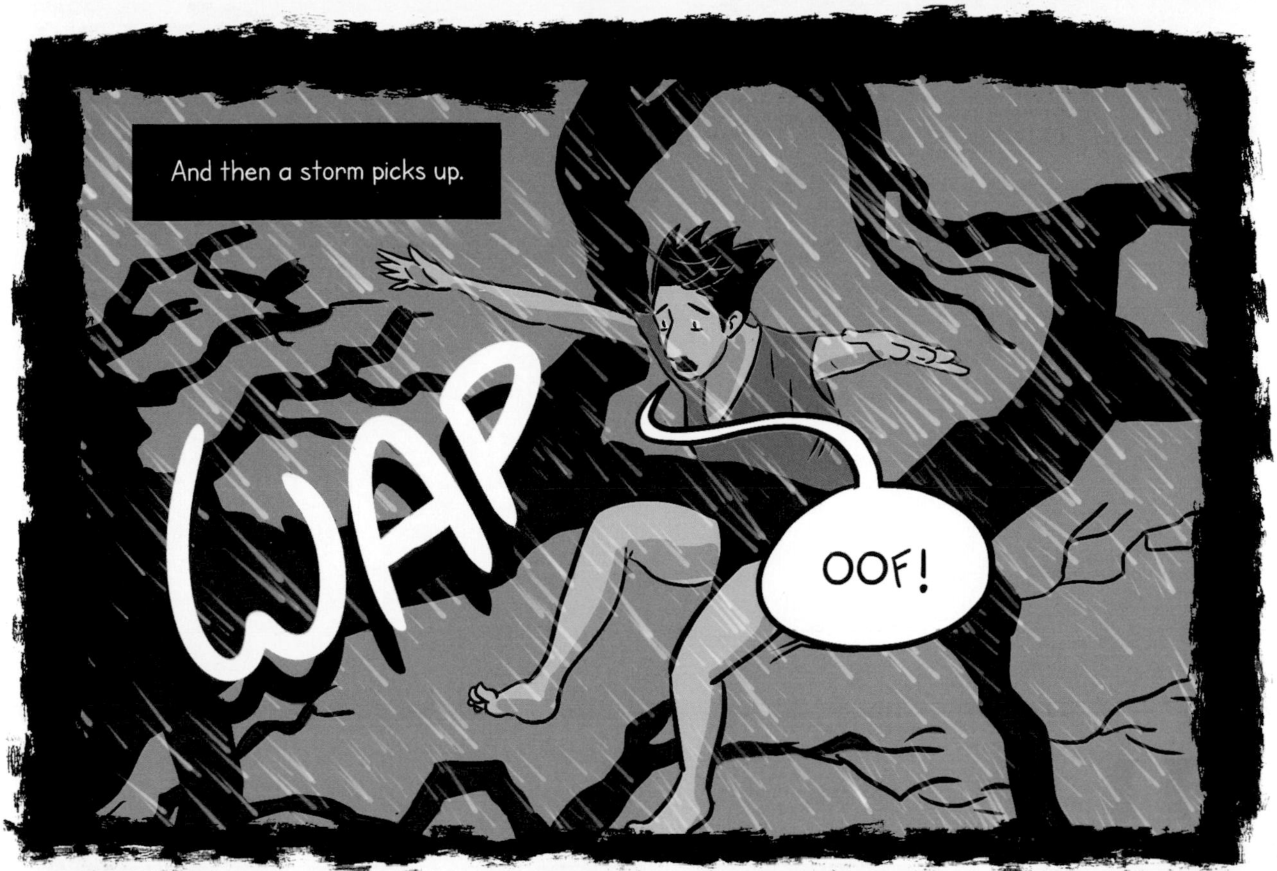
And then a storm picks up.
WAP
OOF!

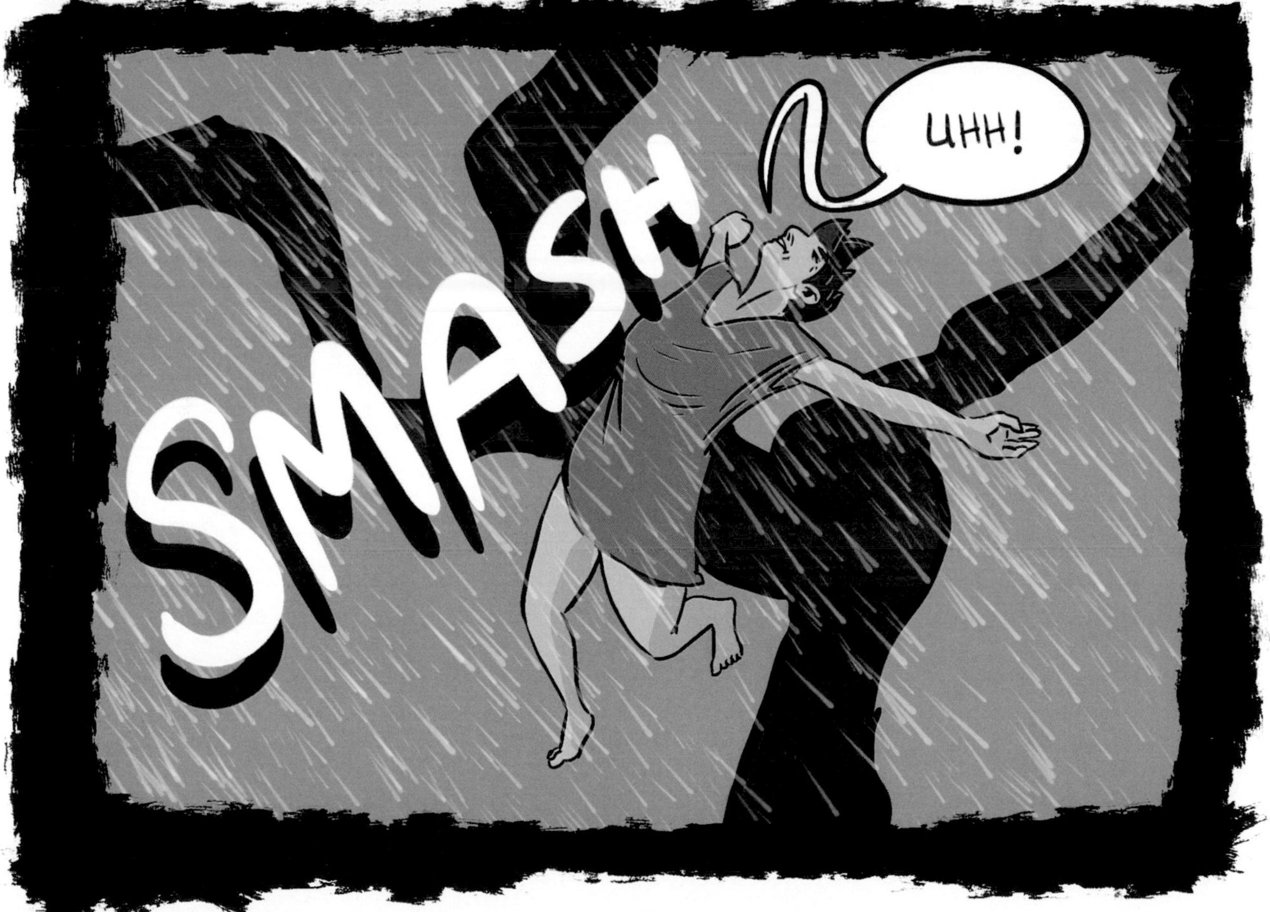
SMASH
UHH!

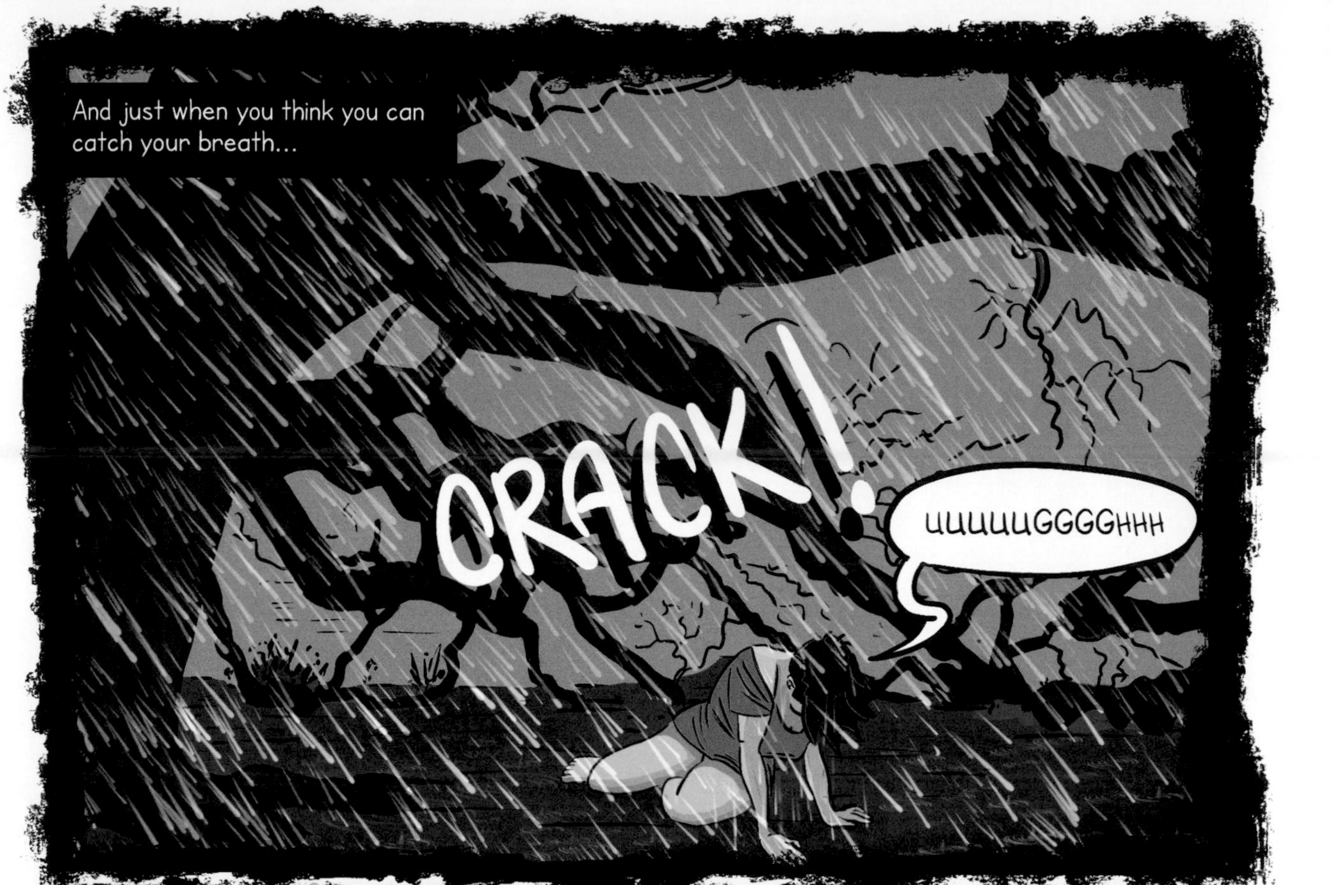
And just when you think you can catch your breath...
CRACK!
UUUUUGGGGHHH

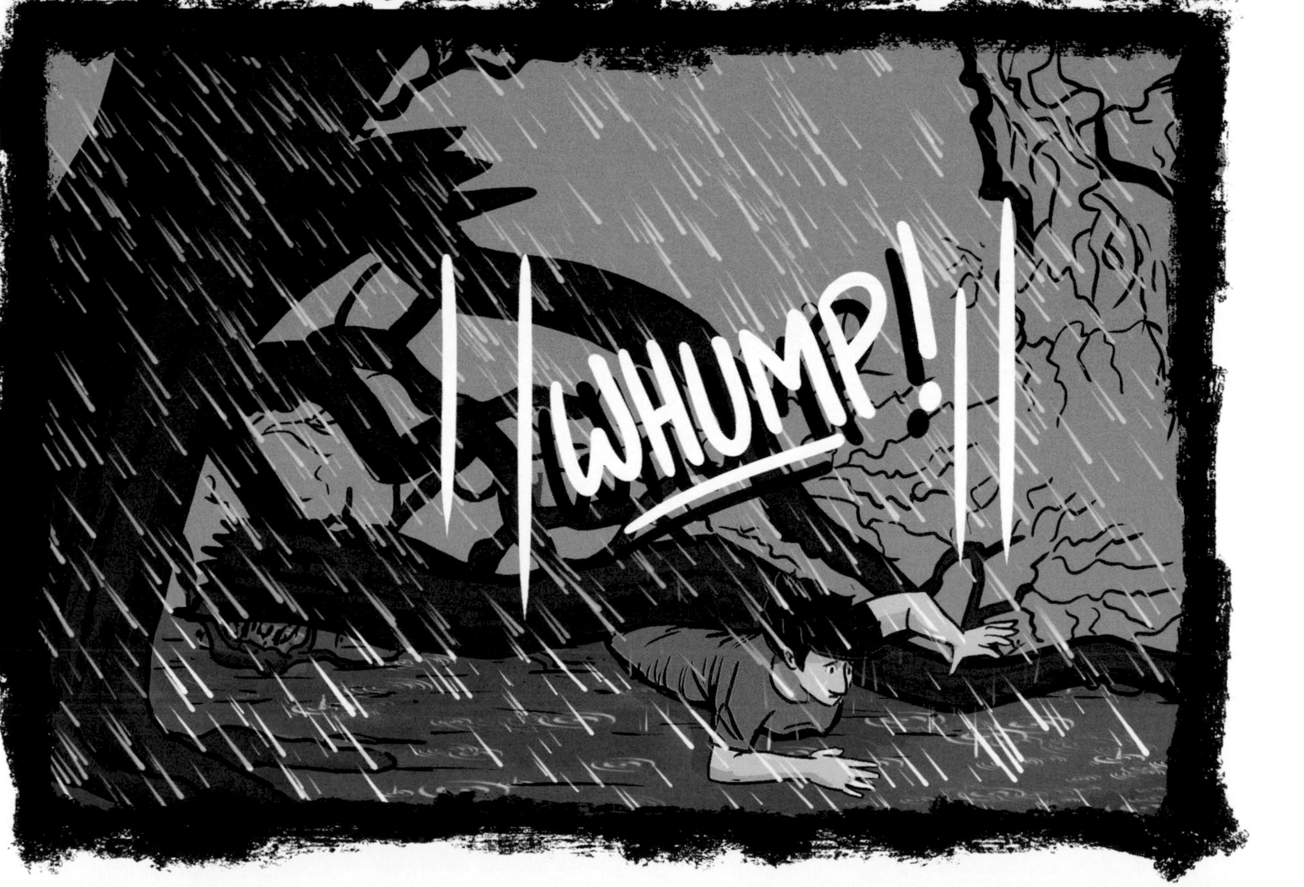
WHUMP!

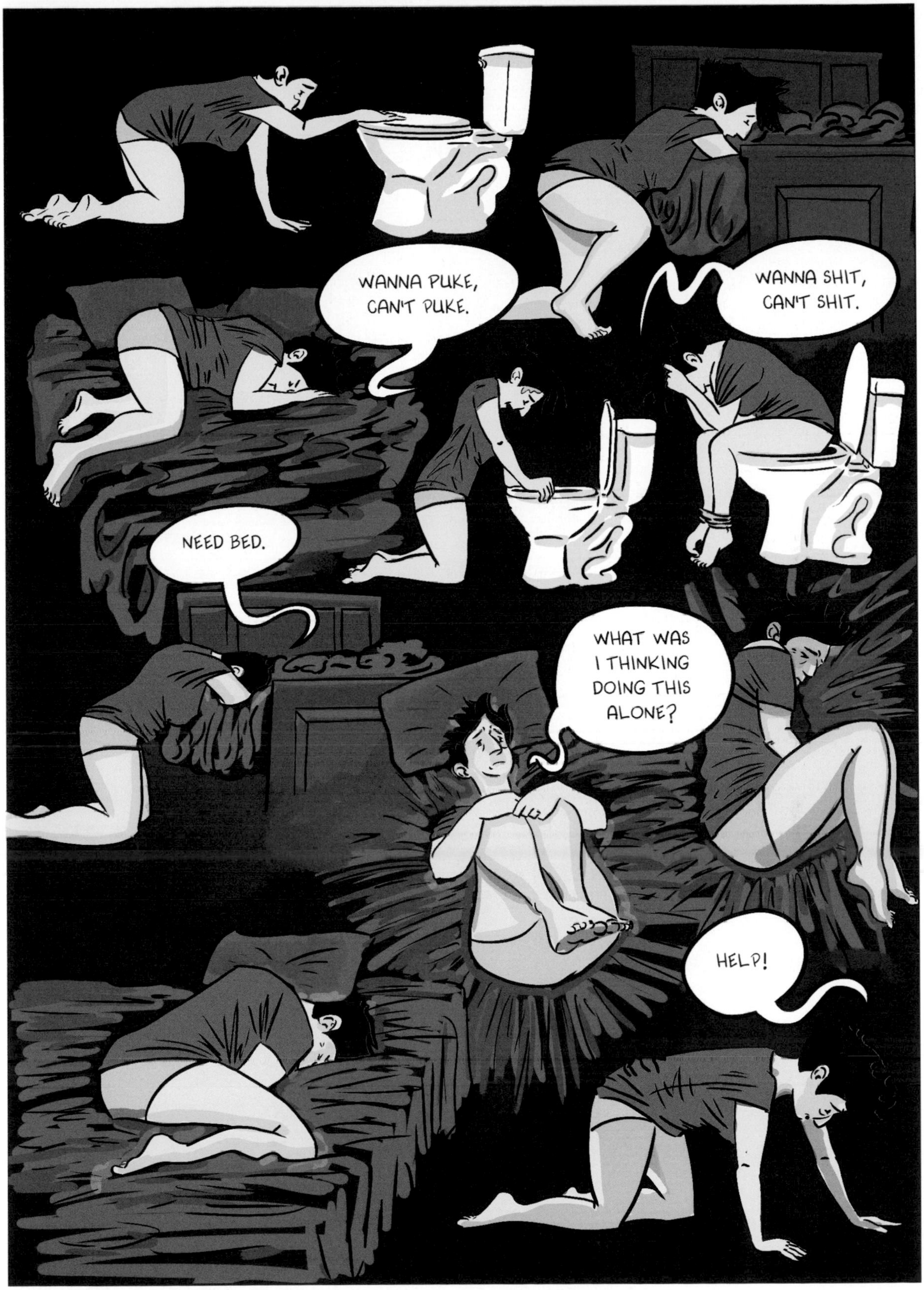
WANNA PUKE, CAN'T PUKE.
WANNA SHIT, CAN'T SHIT.
NEED BED.
WHAT WAS I THINKING DOING THIS ALONE?
HELP!

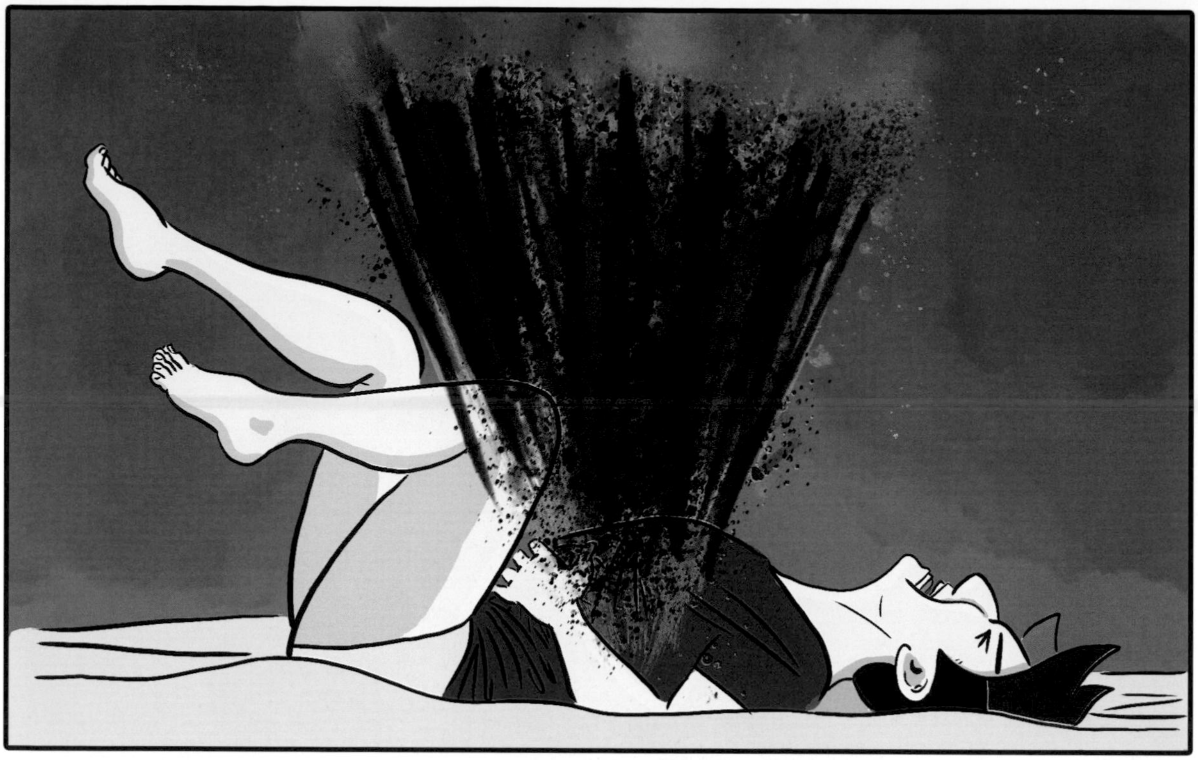

I delayed going to the hospital for as long as I could because I did not want to be writhing in agony in a stark, turbulent waiting room for hours on end. I had also been hoping that the pain would eventually subside. But at 3 a.m., I couldn't take it anymore.

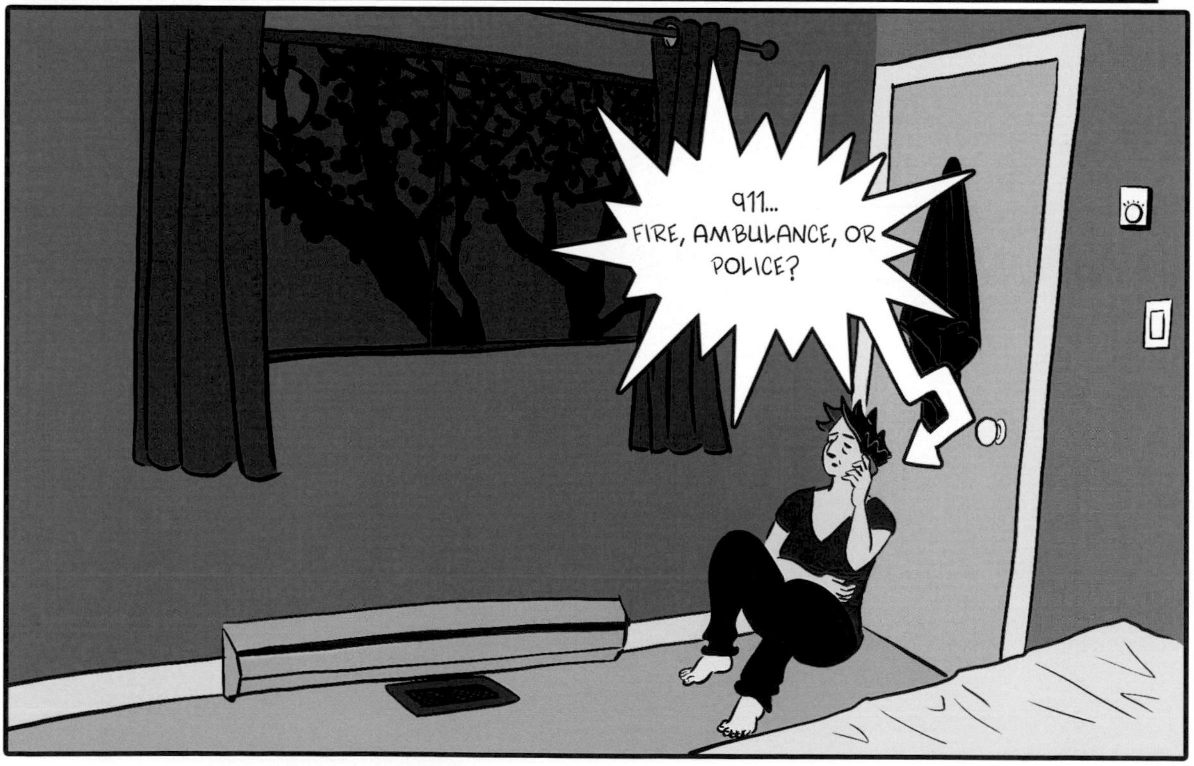
911... FIRE, AMBULANCE, OR POLICE?

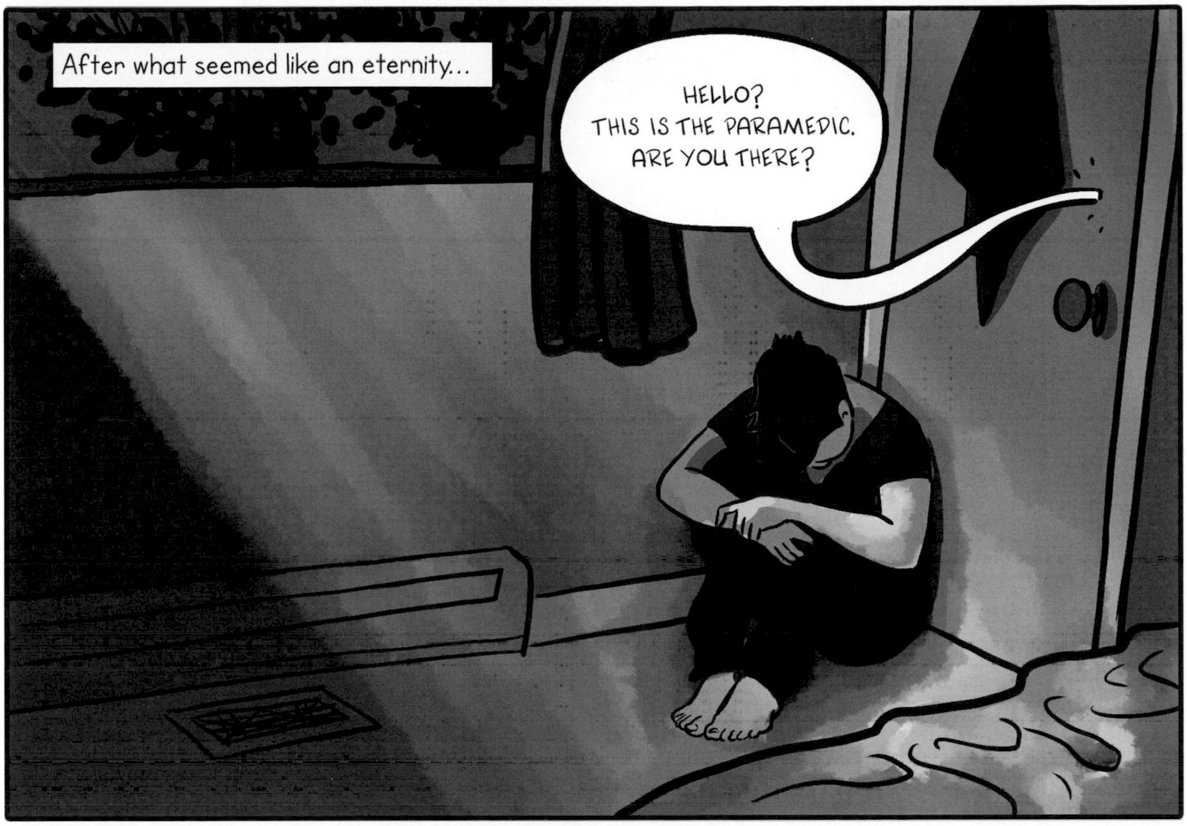
After what seemed like an eternity...
HELLO? THIS IS THE PARAMEDIC. ARE YOU THERE?

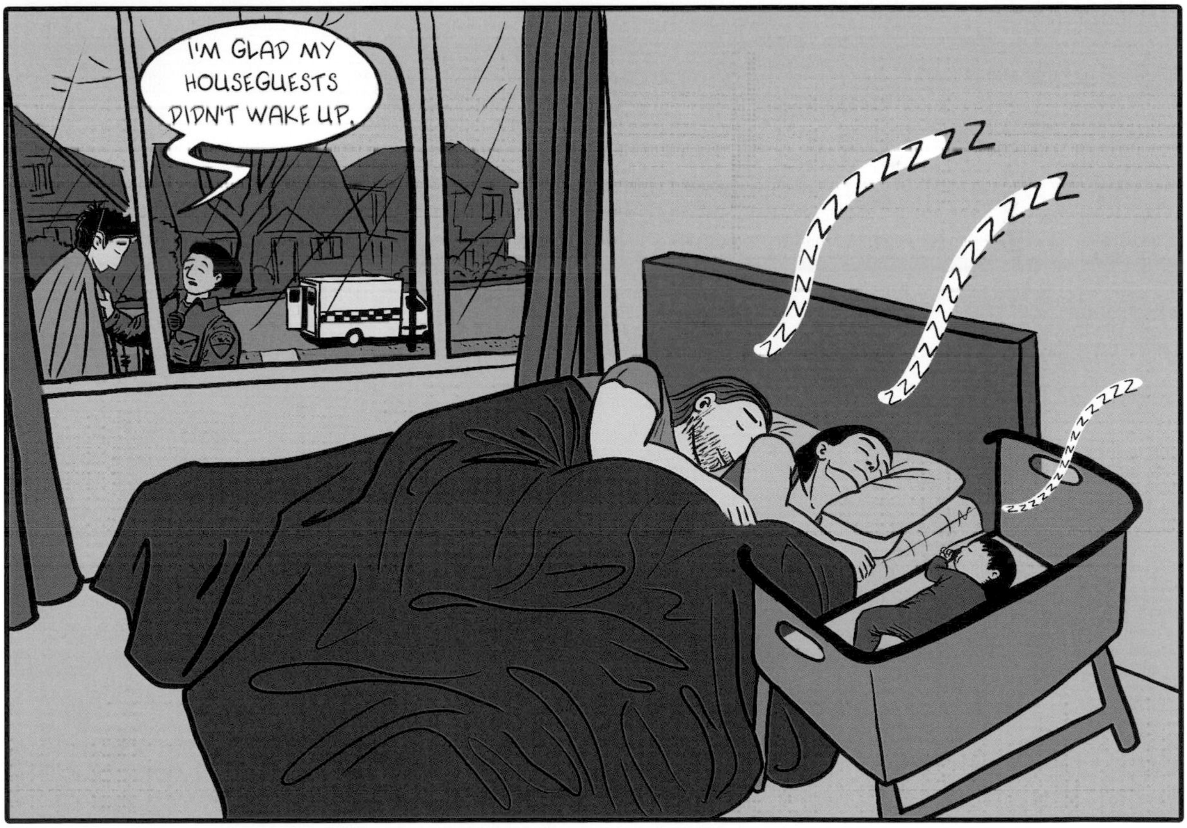
I'M GLAD MY HOUSEGUESTS DIDN'T WAKE UP.
ZZZZZZZZZZZZZ

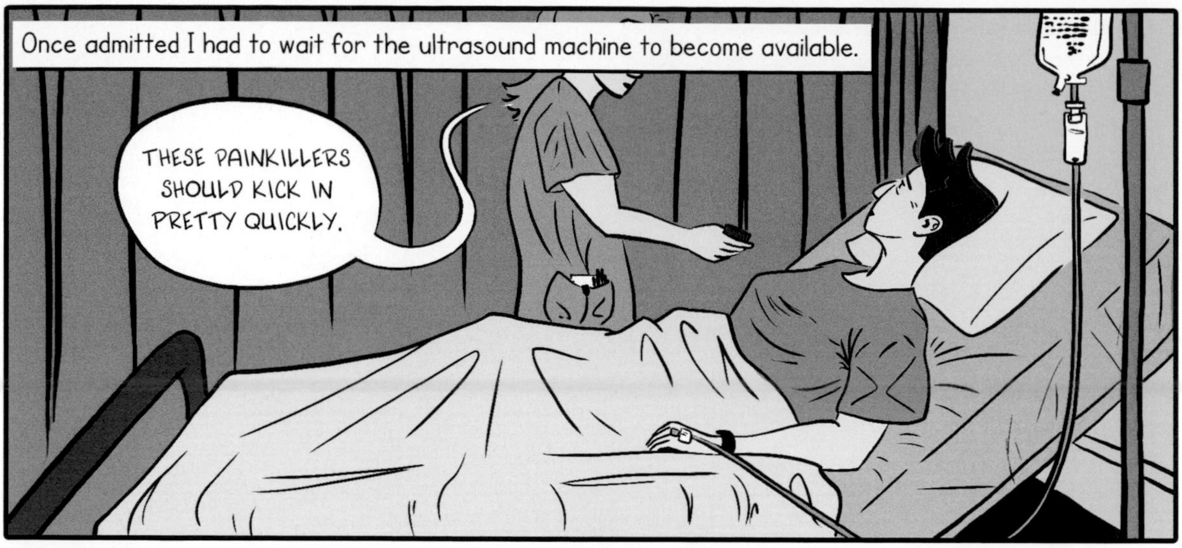
Once admitted I had to wait for the ultrasound machine to become available.
THESE PAINKILLERS SHOULD KICK IN PRETTY QUICKLY.

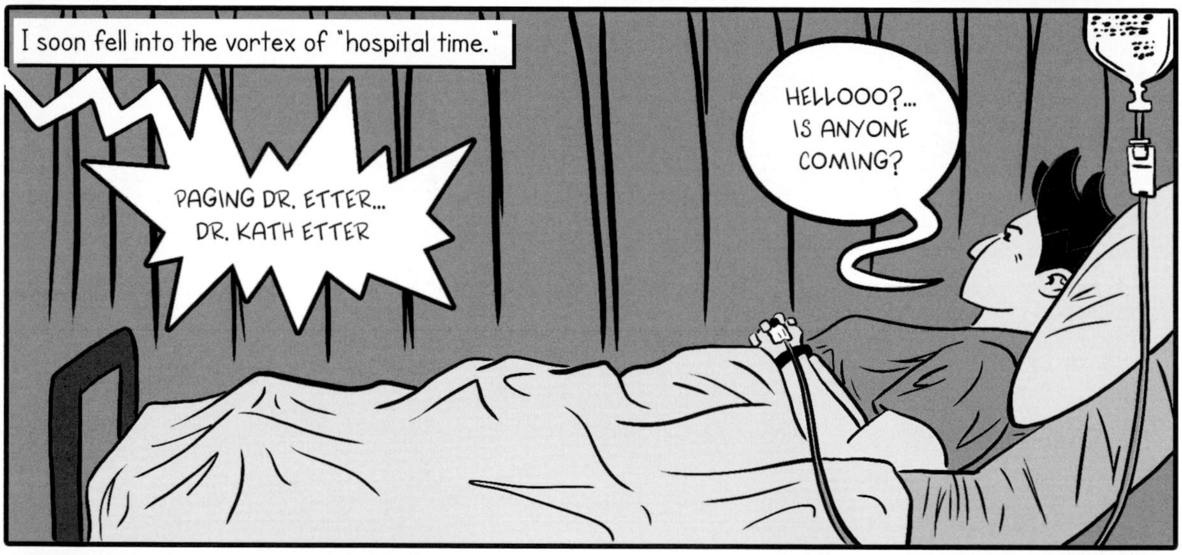
I soon fell into the vortex of "hospital time."
PAGING DR. ETTER... DR. KATH ETTER
HELLOOO?... IS ANYONE COMING?

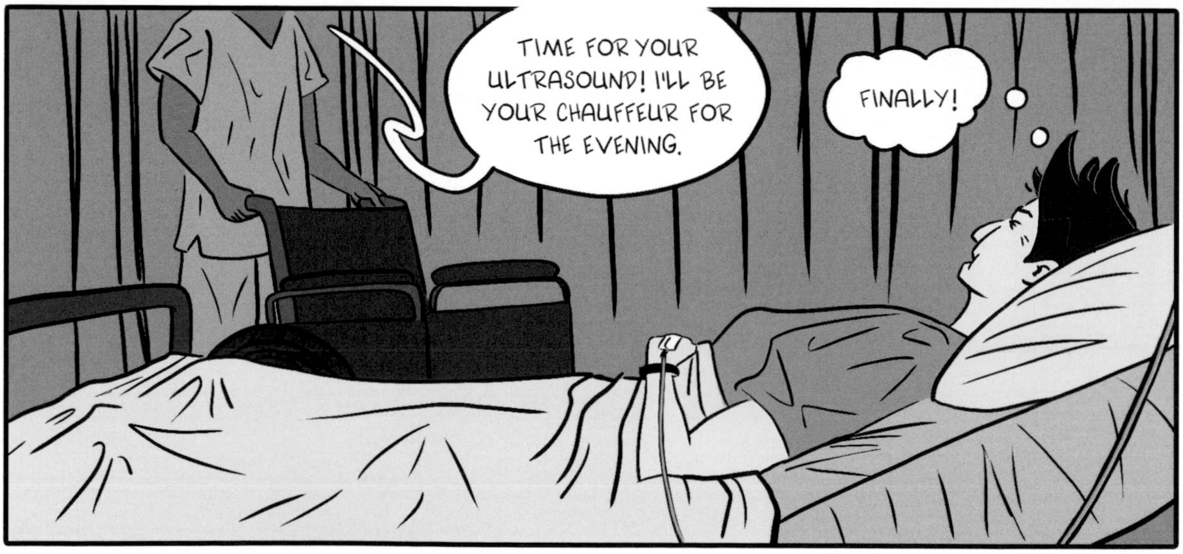
TIME FOR YOUR ULTRASOUND! I'LL BE YOUR CHAUFFEUR FOR THE EVENING.
FINALLY!

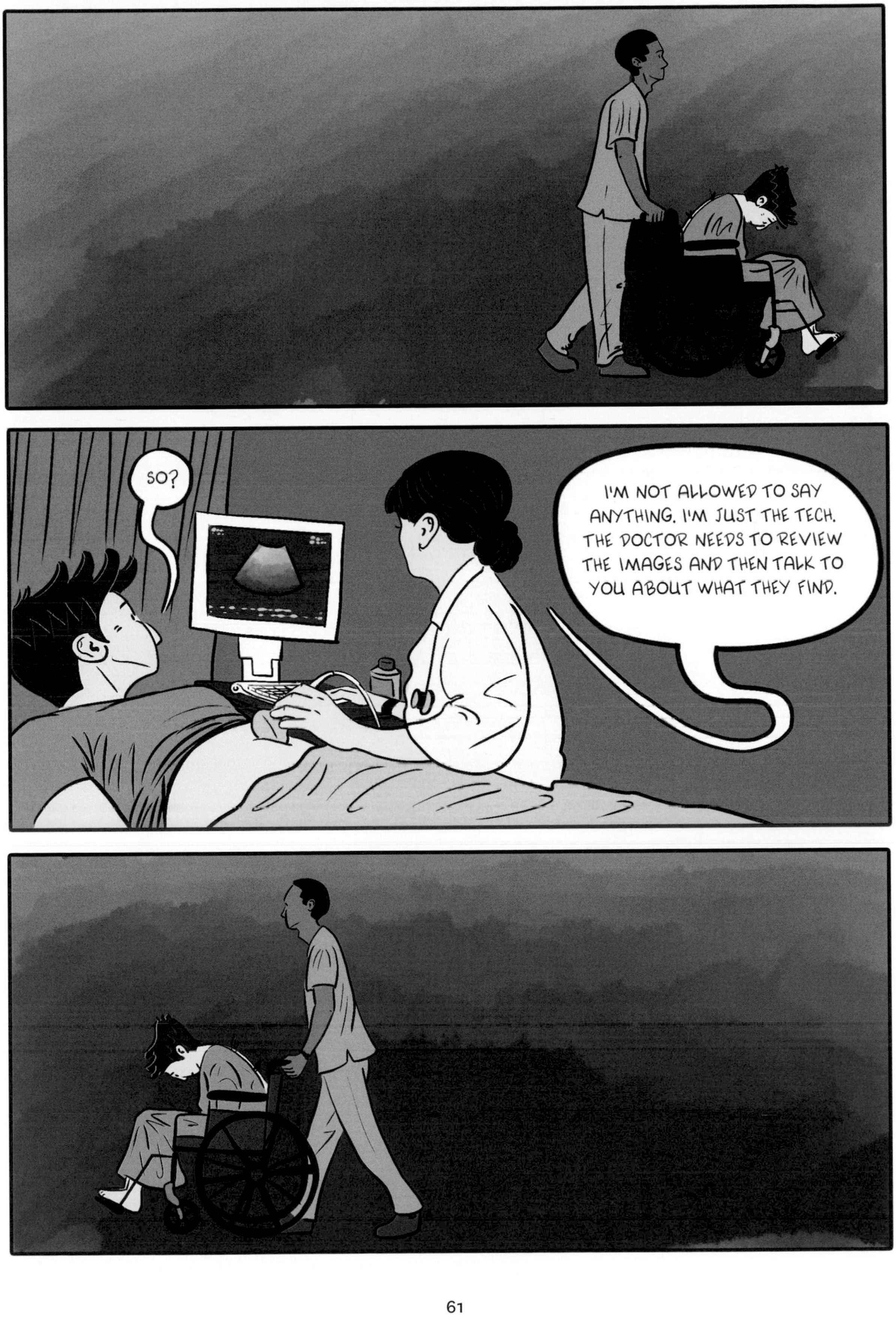
SO?
I'M NOT ALLOWED TO SAY ANYTHING. I'M JUST THE TECH. THE DOCTOR NEEDS TO REVIEW THE IMAGES AND THEN TALK TO YOU ABOUT WHAT THEY FIND.

When the doctor showed up hours later, he announced there was no more baby. My uterus was empty.

I'm not sure how I found the strength to call Johanna to pick me up from the hospital, nor how I managed to wait for her on a busy downtown street without disintegrating. I was numb, trembling, crying, in shock, and experiencing a quality of sadness that I'd never thought possible.

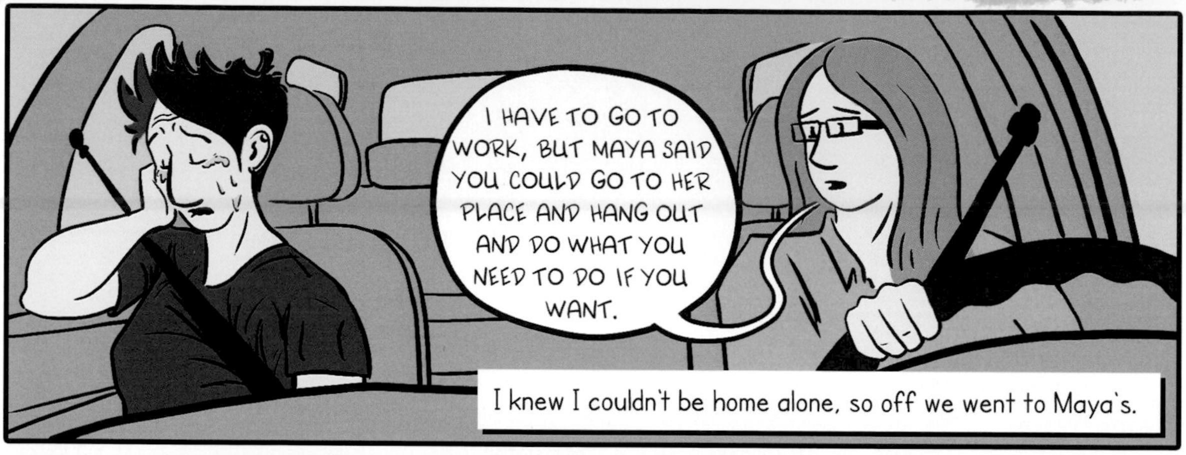
I HAVE TO GO TO WORK, BUT MAYA SAID YOU COULD GO TO HER PLACE AND HANG OUT AND DO WHAT YOU NEED TO DO IF YOU WANT.
I knew I couldn't be home alone, so off we went to Maya's.

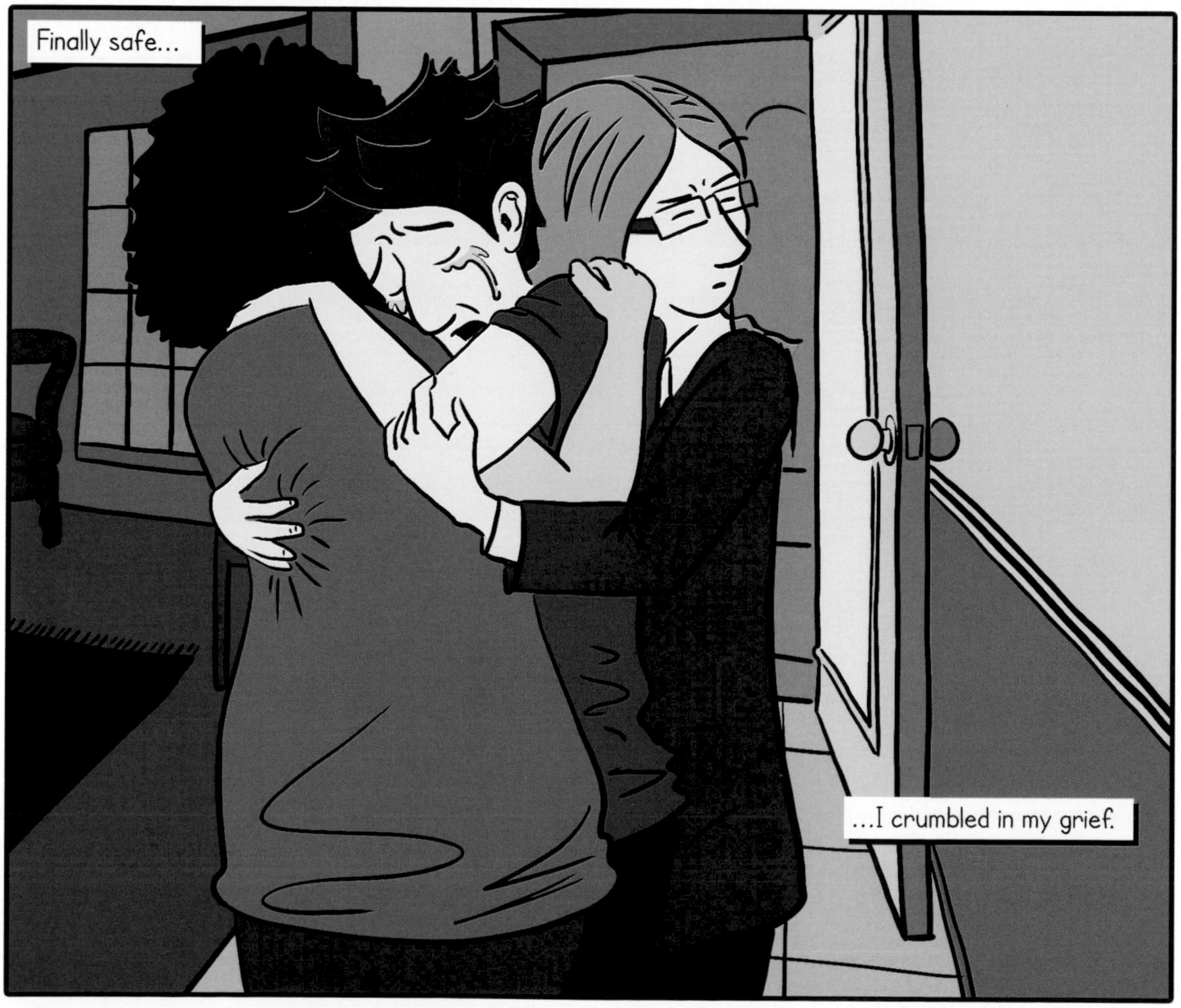
Finally safe...
...I crumbled in my grief.

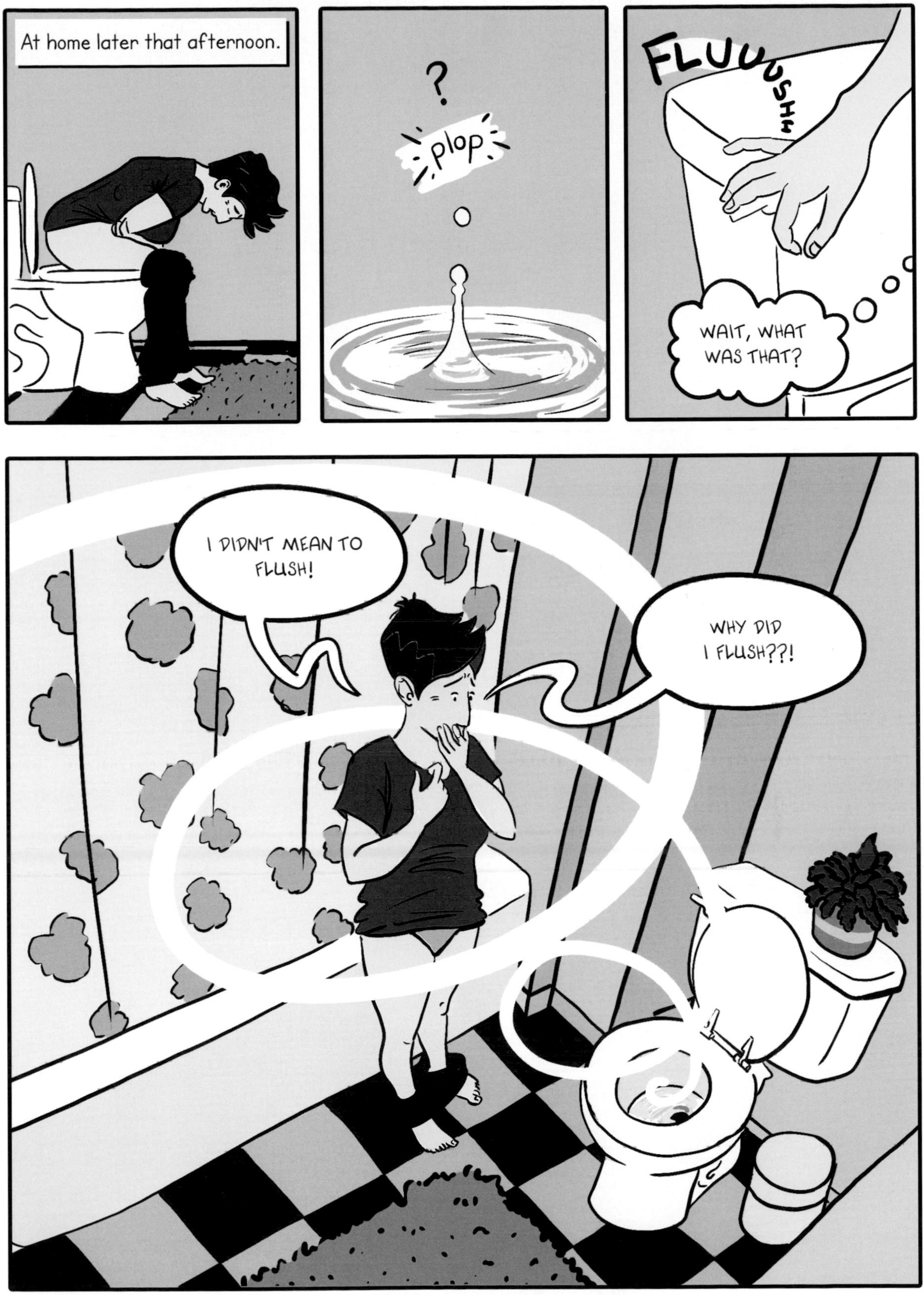
At home later that afternoon.
?
plop
FLUUUSHH
WAIT, WHAT WAS THAT?
I DIDN'T MEAN TO FLUSH!
WHY DID I FLUSH??!

No one EVER told me that this can happen.

And it does...often.

I was now one of the countless women who have not only endured the physical loss of their baby but have also then been faced with the confusion, humiliation, shame, horror, and despair that the child they so wanted is now floating in a toilet bowl—either to be fished out to be dealt with some other way (e.g., burial or medical autopsy) or flushed.

It would take all my courage, strength, fortitude, and willpower to move through and past that realization and go on with my life.

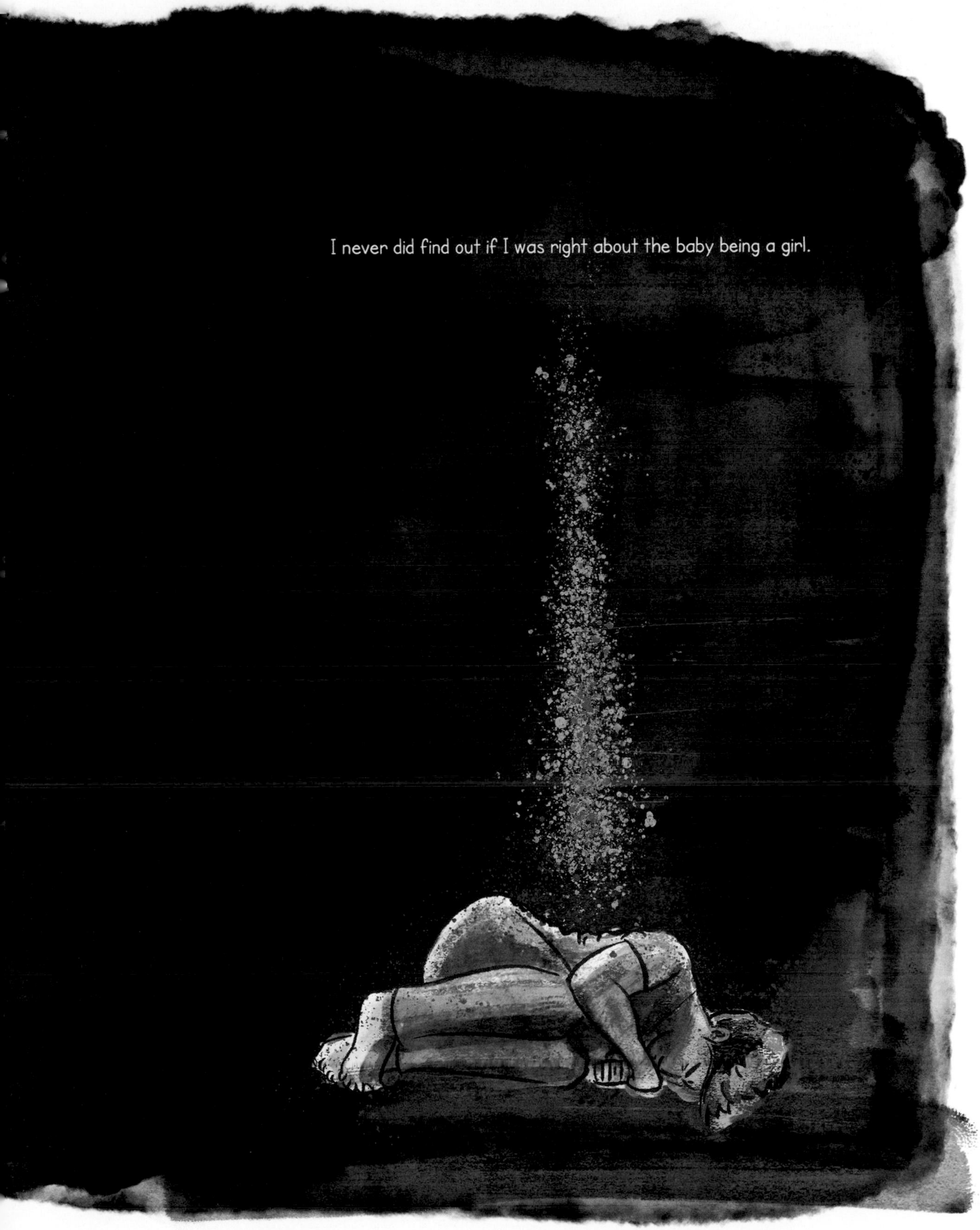
I never did find out if I was right about the baby being a girl.

Chapter 2

Insemination Ingemination

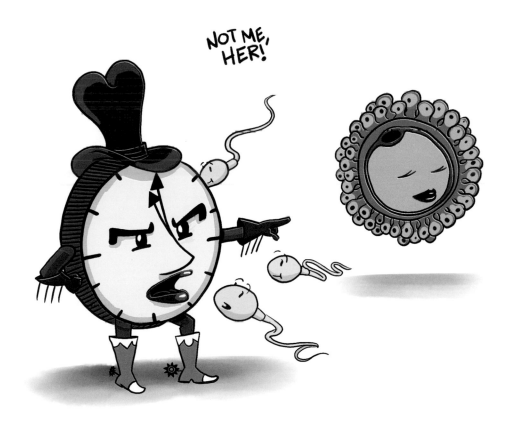

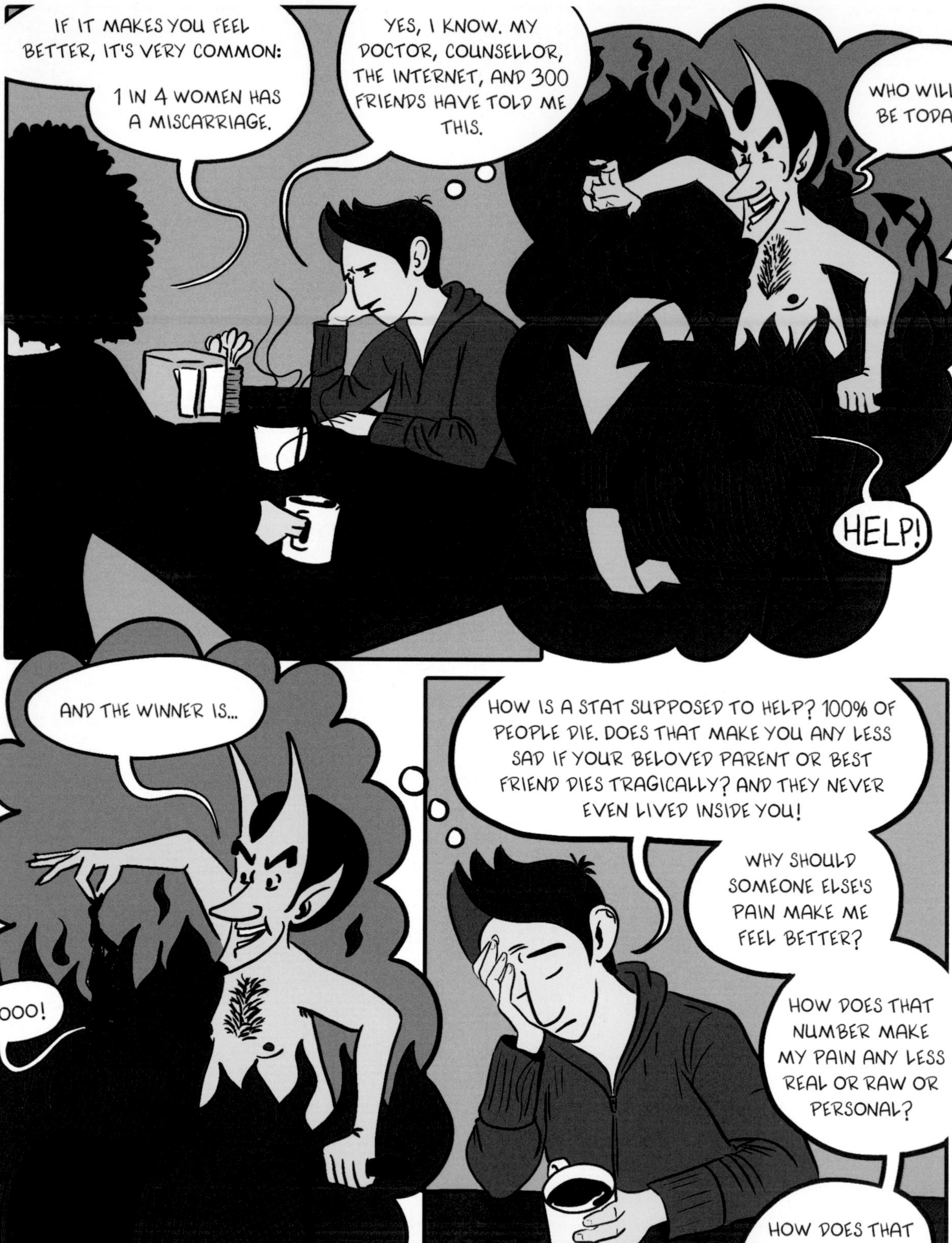
IF IT MAKES YOU FEEL BETTER, IT'S VERY COMMON:
1 IN 4 WOMEN HAS A MISCARRIAGE.
YES, I KNOW. MY DOCTOR, COUNSELLOR, THE INTERNET, AND 300 FRIENDS HAVE TOLD ME THIS.
WHO WILL IT BE TODAY?
HELP!
AND THE WINNER IS...
NOOO!
HOW IS A STAT SUPPOSED TO HELP? 100% OF PEOPLE DIE. DOES THAT MAKE YOU ANY LESS SAD IF YOUR BELOVED PARENT OR BEST FRIEND DIES TRAGICALLY? AND THEY NEVER EVEN LIVED INSIDE YOU!
WHY SHOULD SOMEONE ELSE'S PAIN MAKE ME FEEL BETTER?
HOW DOES THAT NUMBER MAKE MY PAIN ANY LESS REAL OR RAW OR PERSONAL?
HOW DOES THAT MAKE IT ANY MORE FAIR?

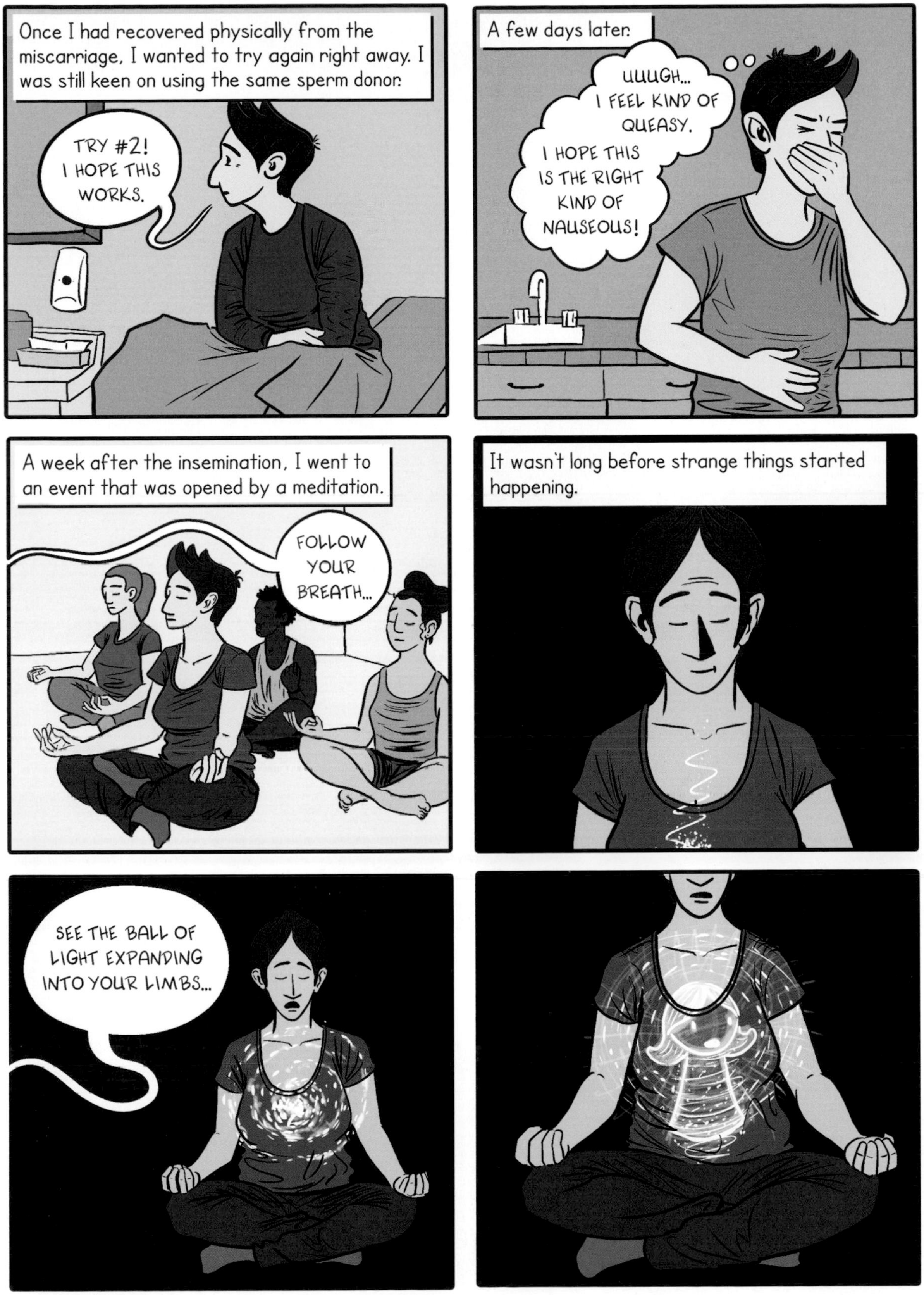
Once I had recovered physically from the miscarriage, I wanted to try again right away. I was still keen on using the same sperm donor.
TRY #2! I HOPE THIS WORKS.
A few days later.
UUUGH... I FEEL KIND OF QUEASY.
I HOPE THIS IS THE RIGHT KIND OF NAUSEOUS!
A week after the insemination, I went to an event that was opened by a meditation.
FOLLOW YOUR BREATH...
It wasn't long before strange things started happening.
SEE THE BALL OF LIGHT EXPANDING INTO YOUR LIMBS...

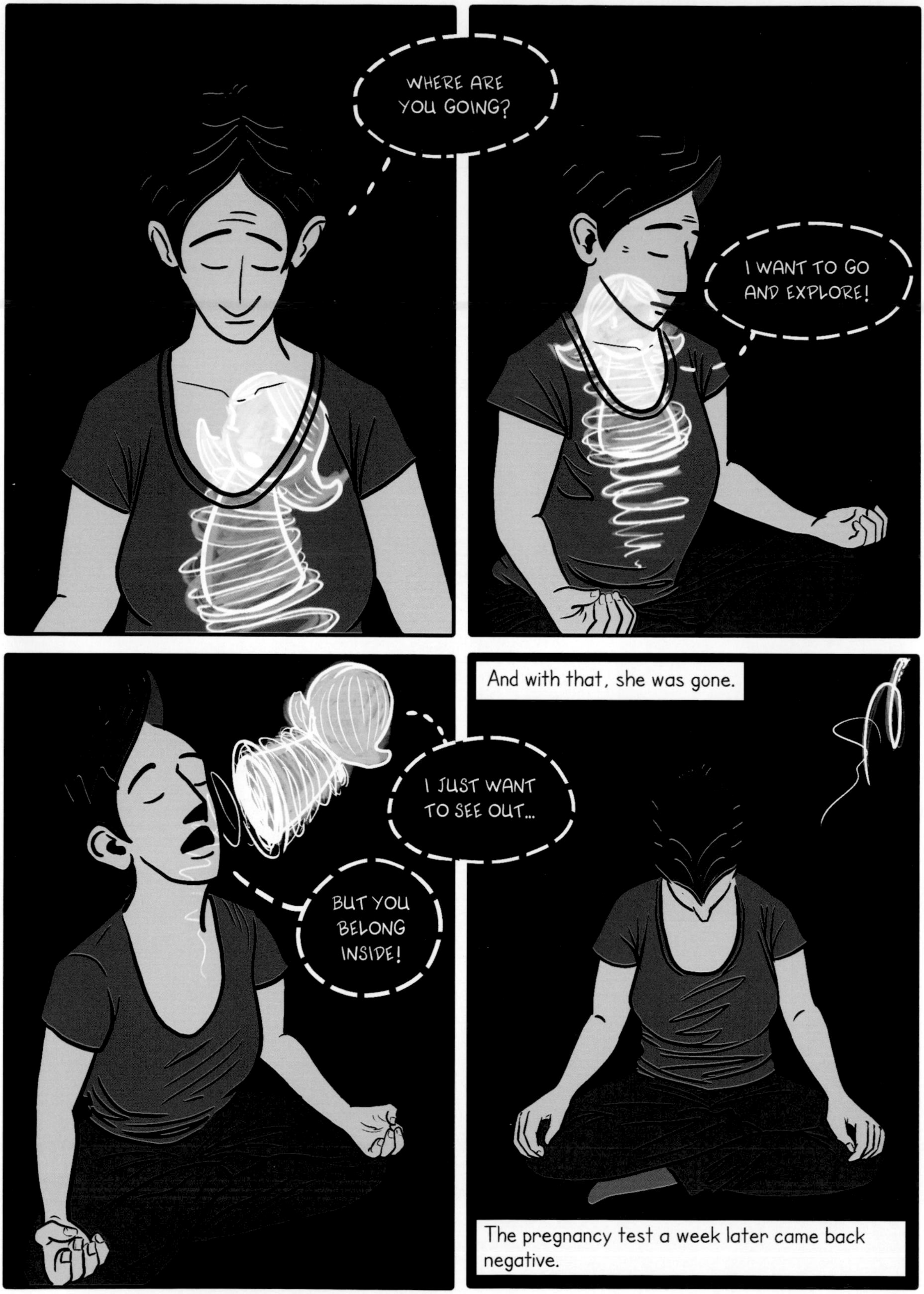
WHERE ARE YOU GOING?
I WANT TO GO AND EXPLORE!
I JUST WANT TO SEE OUT...
BUT YOU BELONG INSIDE!
And with that, she was gone.
The pregnancy test a week later came back negative.

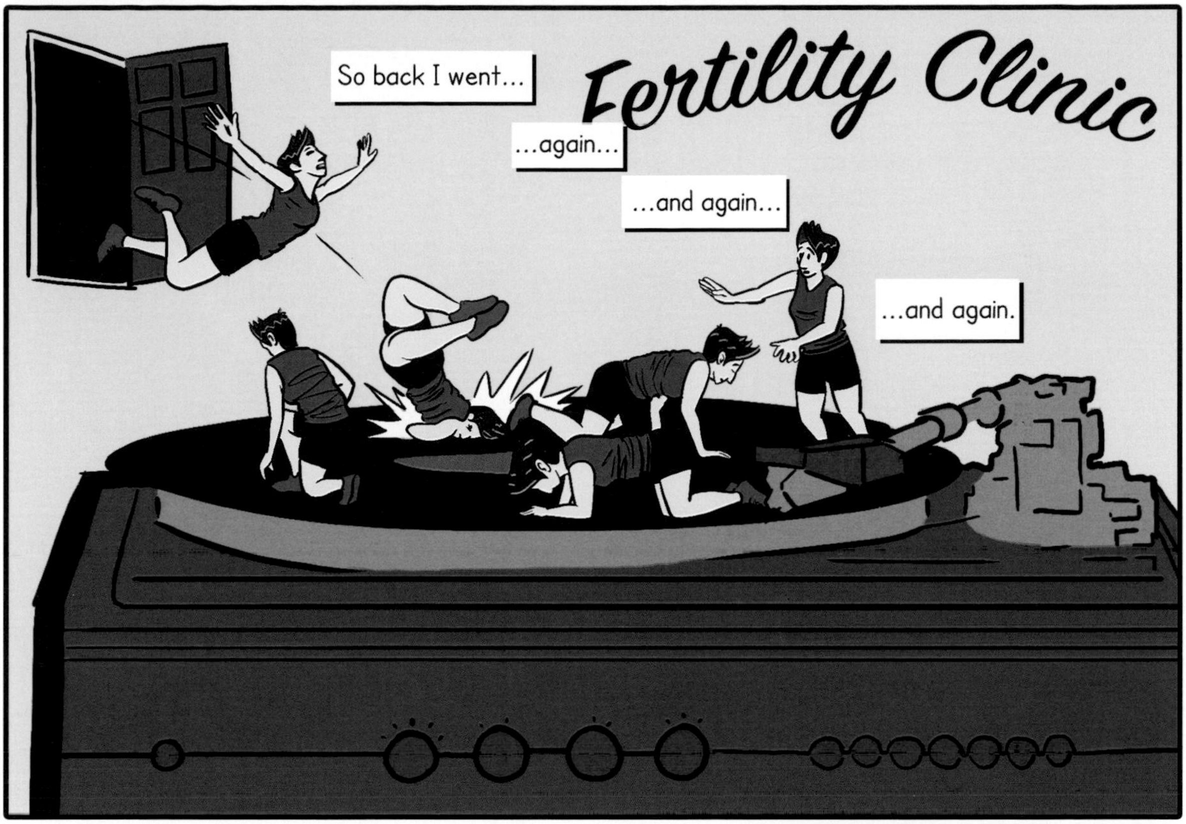
So back I went...
Fertility Clinic
...again...
...and again...
...and again.

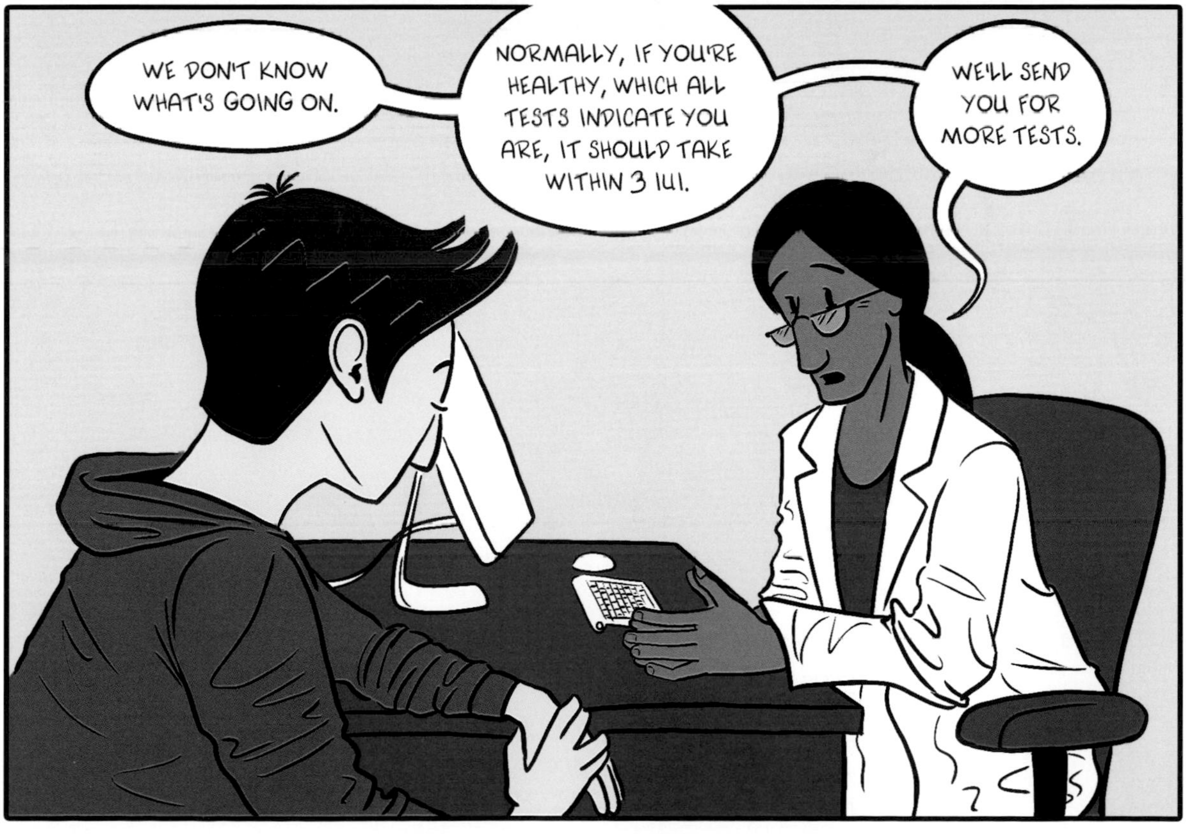
WE DON'T KNOW WHAT'S GOING ON.
NORMALLY, IF YOU'RE HEALTHY, WHICH ALL TESTS INDICATE YOU ARE, IT SHOULD TAKE WITHIN 3 IUI.
WE'LL SEND YOU FOR MORE TESTS.

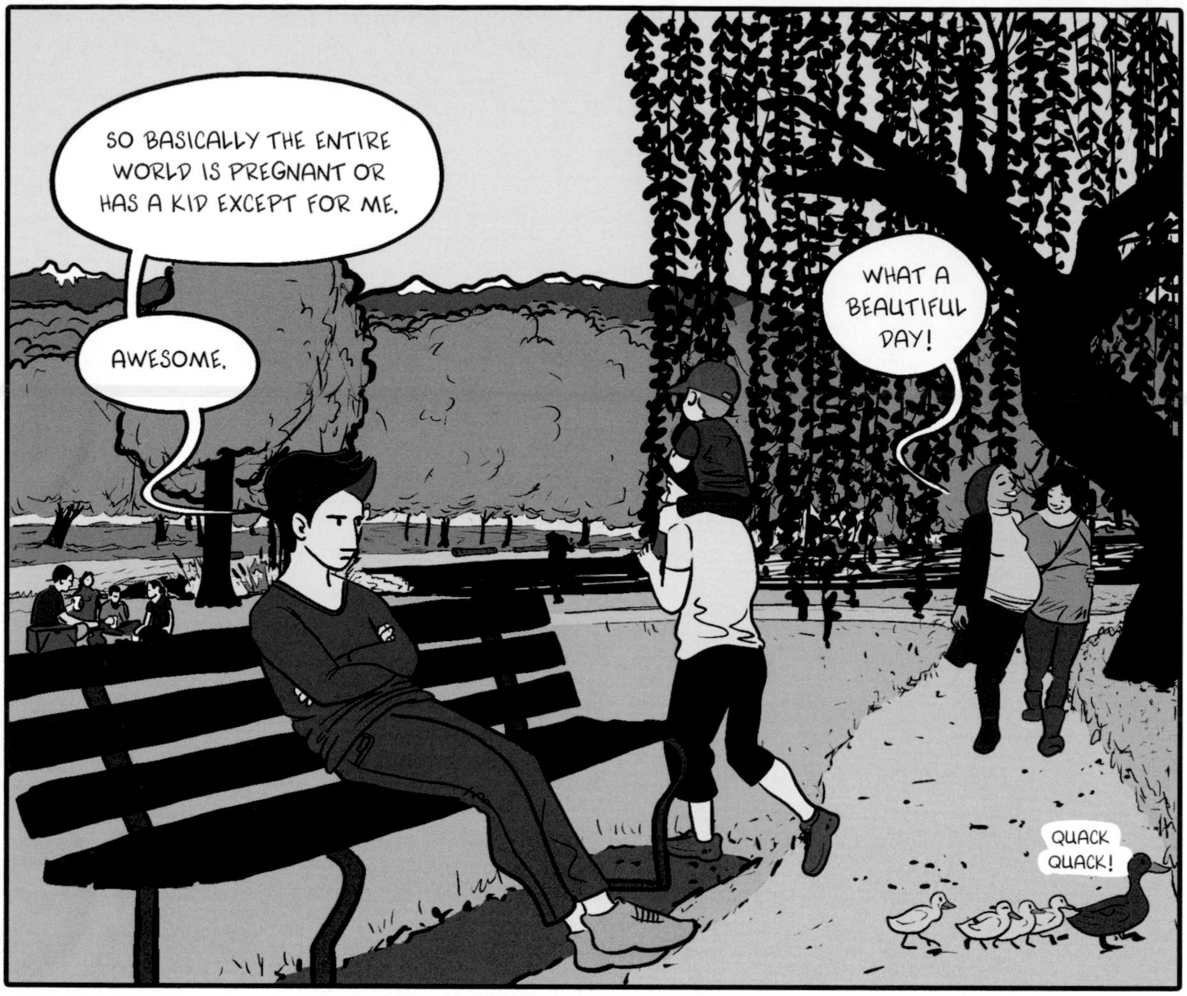
SO BASICALLY THE ENTIRE WORLD IS PREGNANT OR HAS A KID EXCEPT FOR ME.
AWESOME.
WHAT A BEAUTIFUL DAY!
QUACK QUACK!

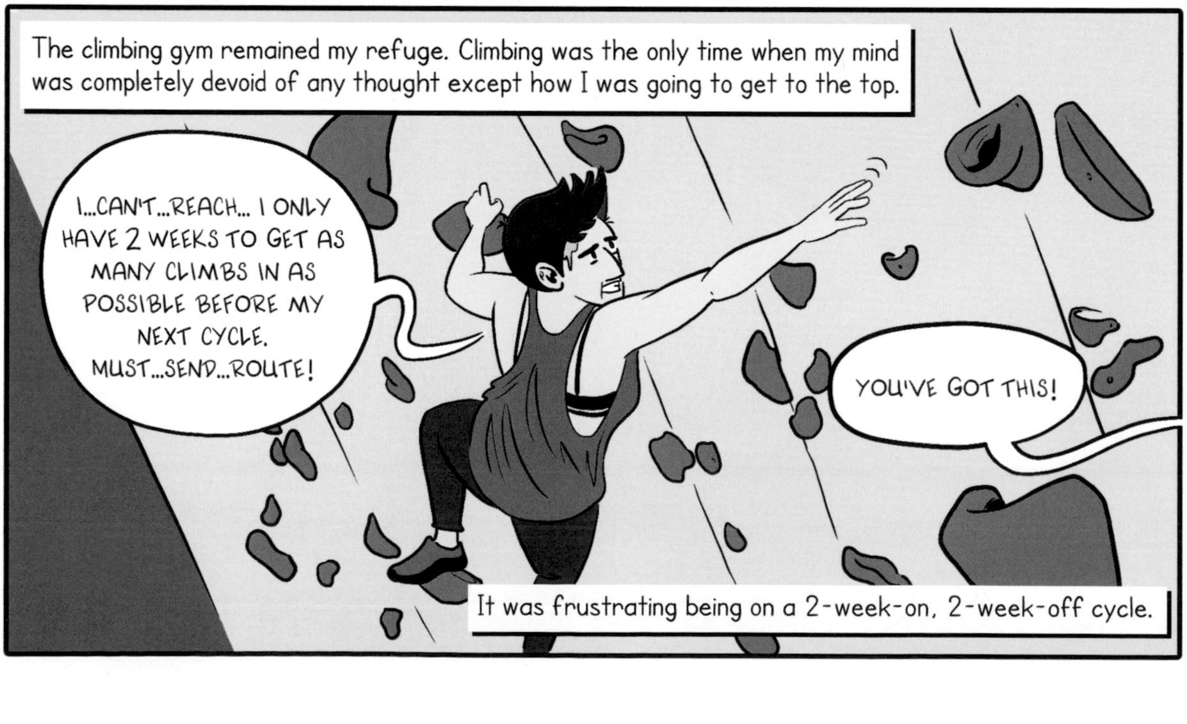
The climbing gym remained my refuge. Climbing was the only time when my mind was completely devoid of any thought except how I was going to get to the top.
I...CAN'T...REACH... I ONLY HAVE 2 WEEKS TO GET AS MANY CLIMBS IN AS POSSIBLE BEFORE MY NEXT CYCLE. MUST...SEND...ROUTE!
YOU'VE GOT THIS!
It was frustrating being on a 2-week-on, 2-week-off cycle.

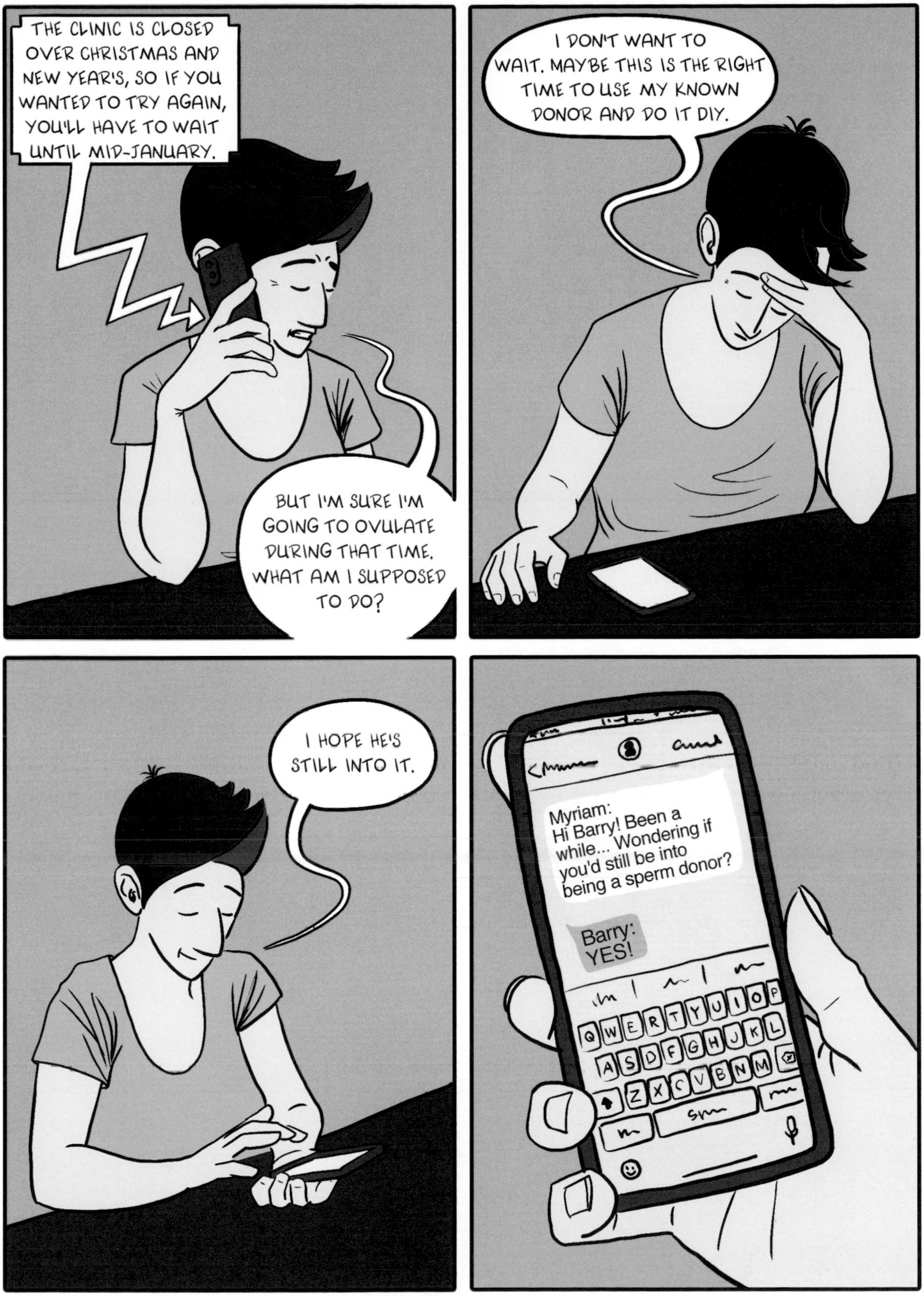
THE CLINIC IS CLOSED OVER CHRISTMAS AND NEW YEAR'S, SO IF YOU WANTED TO TRY AGAIN, YOU'LL HAVE TO WAIT UNTIL MID-JANUARY.
BUT I'M SURE I'M GOING TO OVULATE DURING THAT TIME. WHAT AM I SUPPOSED TO DO?
I DON'T WANT TO WAIT. MAYBE THIS IS THE RIGHT TIME TO USE MY KNOWN DONOR AND DO IT DIY.
I HOPE HE'S STILL INTO IT.
Myriam:
Hi Barry! Been a while... Wondering if you'd still be into being a sperm donor?
Barry:
YES!

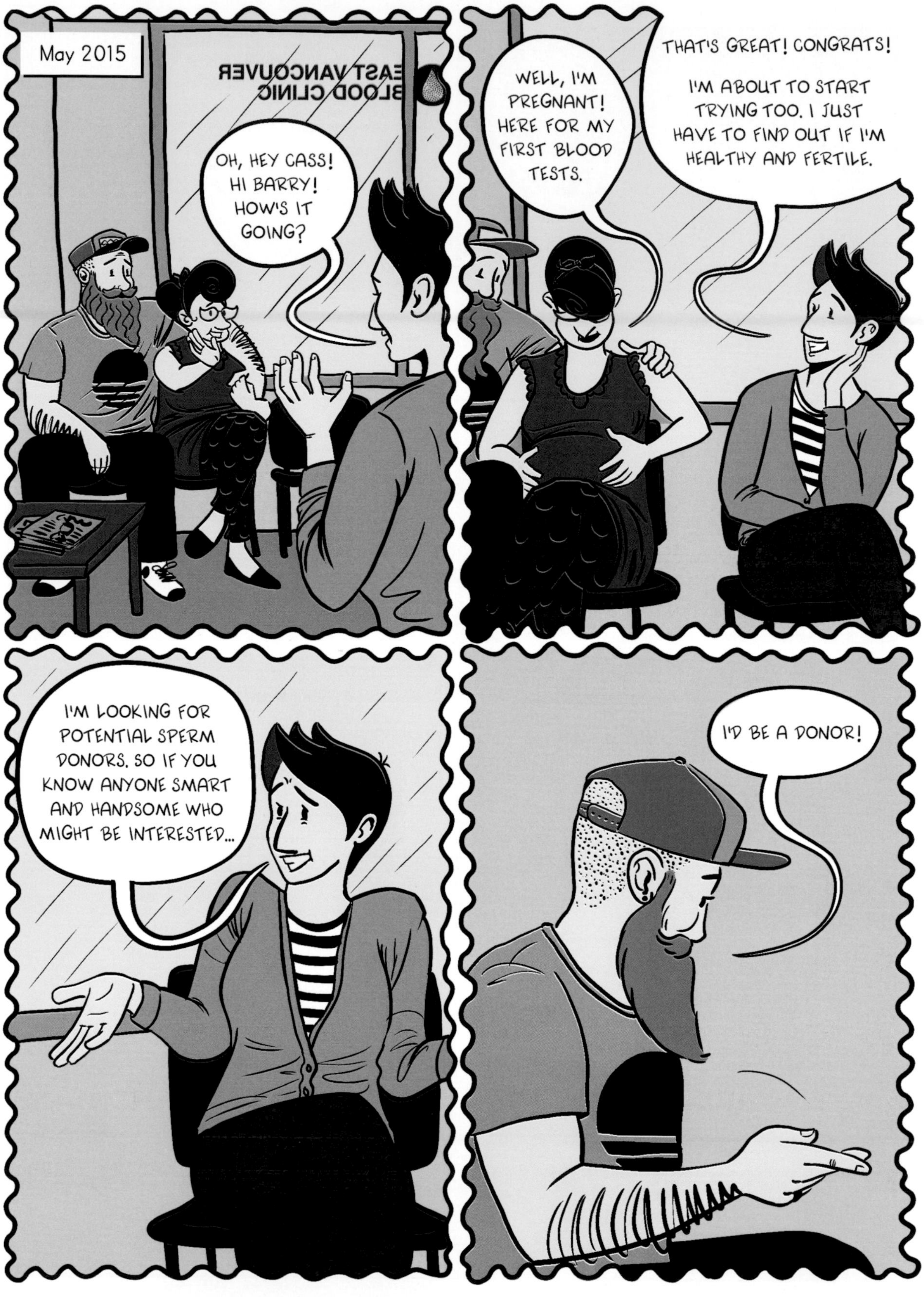
May 2015
EAST VANCOUVER BLOOD CLINIC
OH, HEY CASS! HI BARRY! HOW'S IT GOING?
WELL, I'M PREGNANT! HERE FOR MY FIRST BLOOD TESTS.
THAT'S GREAT! CONGRATS!
I'M ABOUT TO START TRYING TOO. I JUST HAVE TO FIND OUT IF I'M HEALTHY AND FERTILE.
I'M LOOKING FOR POTENTIAL SPERM DONORS. SO IF YOU KNOW ANYONE SMART AND HANDSOME WHO MIGHT BE INTERESTED...
I'D BE A DONOR!

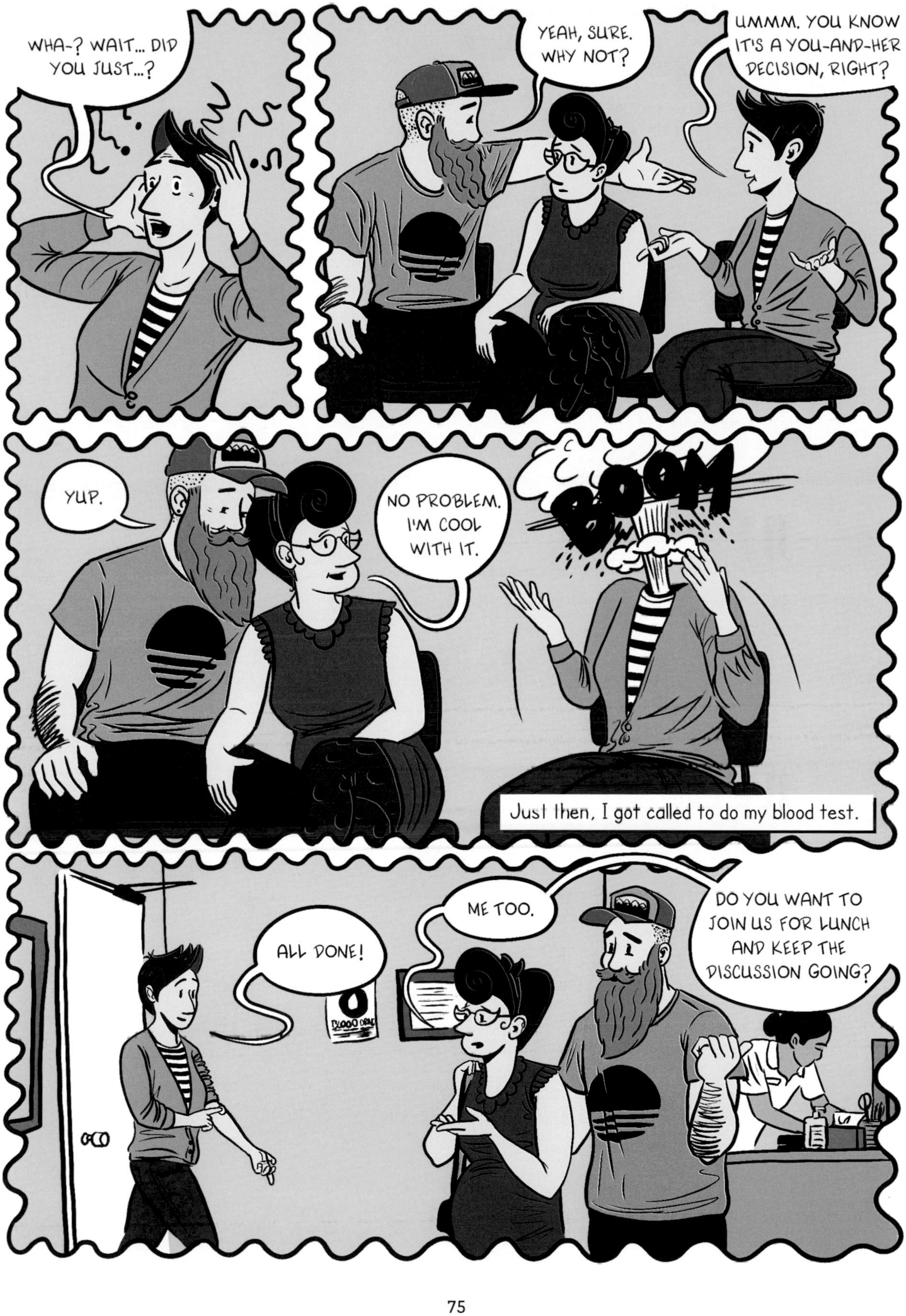
WHA-? WAIT... DID YOU JUST...?
YEAH, SURE. WHY NOT?
UMMM. YOU KNOW IT'S A YOU-AND-HER DECISION, RIGHT?
YUP.
NO PROBLEM. I'M COOL WITH IT.
BOOM
Just then, I got called to do my blood test.
ALL DONE!
ME TOO.
DO YOU WANT TO JOIN US FOR LUNCH AND KEEP THE DISCUSSION GOING?

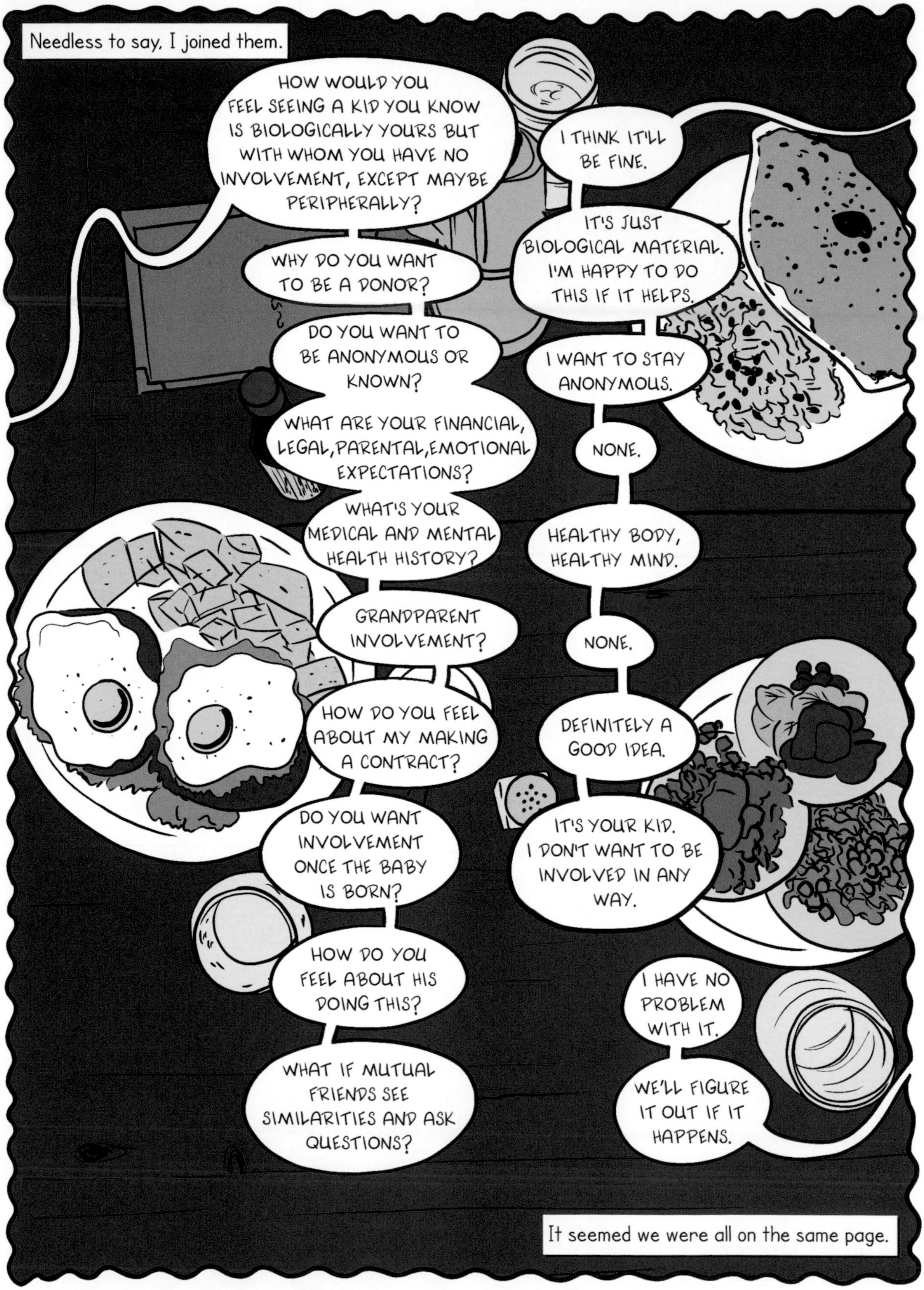
Needless to say, I joined them.
HOW WOULD YOU FEEL SEEING A KID YOU KNOW IS BIOLOGICALLY YOURS BUT WITH WHOM YOU HAVE NO INVOLVEMENT, EXCEPT MAYBE PERIPHERALLY?
I THINK IT'LL BE FINE.
WHY DO YOU WANT TO BE A DONOR?
IT'S JUST BIOLOGICAL MATERIAL. I'M HAPPY TO DO THIS IF IT HELPS.
DO YOU WANT TO BE ANONYMOUS OR KNOWN?
I WANT TO STAY ANONYMOUS.
WHAT ARE YOUR FINANCIAL, LEGAL, PARENTAL, EMOTIONAL EXPECTATIONS?
NONE.
WHAT'S YOUR MEDICAL AND MENTAL HEALTH HISTORY?
HEALTHY BODY, HEALTHY MIND.
GRANDPARENT INVOLVEMENT?
NONE.
HOW DO YOU FEEL ABOUT MY MAKING A CONTRACT?
DEFINITELY A GOOD IDEA.
DO YOU WANT INVOLVEMENT ONCE THE BABY IS BORN?
IT'S YOUR KID. I DON'T WANT TO BE INVOLVED IN ANY WAY.
HOW DO YOU FEEL ABOUT HIS DOING THIS?
I HAVE NO PROBLEM WITH IT.
WHAT IF MUTUAL FRIENDS SEE SIMILARITIES AND ASK QUESTIONS?
WE'LL FIGURE IT OUT IF IT HAPPENS.
It seemed we were all on the same page.

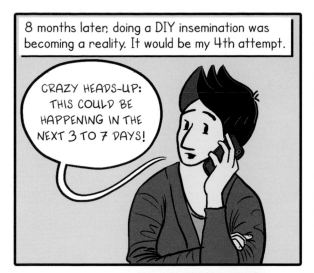

8 months later, doing a DIY insemination was becoming a reality. It would be my 4th attempt.

CRAZY HEADS-UP: THIS COULD BE HAPPENING IN THE NEXT 3 TO 7 DAYS!

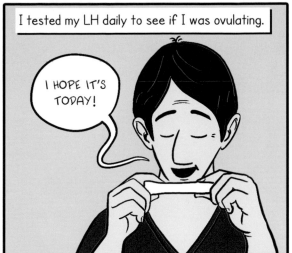

I tested my LH daily to see if I was ovulating.

I HOPE IT'S TODAY!

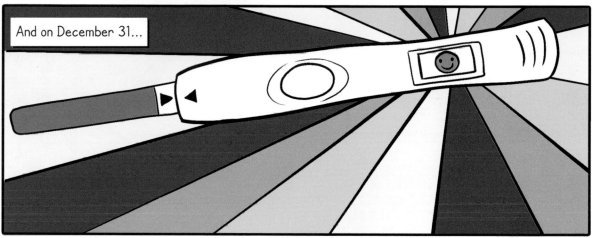

And on December 31...

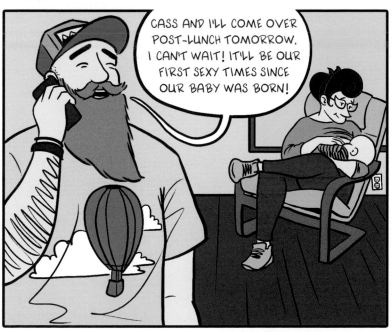

CASS AND I'LL COME OVER POST-LUNCH TOMORROW. I CAN'T WAIT! IT'LL BE OUR FIRST SEXY TIMES SINCE OUR BABY WAS BORN!

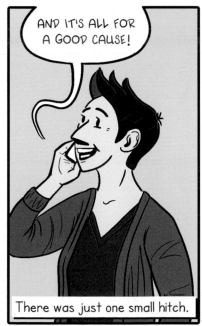

AND IT'S ALL FOR A GOOD CAUSE!

There was just one small hitch.

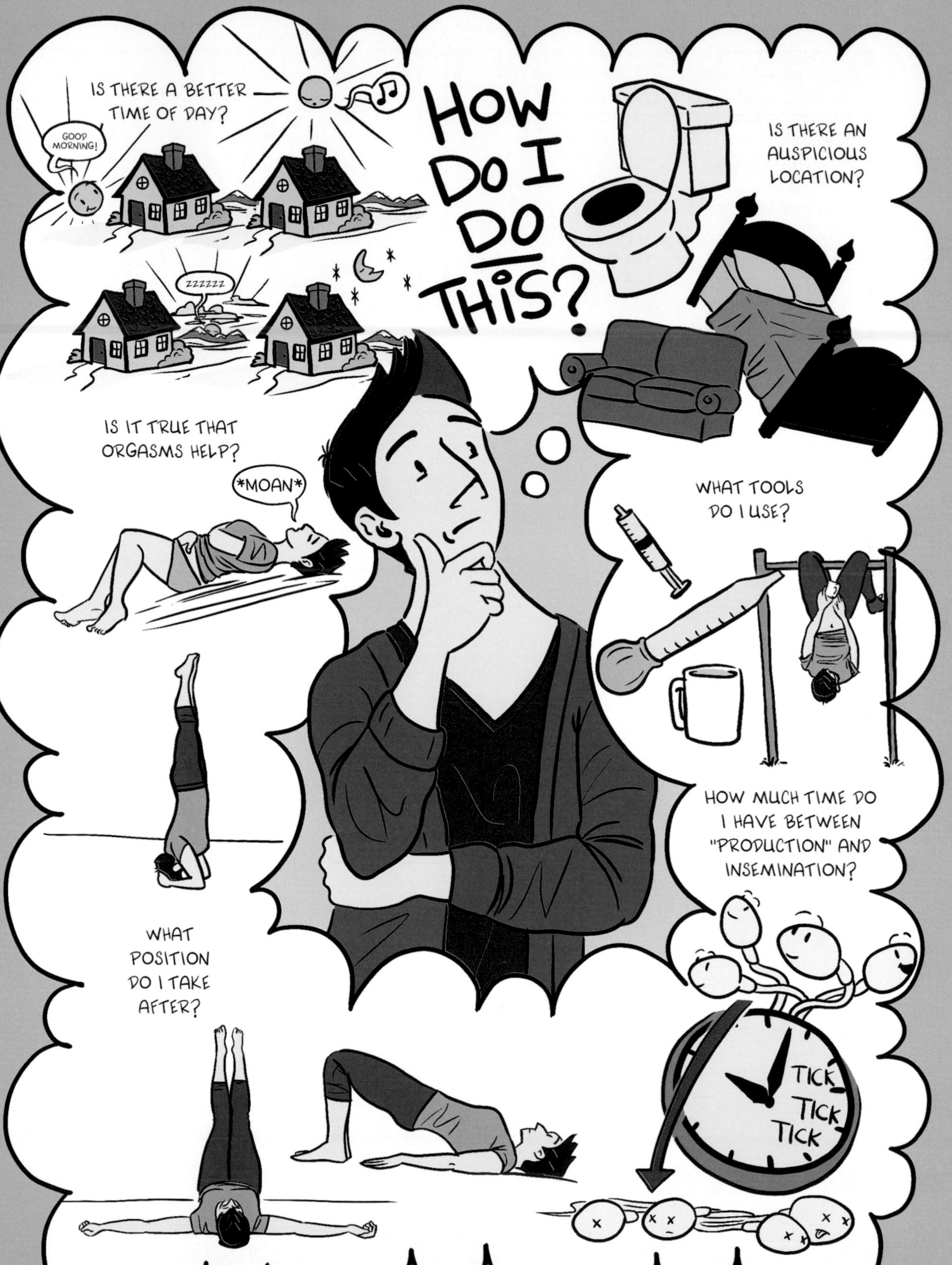
HOW DO I DO THIS?
IS THERE A BETTER TIME OF DAY?
GOOD MORNING!
ZZZZZZ
IS THERE AN AUSPICIOUS LOCATION?
IS IT TRUE THAT ORGASMS HELP?
MOAN
WHAT TOOLS DO I USE?
HOW MUCH TIME DO I HAVE BETWEEN "PRODUCTION" AND INSEMINATION?
WHAT POSITION DO I TAKE AFTER?
TICK
TICK
TICK

The solution? Call the one person I knew who had successfully gotten pregnant going the turkey-basting route. Both her kids were conceived in one try each, so she must have done something right.

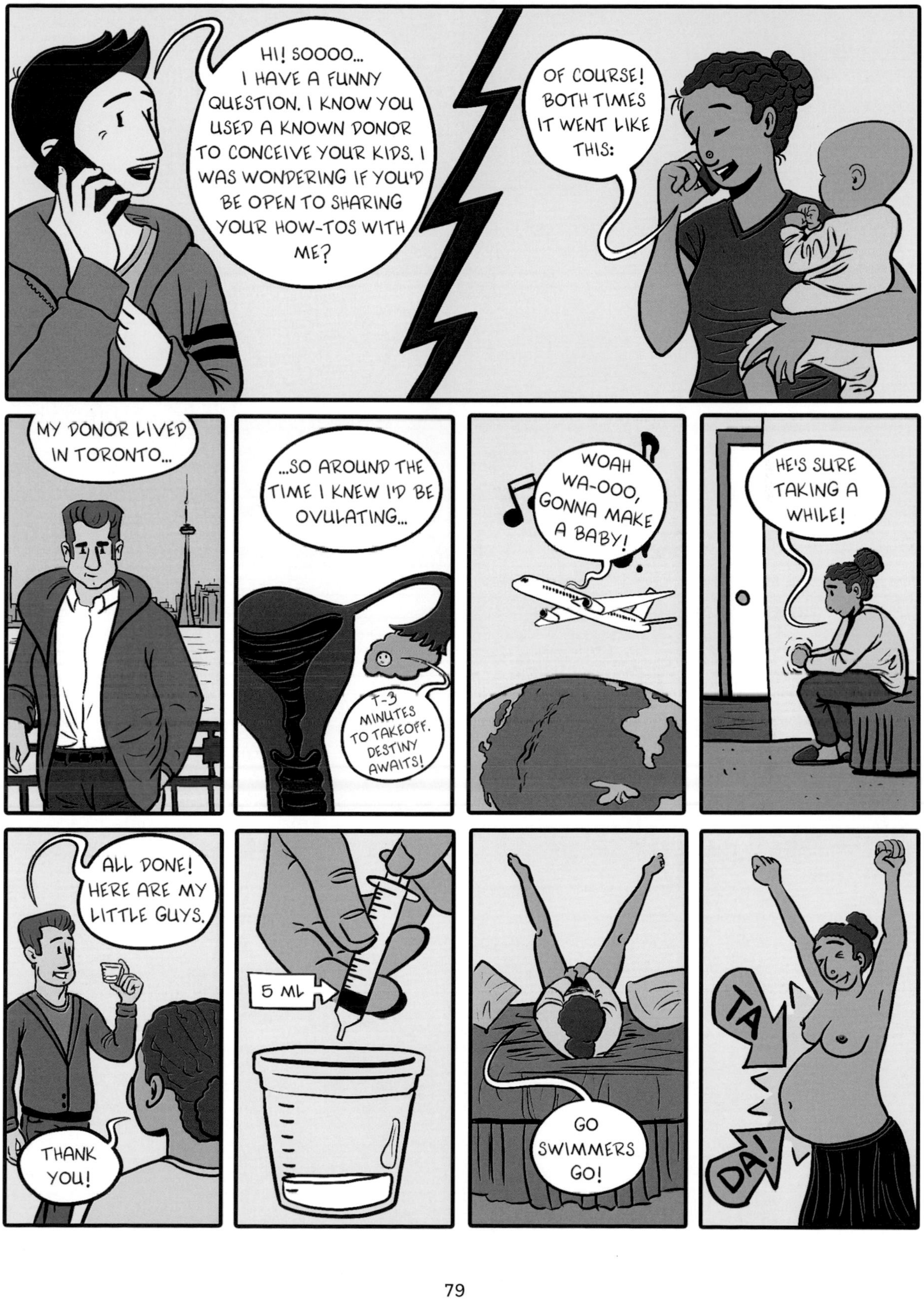

HI! SOOOO... I HAVE A FUNNY QUESTION. I KNOW YOU USED A KNOWN DONOR TO CONCEIVE YOUR KIDS. I WAS WONDERING IF YOU'D BE OPEN TO SHARING YOUR HOW-TOS WITH ME?
OF COURSE! BOTH TIMES IT WENT LIKE THIS:
MY DONOR LIVED IN TORONTO...
...SO AROUND THE TIME I KNEW I'D BE OVULATING...
T-3 MINUTES TO TAKEOFF. DESTINY AWAITS!
WOAH WA-OOO, GONNA MAKE A BABY!
HE'S SURE TAKING A WHILE!
ALL DONE! HERE ARE MY LITTLE GUYS.
THANK YOU!
5 ML
GO SWIMMERS GO!
TA
DA!

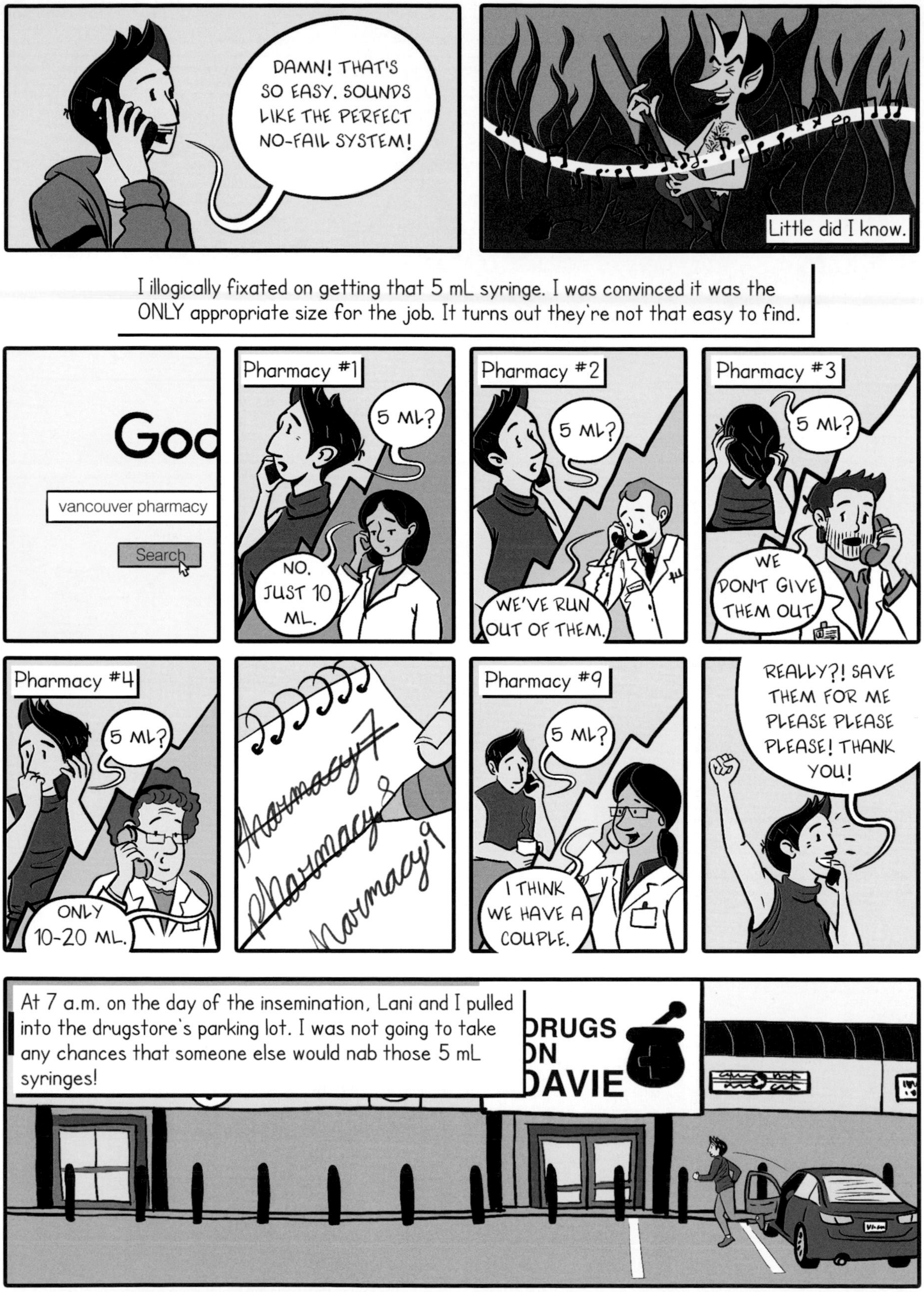
DAMN! THAT'S SO EASY. SOUNDS LIKE THE PERFECT NO-FAIL SYSTEM!
Little did I know.
I illogically fixated on getting that 5 mL syringe. I was convinced it was the ONLY appropriate size for the job. It turns out they're not that easy to find.
Goo
vancouver pharmacy
Search
Pharmacy #1
5 ML?
NO. JUST 10 ML.
Pharmacy #2
5 ML?
WE'VE RUN OUT OF THEM.
Pharmacy #3
5 ML?
WE DON'T GIVE THEM OUT.
Pharmacy #4
5 ML?
ONLY 10-20 ML.
Pharmacy 7
Pharmacy 8
Pharmacy 9
Pharmacy #9
5 ML?
I THINK WE HAVE A COUPLE.
REALLY?! SAVE THEM FOR ME PLEASE PLEASE PLEASE! THANK YOU!
At 7 a.m. on the day of the insemination, Lani and I pulled into the drugstore's parking lot. I was not going to take any chances that someone else would nab those 5 mL syringes!
DRUGS ON DAVIE

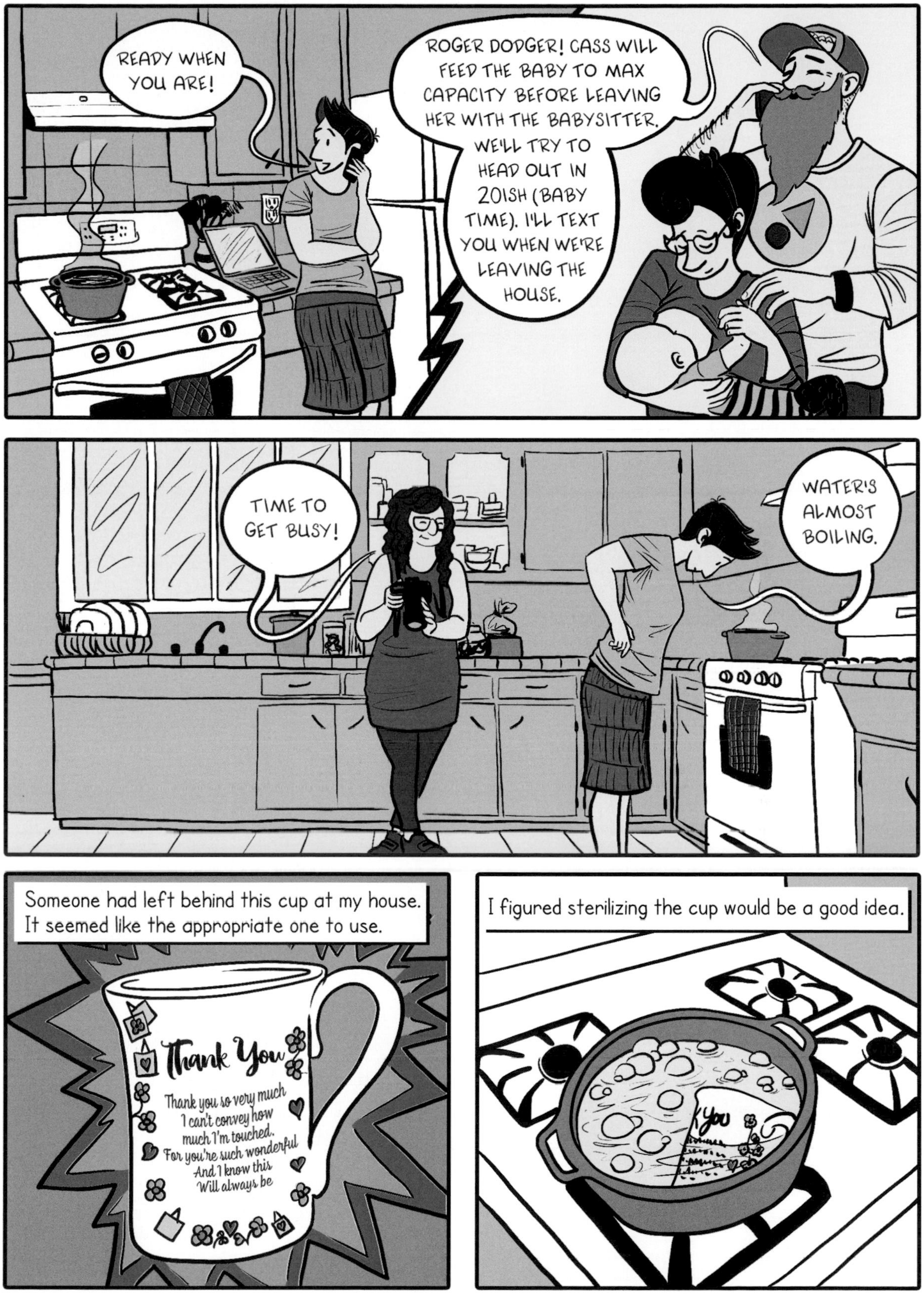
READY WHEN YOU ARE!
ROGER DODGER! CASS WILL FEED THE BABY TO MAX CAPACITY BEFORE LEAVING HER WITH THE BABYSITTER. WE'LL TRY TO HEAD OUT IN 20ISH (BABY TIME). I'LL TEXT YOU WHEN WE'RE LEAVING THE HOUSE.
TIME TO GET BUSY!
WATER'S ALMOST BOILING.
Someone had left behind this cup at my house. It seemed like the appropriate one to use.
Thank You
Thank you so very much
I can't convey how
much I'm touched.
For you're such wonderful
And I know this
Will always be
I figured sterilizing the cup would be a good idea.

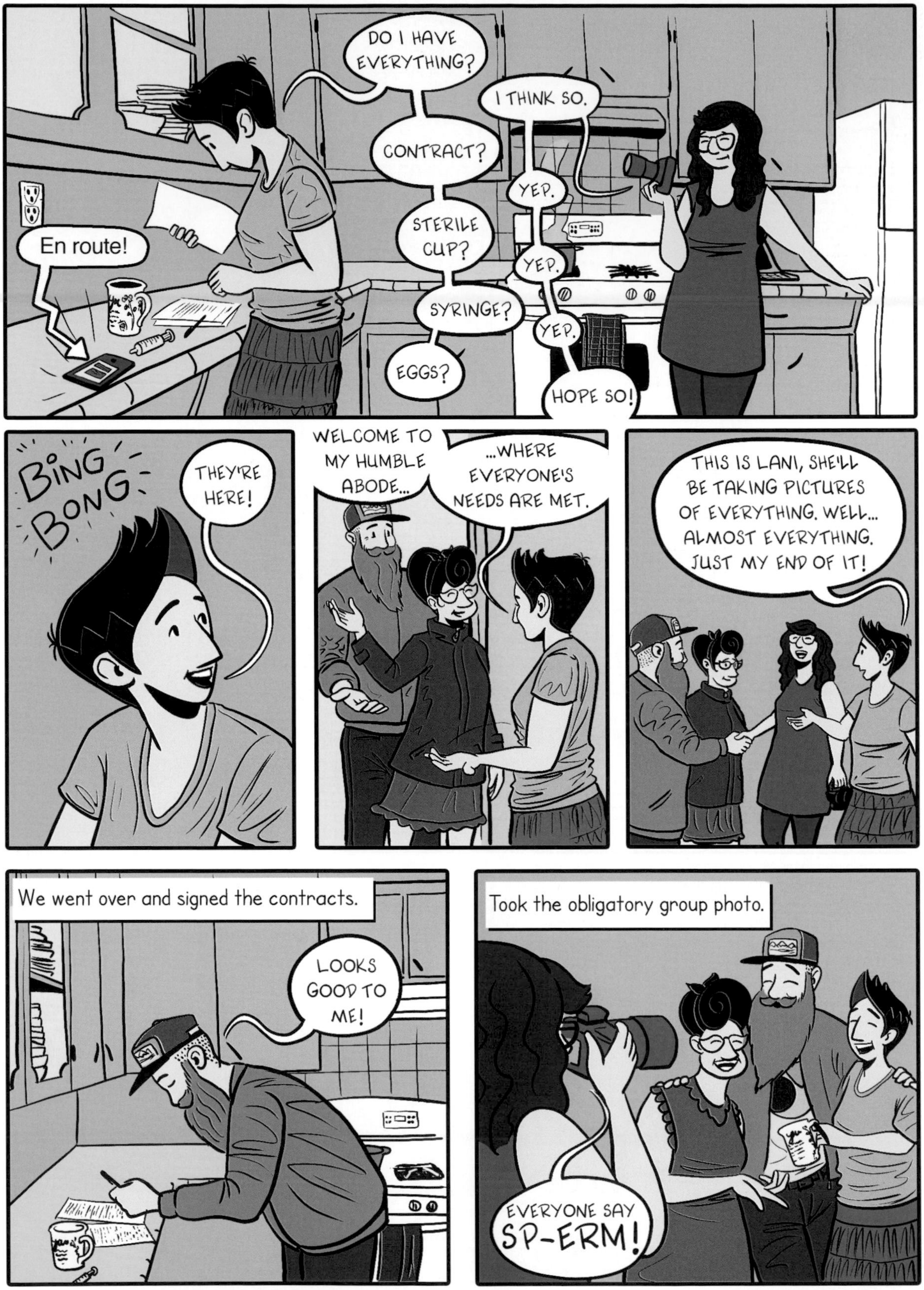
DO I HAVE EVERYTHING?
I THINK SO.
CONTRACT?
YEP.
STERILE CUP?
YEP.
SYRINGE?
YEP.
EGGS?
HOPE SO!
En route!
BING BONG
THEY'RE HERE!
WELCOME TO MY HUMBLE ABODE...
...WHERE EVERYONE'S NEEDS ARE MET.
THIS IS LANI, SHE'LL BE TAKING PICTURES OF EVERYTHING. WELL... ALMOST EVERYTHING. JUST MY END OF IT!
We went over and signed the contracts.
LOOKS GOOD TO ME!
Took the obligatory group photo.
EVERYONE SAY SP-ERM!

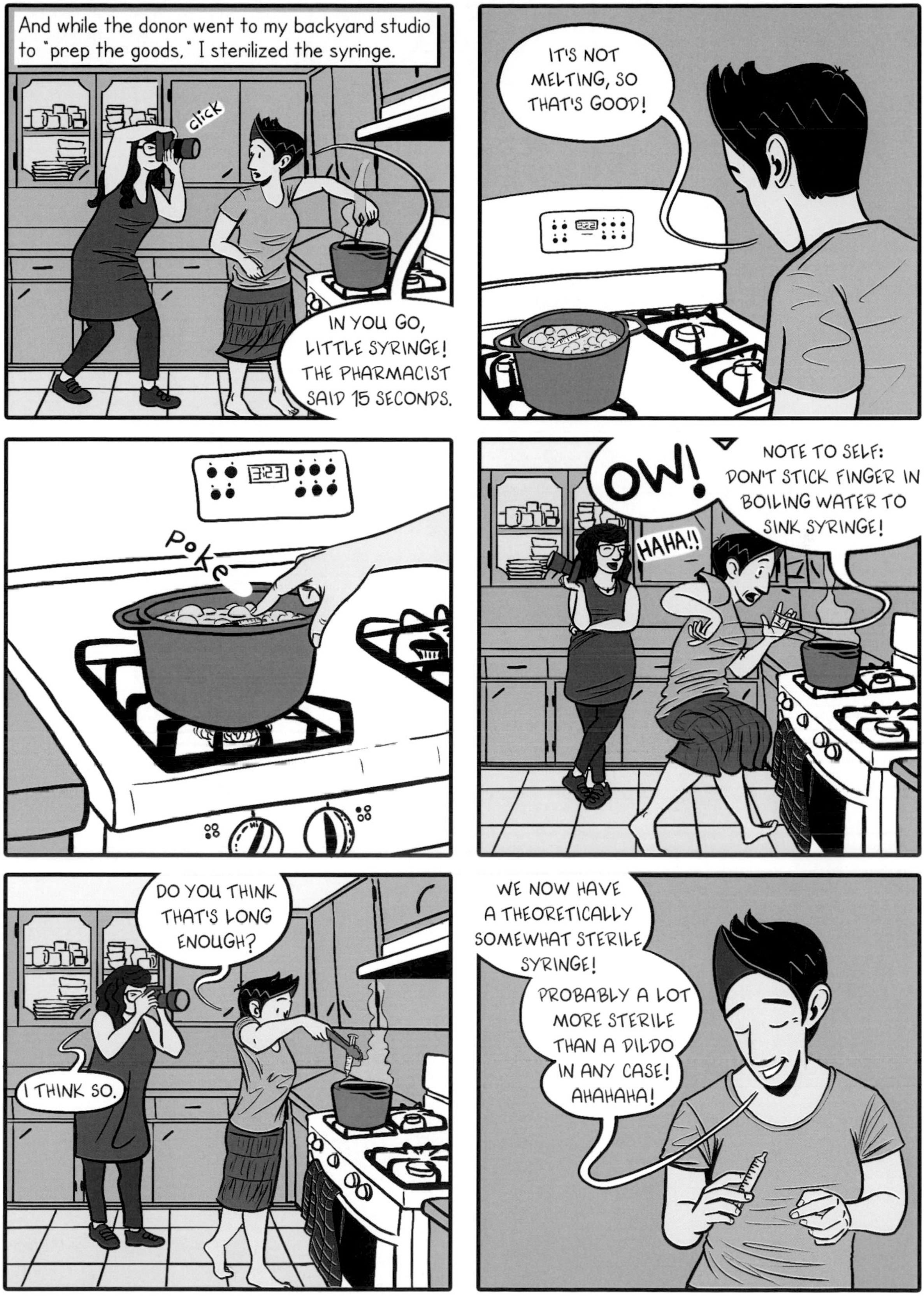
And while the donor went to my backyard studio to "prep the goods," I sterilized the syringe.
click
IN YOU GO, LITTLE SYRINGE! THE PHARMACIST SAID 15 SECONDS.
IT'S NOT MELTING, SO THAT'S GOOD!
Poke
OW!
NOTE TO SELF: DON'T STICK FINGER IN BOILING WATER TO SINK SYRINGE!
HAHA!!
DO YOU THINK THAT'S LONG ENOUGH?
I THINK SO.
WE NOW HAVE A THEORETICALLY SOMEWHAT STERILE SYRINGE!
PROBABLY A LOT MORE STERILE THAN A DILDO IN ANY CASE! AHAHAHA!

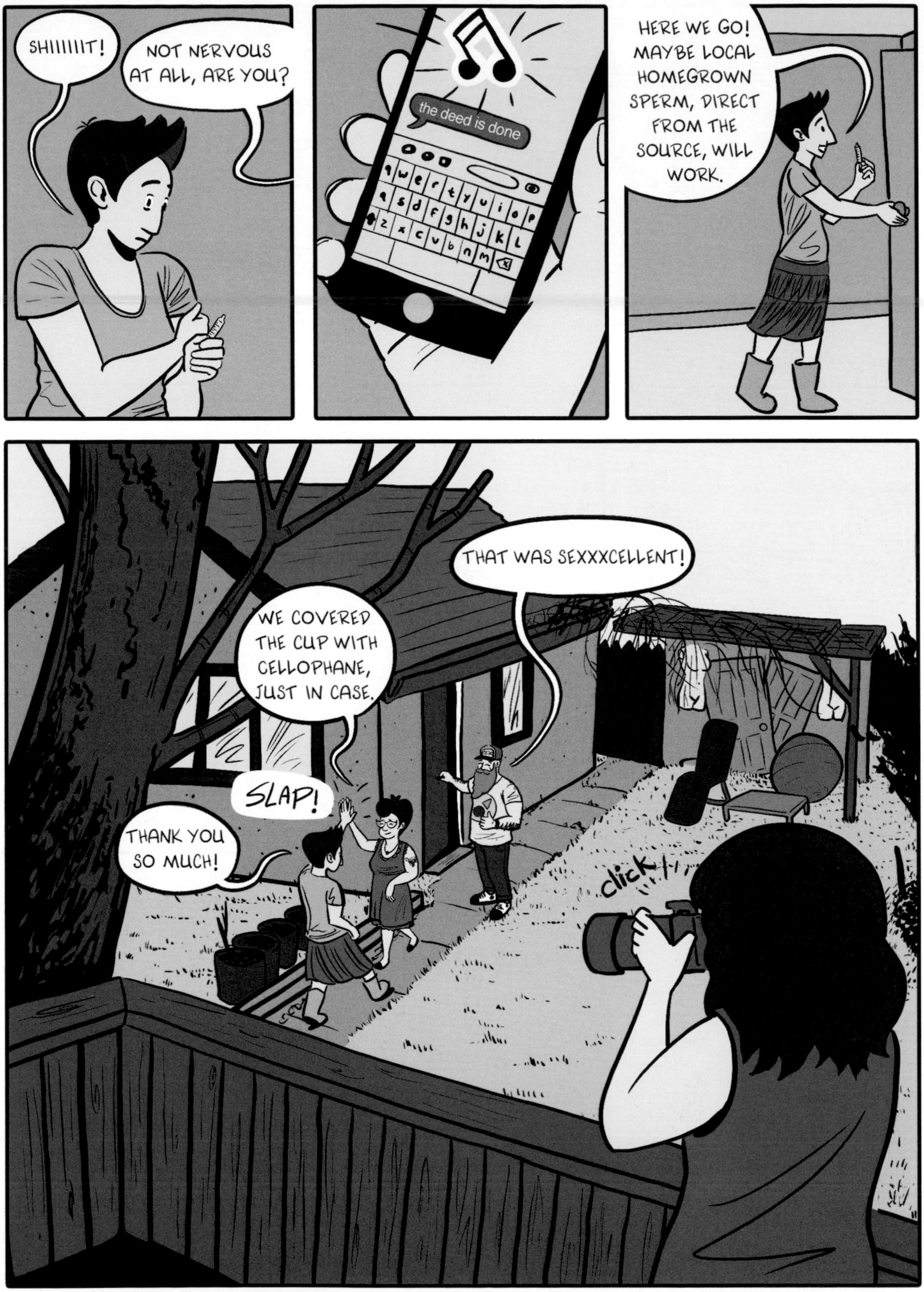
SHIIIIIIT!
NOT NERVOUS AT ALL, ARE YOU?
the deed is done
HERE WE GO! MAYBE LOCAL HOMEGROWN SPERM, DIRECT FROM THE SOURCE, WILL WORK.
THAT WAS SEXXXCELLENT!
WE COVERED THE CUP WITH CELLOPHANE, JUST IN CASE.
SLAP!
THANK YOU SO MUCH!
click

I CAN'T BELIEVE THIS IS ACTUALLY HAPPENING!
Thank You
Thank you so very much
I can't convey how
much I'm touched.
For you're such wonderful
And I know this
Will always be
THERE IT IS!
HERE WE GO!
THERE'S A FAIR AMOUNT. I'M GLAD HE HAD GOOD AIM. THIS SHOULD BE EASY!
COME ON, YOU. GET IN THERE!
I THINK I GOT IT ALL.

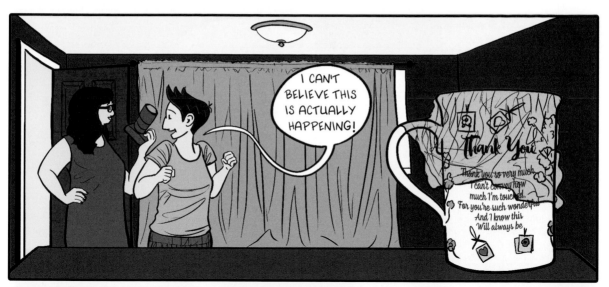

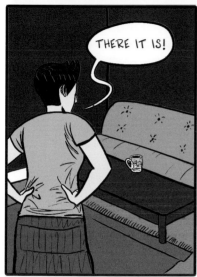

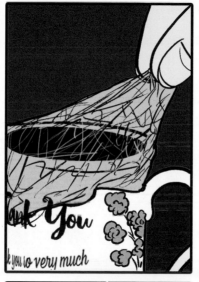

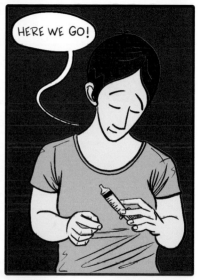

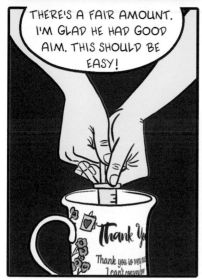

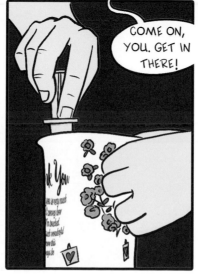

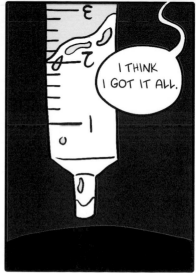

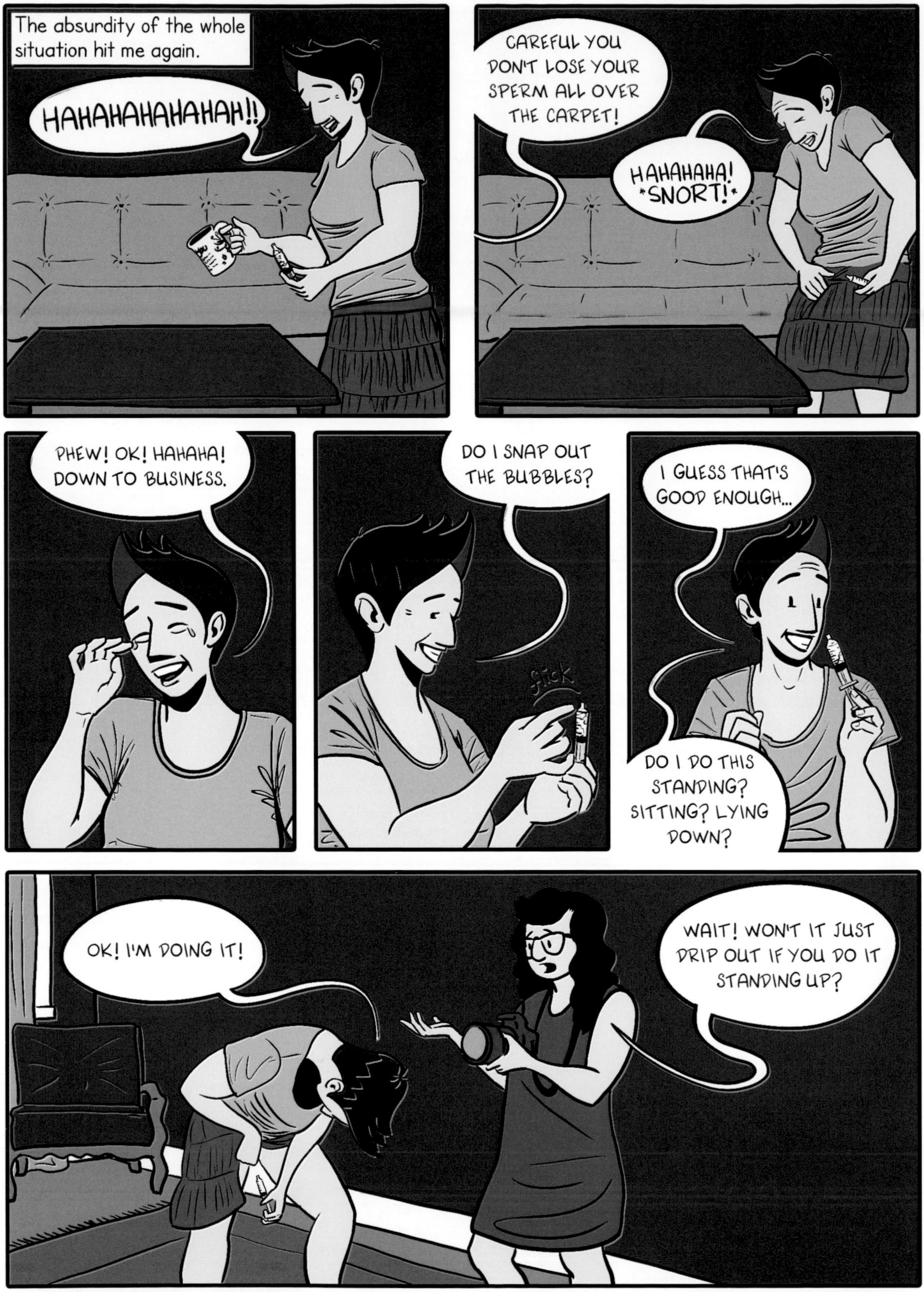
The absurdity of the whole situation hit me again.
HAHAHAHAHAHAH!!
CAREFUL YOU DON'T LOSE YOUR SPERM ALL OVER THE CARPET!
HAHAHAHA! *SNORT!*
PHEW! OK! HAHAHA! DOWN TO BUSINESS.
DO I SNAP OUT THE BUBBLES?
flick
I GUESS THAT'S GOOD ENOUGH...
DO I DO THIS STANDING? SITTING? LYING DOWN?
OK! I'M DOING IT!
WAIT! WON'T IT JUST DRIP OUT IF YOU DO IT STANDING UP?

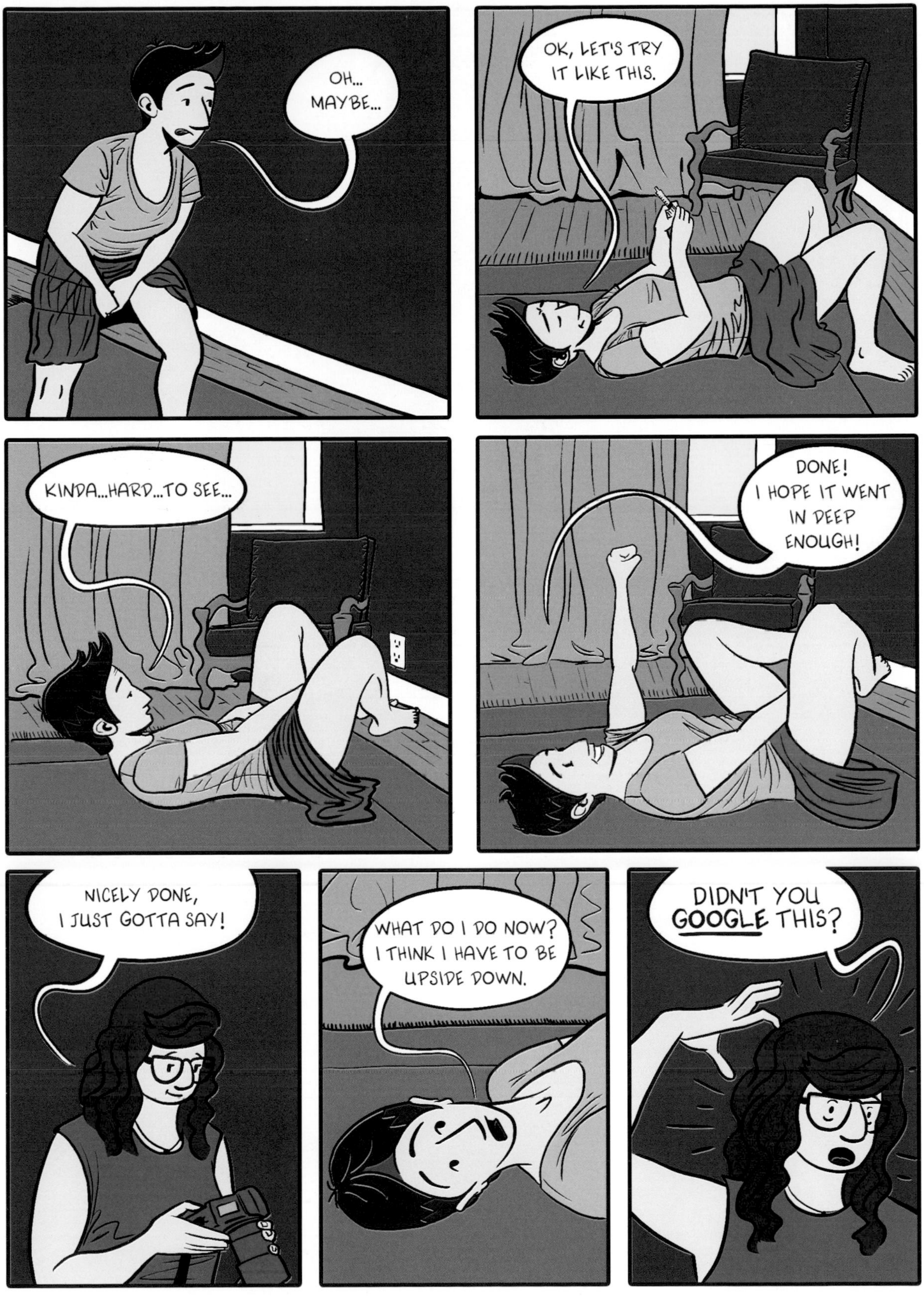
OH... MAYBE...
OK, LET'S TRY IT LIKE THIS.
KINDA...HARD...TO SEE...
DONE! I HOPE IT WENT IN DEEP ENOUGH!
NICELY DONE, I JUST GOTTA SAY!
WHAT DO I DO NOW? I THINK I HAVE TO BE UPSIDE DOWN.
DIDN'T YOU GOOGLE THIS?

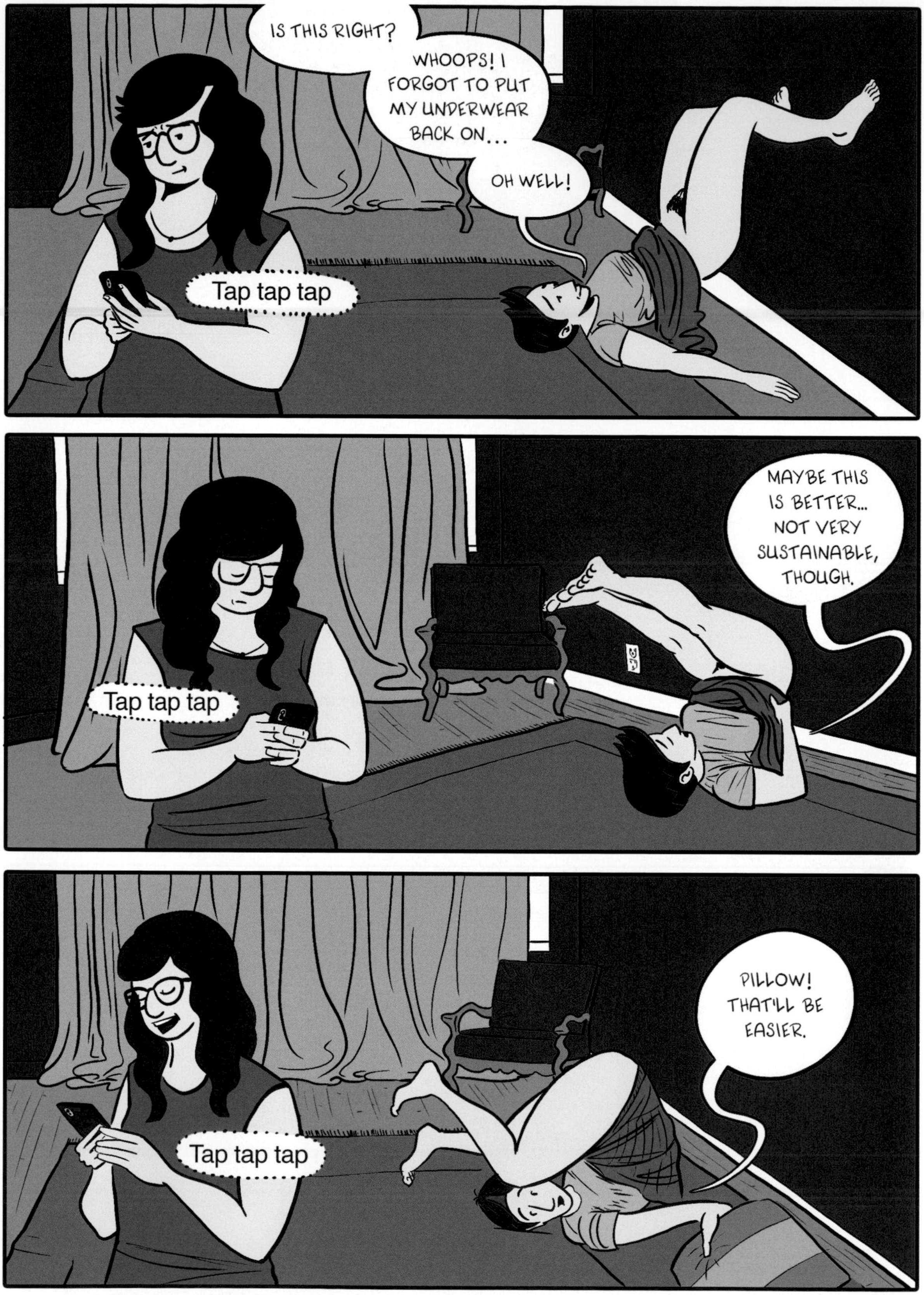
IS THIS RIGHT?
WHOOPS! I FORGOT TO PUT MY UNDERWEAR BACK ON...
OH WELL!
Tap tap tap
Tap tap tap
MAYBE THIS IS BETTER... NOT VERY SUSTAINABLE, THOUGH.
Tap tap tap
PILLOW! THAT'LL BE EASIER.

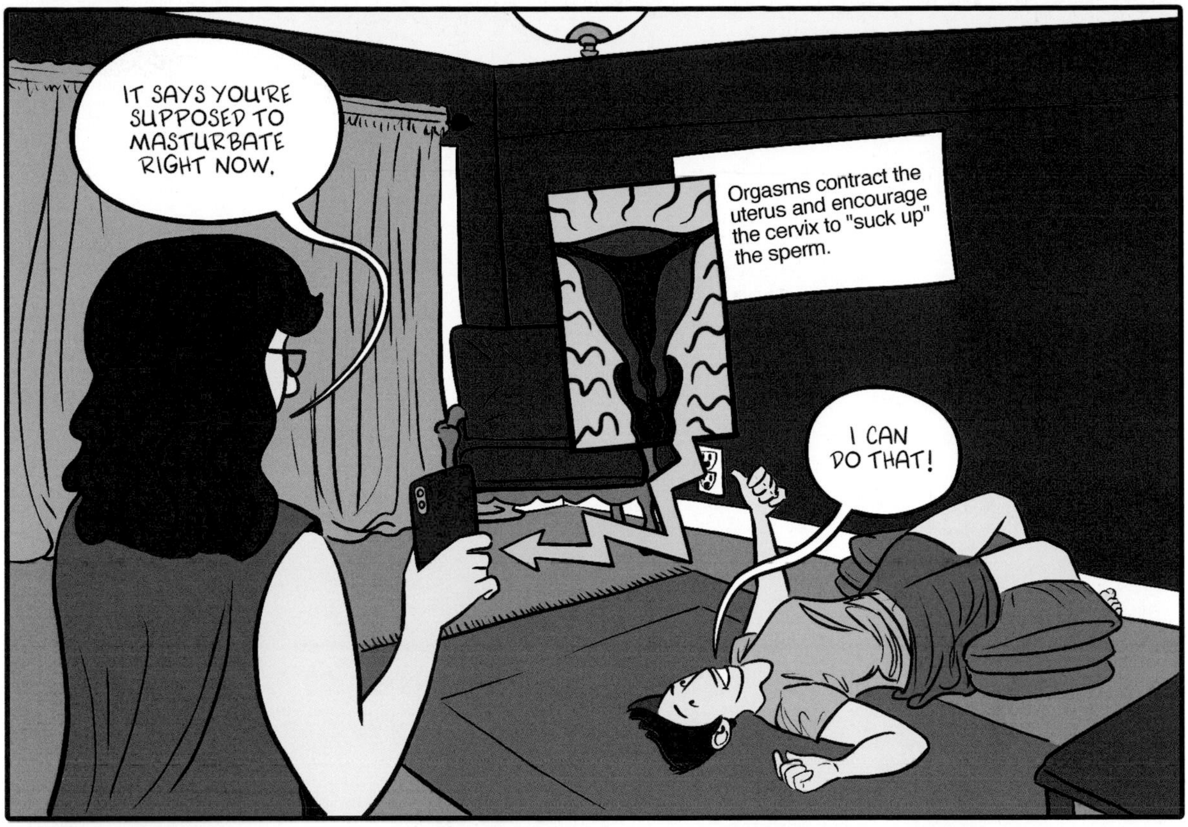
IT SAYS YOU'RE SUPPOSED TO MASTURBATE RIGHT NOW.
Orgasms contract the uterus and encourage the cervix to "suck up" the sperm.
I CAN DO THAT!

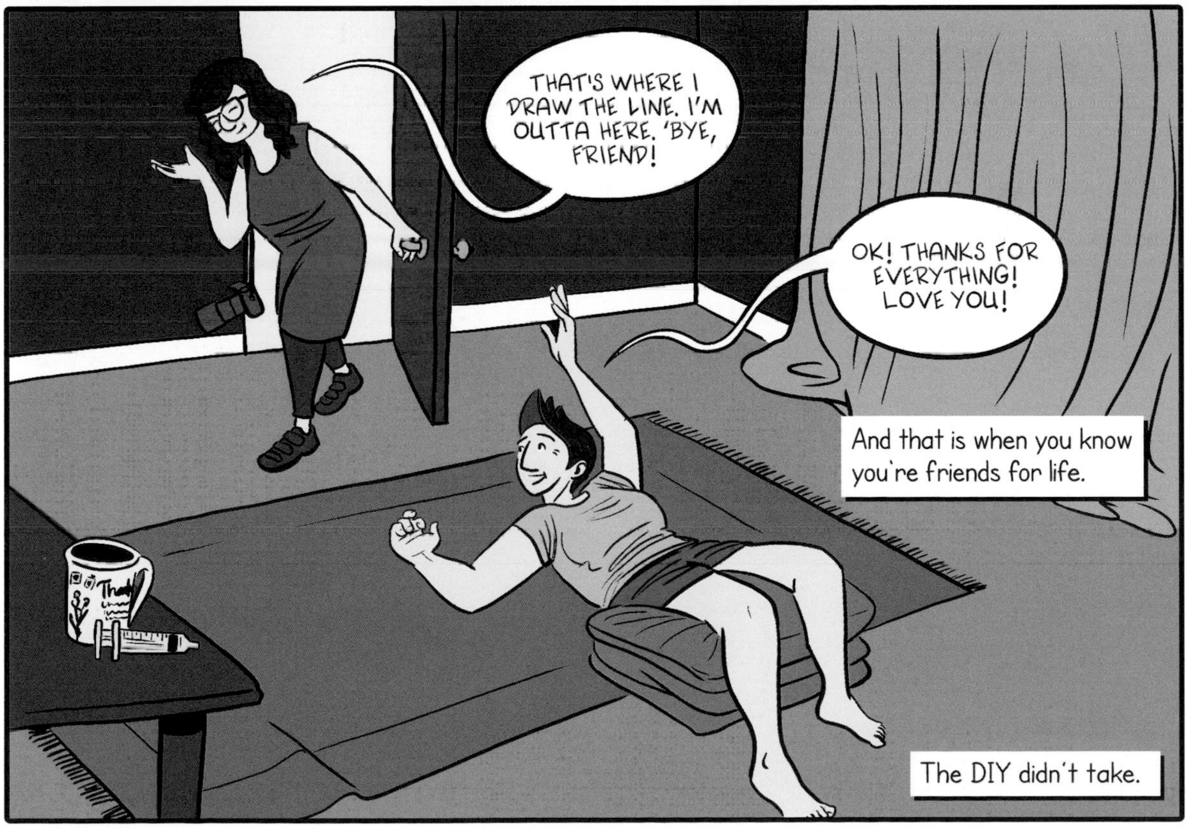
THAT'S WHERE I DRAW THE LINE. I'M OUTTA HERE. 'BYE, FRIEND!
OK! THANKS FOR EVERYTHING! LOVE YOU!
And that is when you know you're friends for life.
The DIY didn't take.

Chapter 3

Azariah

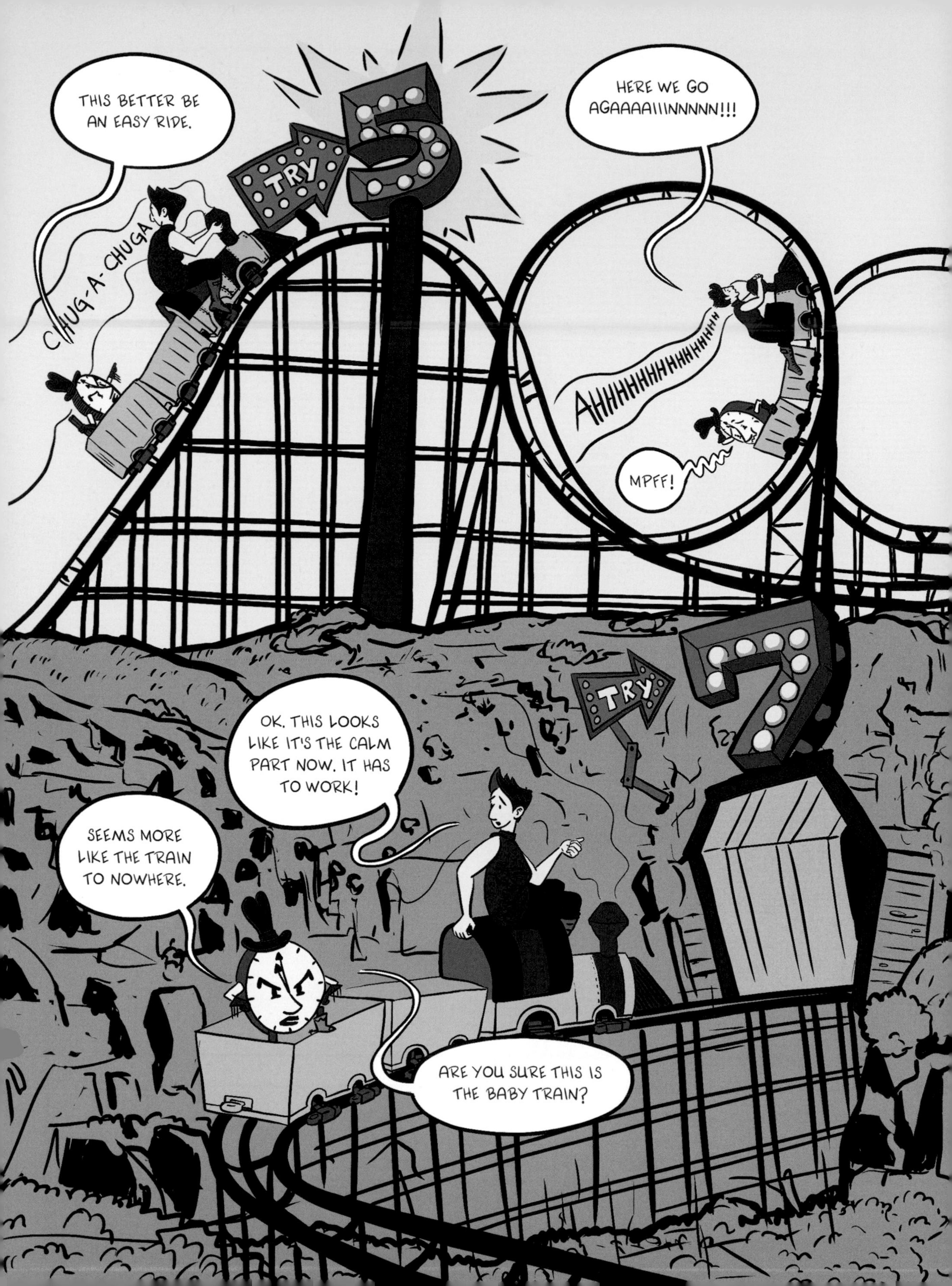
THIS BETTER BE AN EASY RIDE.
TRY
5
CHUG-A-CHUGA
HERE WE GO AGAAAAIIINNNNN!!!
AHHHHHHHHHHHHHHH
MPFF!
TRY
7
OK. THIS LOOKS LIKE IT'S THE CALM PART NOW. IT HAS TO WORK!
SEEMS MORE LIKE THE TRAIN TO NOWHERE.
ARE YOU SURE THIS IS THE BABY TRAIN?

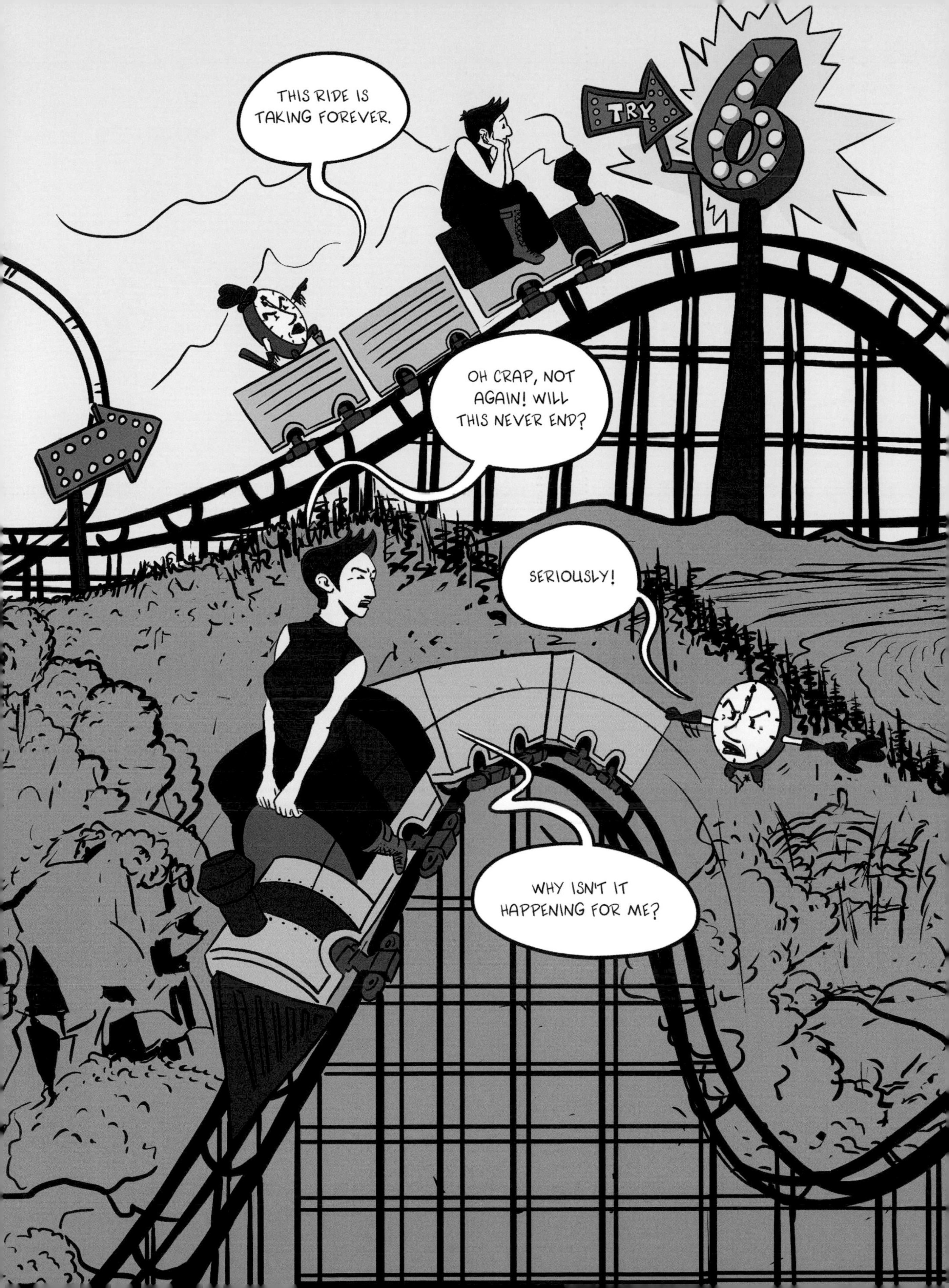
THIS RIDE IS TAKING FOREVER.
TRY 6
OH CRAP, NOT AGAIN! WILL THIS NEVER END?
SERIOUSLY!
WHY ISN'T IT HAPPENING FOR ME?

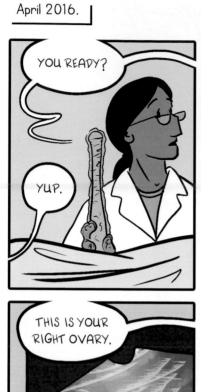

YOU READY?

YUP.

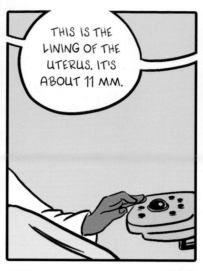

THIS IS THE LINING OF THE UTERUS. IT'S ABOUT 11 MM.

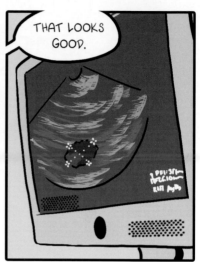

THAT LOOKS GOOD.

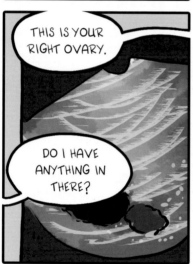

THIS IS YOUR RIGHT OVARY.

DO I HAVE ANYTHING IN THERE?

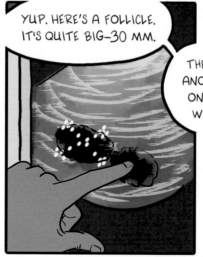

YUP. HERE'S A FOLLICLE. IT'S QUITE BIG—30 MM.

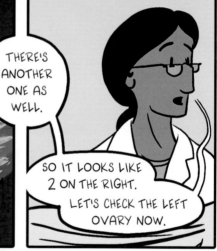

THERE'S ANOTHER ONE AS WELL.

SO IT LOOKS LIKE 2 ON THE RIGHT.

LET'S CHECK THE LEFT OVARY NOW.

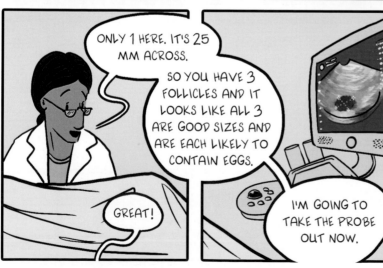

ONLY 1 HERE. IT'S 25 MM ACROSS.

SO YOU HAVE 3 FOLLICLES AND IT LOOKS LIKE ALL 3 ARE GOOD SIZES AND ARE EACH LIKELY TO CONTAIN EGGS.

GREAT!

I'M GOING TO TAKE THE PROBE OUT NOW.

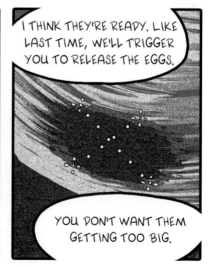

I THINK THEY'RE READY. LIKE LAST TIME, WE'LL TRIGGER YOU TO RELEASE THE EGGS.

YOU DON'T WANT THEM GETTING TOO BIG.

For the first few IUIs, they relied on the supposed accuracy of the home ovulation tests. This time, they triggered the release of the eggs by injecting hCG into my belly to guarantee that the insemination was timed precisely with my eggs dropping into my Fallopian tubes.

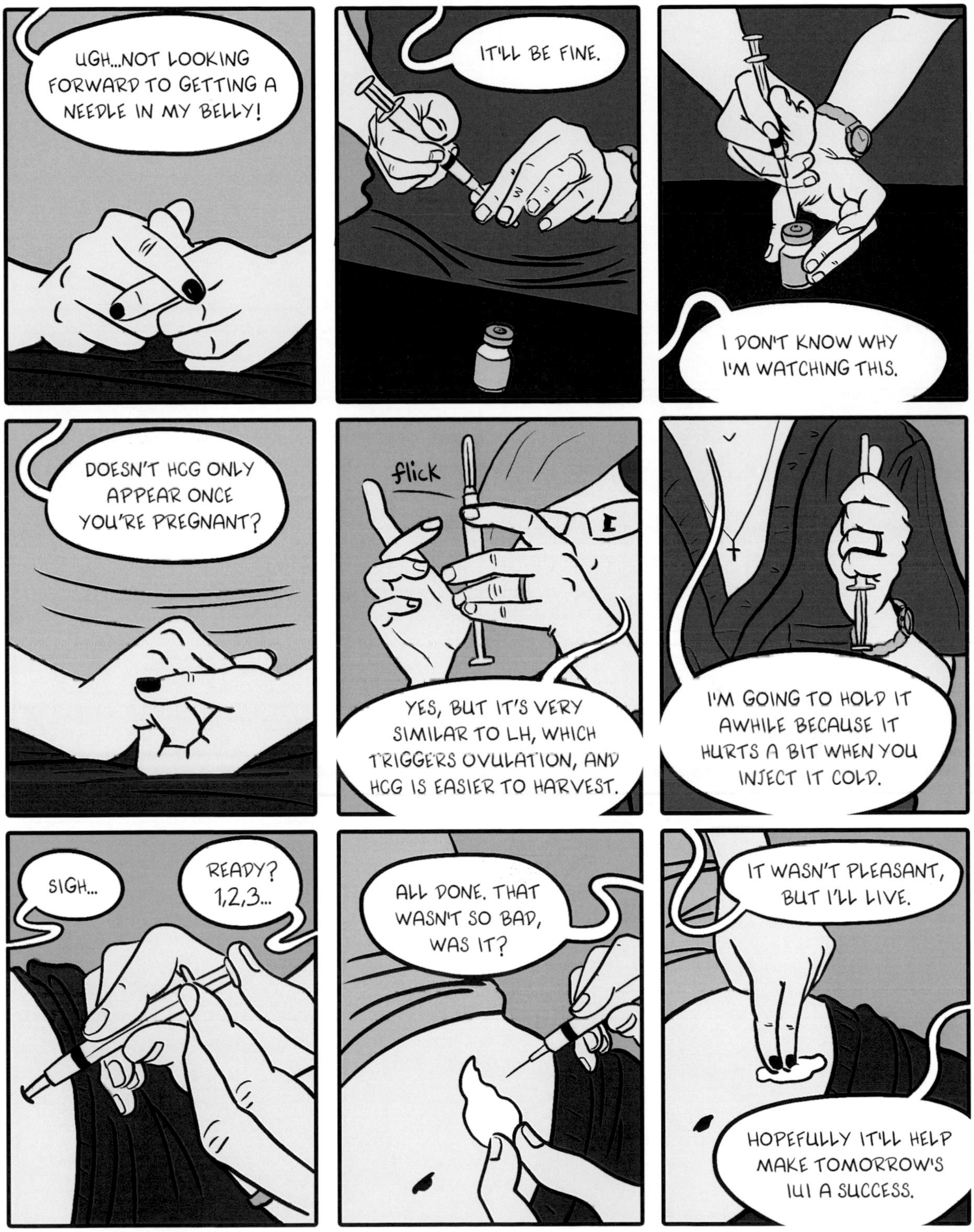
UGH...NOT LOOKING FORWARD TO GETTING A NEEDLE IN MY BELLY!
IT'LL BE FINE.
I DON'T KNOW WHY I'M WATCHING THIS.
DOESN'T HCG ONLY APPEAR ONCE YOU'RE PREGNANT?
flick
YES, BUT IT'S VERY SIMILAR TO LH, WHICH TRIGGERS OVULATION, AND HCG IS EASIER TO HARVEST.
I'M GOING TO HOLD IT AWHILE BECAUSE IT HURTS A BIT WHEN YOU INJECT IT COLD.
SIGH...
READY? 1,2,3...
ALL DONE. THAT WASN'T SO BAD, WAS IT?
IT WASN'T PLEASANT, BUT I'LL LIVE.
HOPEFULLY IT'LL HELP MAKE TOMORROW'S IUI A SUCCESS.

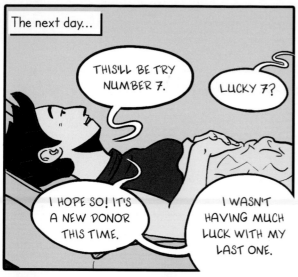

The next day...

THIS'LL BE TRY NUMBER 7.

LUCKY 7?

I HOPE SO! IT'S A NEW DONOR THIS TIME.

I WASN'T HAVING MUCH LUCK WITH MY LAST ONE.

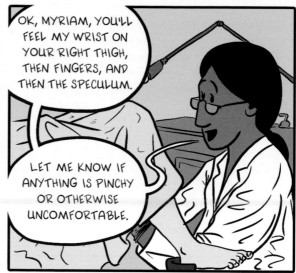

OK, MYRIAM, YOU'LL FEEL MY WRIST ON YOUR RIGHT THIGH, THEN FINGERS, AND THEN THE SPECULUM.

LET ME KNOW IF ANYTHING IS PINCHY OR OTHERWISE UNCOMFORTABLE.

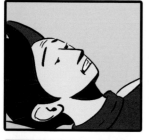

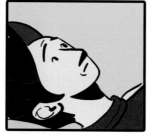

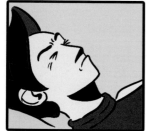

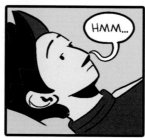

HMM...

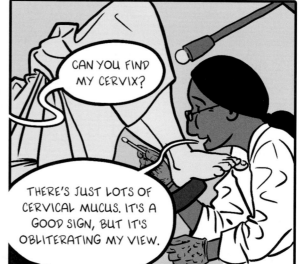

CAN YOU FIND MY CERVIX?

THERE'S JUST LOTS OF CERVICAL MUCUS. IT'S A GOOD SIGN, BUT IT'S OBLITERATING MY VIEW.

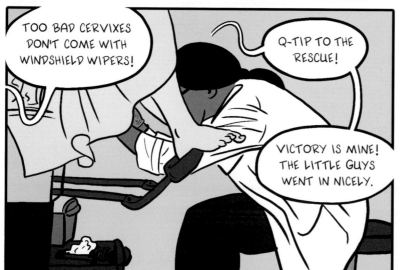

TOO BAD CERVIXES DON'T COME WITH WINDSHIELD WIPERS!

Q-TIP TO THE RESCUE!

VICTORY IS MINE! THE LITTLE GUYS WENT IN NICELY.

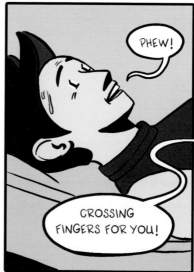

PHEW!

CROSSING FINGERS FOR YOU!

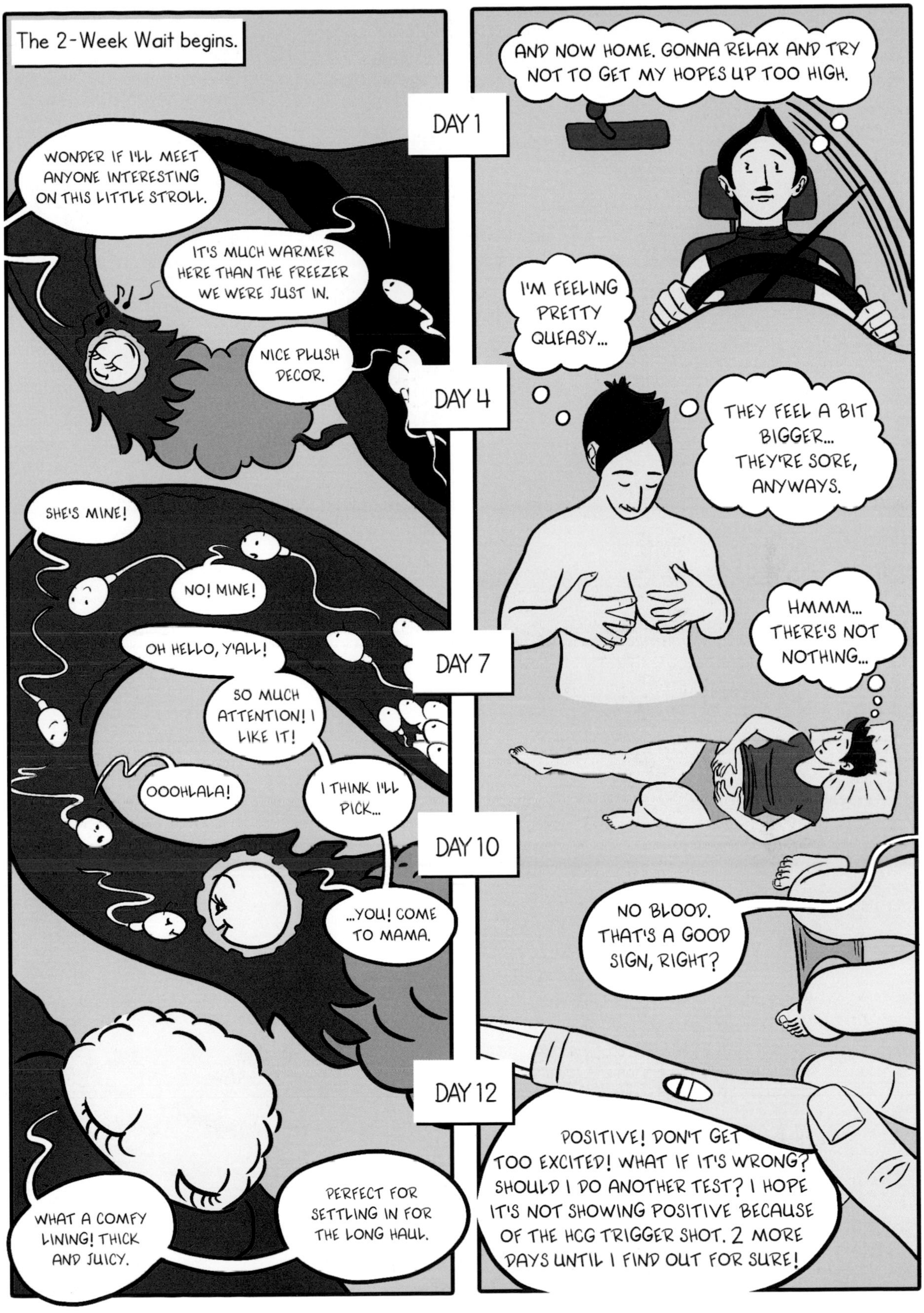
The 2-Week Wait begins.
AND NOW HOME. GONNA RELAX AND TRY NOT TO GET MY HOPES UP TOO HIGH.
DAY 1
WONDER IF I'LL MEET ANYONE INTERESTING ON THIS LITTLE STROLL.
IT'S MUCH WARMER HERE THAN THE FREEZER WE WERE JUST IN.
NICE PLUSH DECOR.
I'M FEELING PRETTY QUEASY...
DAY 4
THEY FEEL A BIT BIGGER... THEY'RE SORE, ANYWAYS.
SHE'S MINE!
NO! MINE!
OH HELLO, Y'ALL!
SO MUCH ATTENTION! I LIKE IT!
DAY 7
HMMM... THERE'S NOT NOTHING...
OOOHLALA!
I THINK I'LL PICK...
DAY 10
...YOU! COME TO MAMA.
NO BLOOD. THAT'S A GOOD SIGN, RIGHT?
DAY 12
WHAT A COMFY LINING! THICK AND JUICY.
PERFECT FOR SETTLING IN FOR THE LONG HAUL.
POSITIVE! DON'T GET TOO EXCITED! WHAT IF IT'S WRONG? SHOULD I DO ANOTHER TEST? I HOPE IT'S NOT SHOWING POSITIVE BECAUSE OF THE HCG TRIGGER SHOT. 2 MORE DAYS UNTIL I FIND OUT FOR SURE!

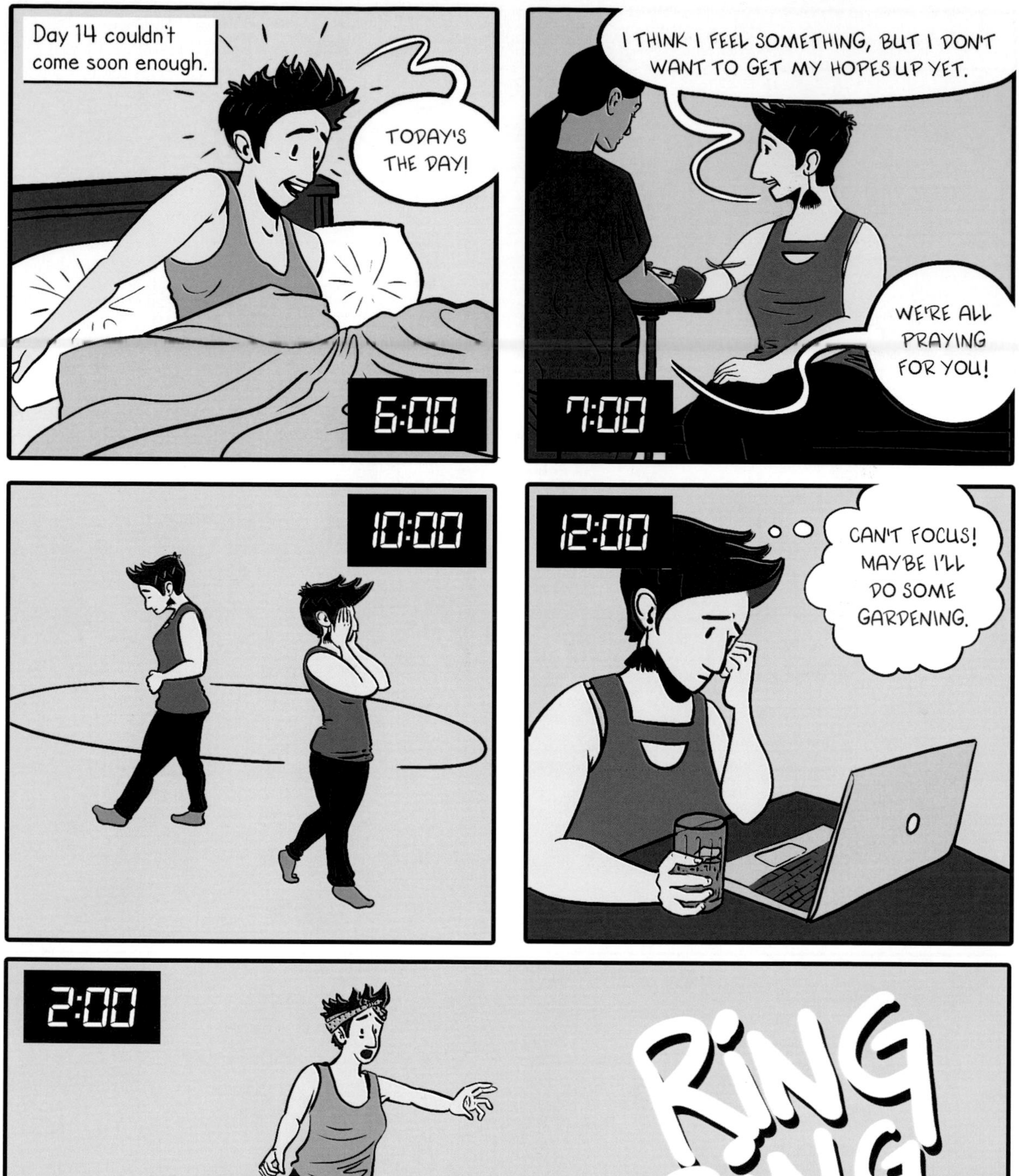
Day 14 couldn't come soon enough.
TODAY'S THE DAY!
6:00
I THINK I FEEL SOMETHING, BUT I DON'T WANT TO GET MY HOPES UP YET.
WE'RE ALL PRAYING FOR YOU!
7:00
10:00
12:00
CAN'T FOCUS! MAYBE I'LL DO SOME GARDENING.
2:00
RING RING

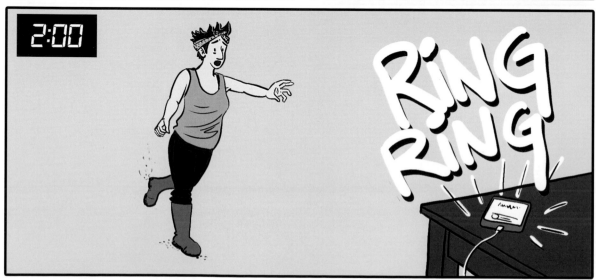

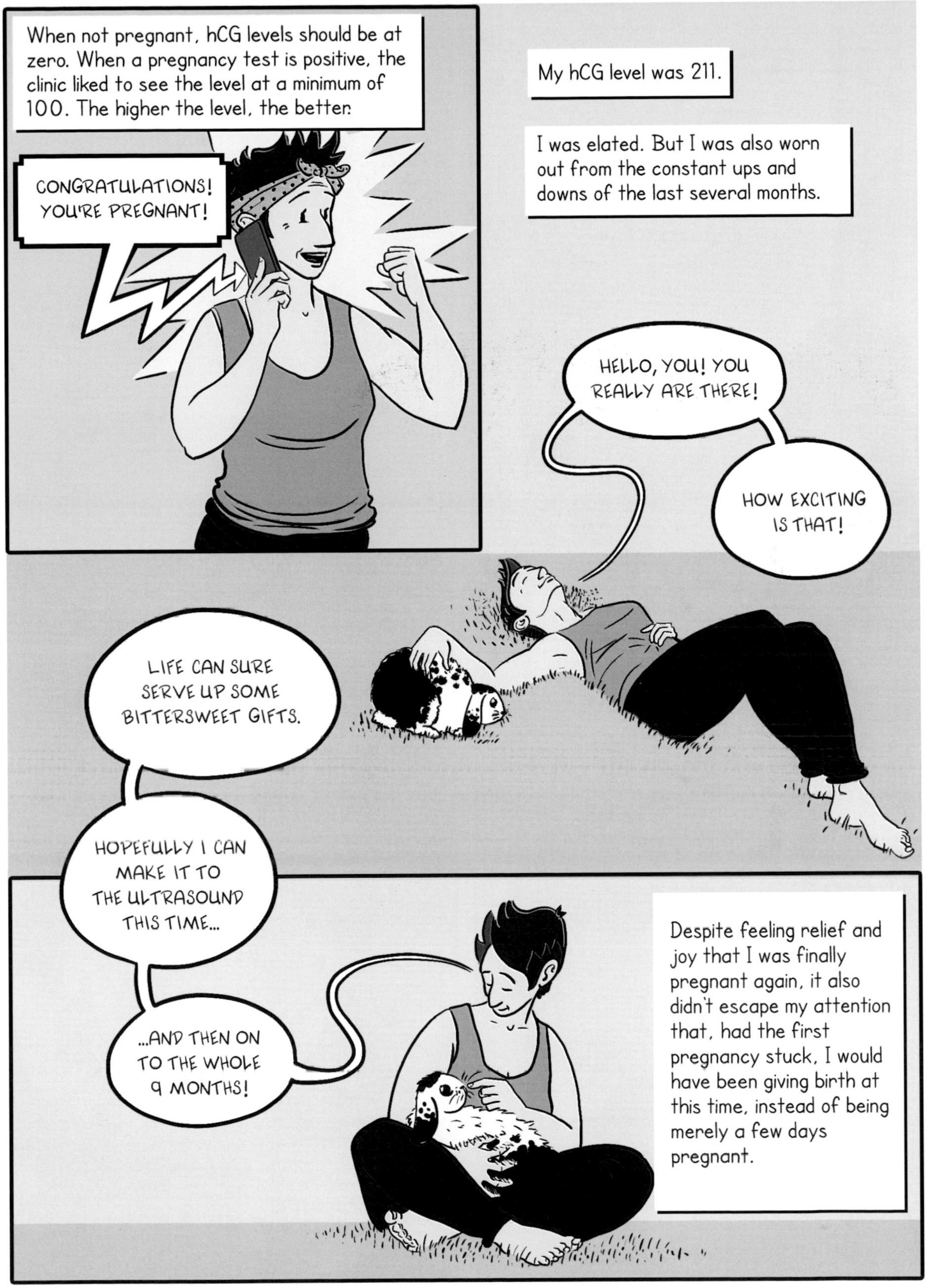
When not pregnant, hCG levels should be at zero. When a pregnancy test is positive, the clinic liked to see the level at a minimum of 100. The higher the level, the better.
CONGRATULATIONS! YOU'RE PREGNANT!
My hCG level was 211.
I was elated. But I was also worn out from the constant ups and downs of the last several months.
HELLO, YOU! YOU REALLY ARE THERE!
HOW EXCITING IS THAT!
LIFE CAN SURE SERVE UP SOME BITTERSWEET GIFTS.
HOPEFULLY I CAN MAKE IT TO THE ULTRASOUND THIS TIME...
...AND THEN ON TO THE WHOLE 9 MONTHS!
Despite feeling relief and joy that I was finally pregnant again, it also didn't escape my attention that, had the first pregnancy stuck, I would have been giving birth at this time, instead of being merely a few days pregnant.

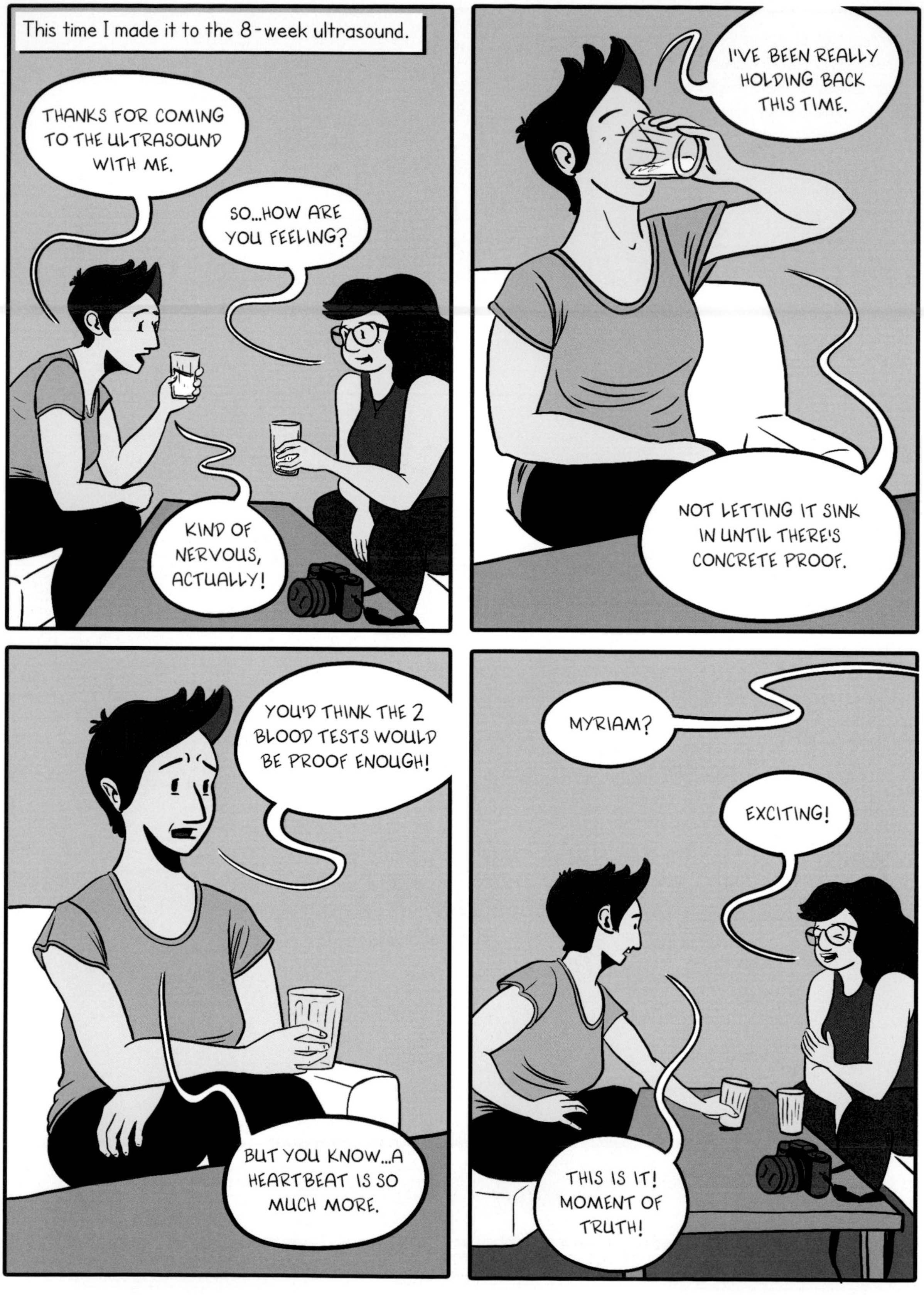
This time I made it to the 8-week ultrasound.
THANKS FOR COMING TO THE ULTRASOUND WITH ME.
SO...HOW ARE YOU FEELING?
KIND OF NERVOUS, ACTUALLY!
I'VE BEEN REALLY HOLDING BACK THIS TIME.
NOT LETTING IT SINK IN UNTIL THERE'S CONCRETE PROOF.
YOU'D THINK THE 2 BLOOD TESTS WOULD BE PROOF ENOUGH!
BUT YOU KNOW...A HEARTBEAT IS SO MUCH MORE.
MYRIAM?
EXCITING!
THIS IS IT! MOMENT OF TRUTH!

THERE IT IS.
THAT'S MY NUGGET!
WHOA!
THERE'S THE HEARTBEAT, 154 BPM. NICE AND FAST. JUST WHAT WE WANT TO SEE.
BOMBOMBOMBOMBOMBOMBOM
CLICK!
LANI! LOOK! THAT'S THE HEAD. AND THERE'S THE BUM!
HEHE!
THEY'VE GOT A BUM!
I KNOW! IT'S SO BEAUTIFUL.

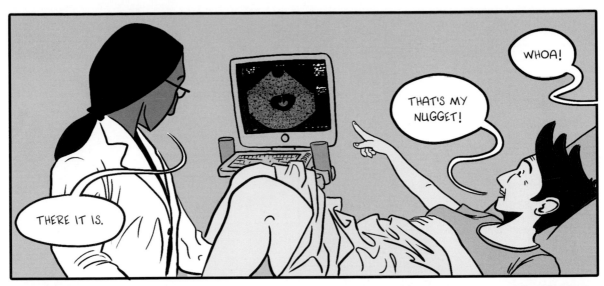

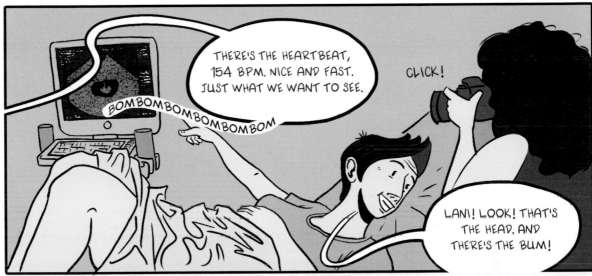

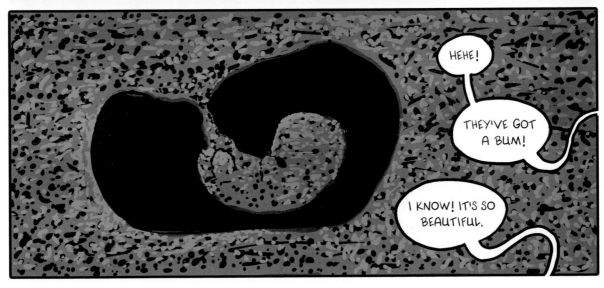

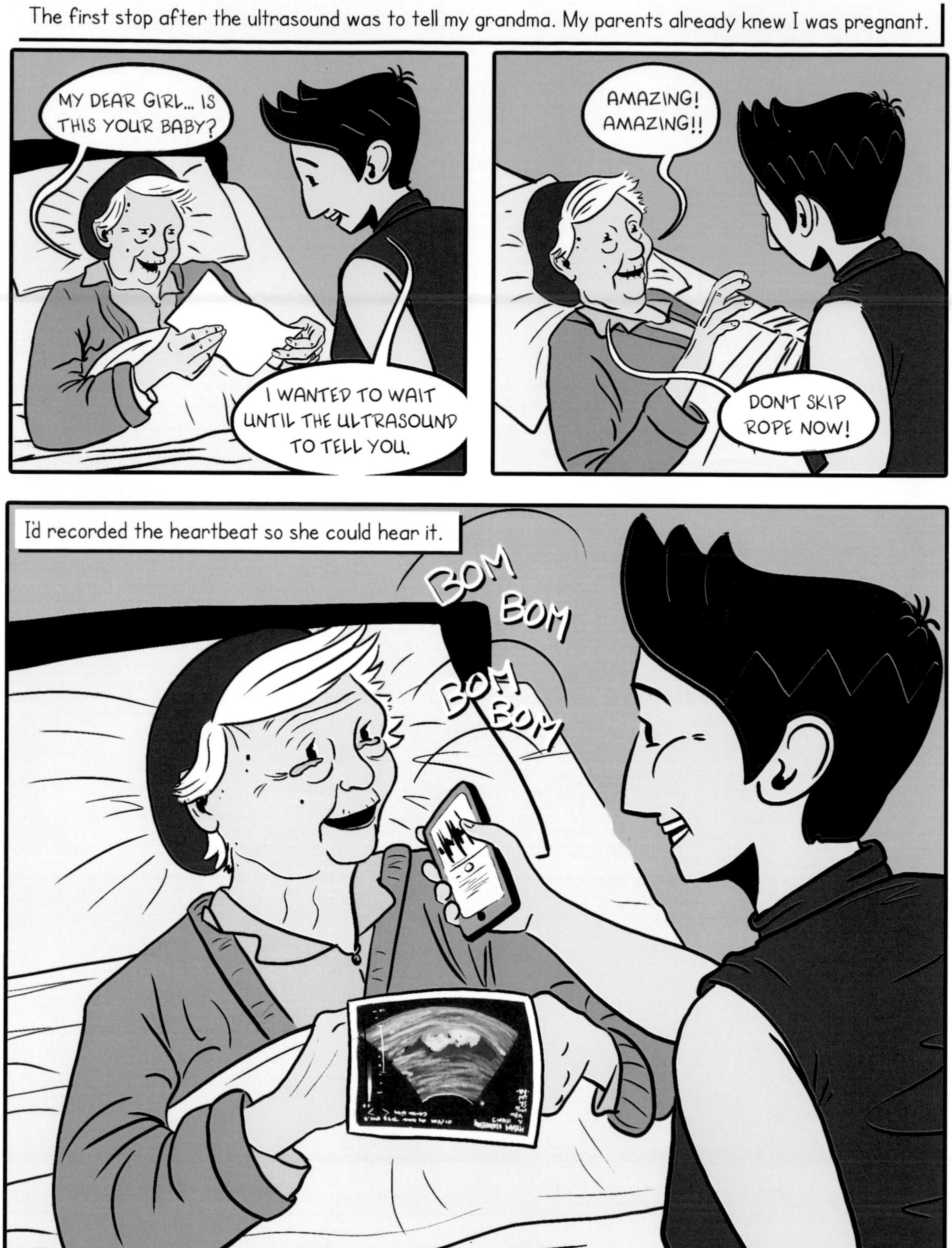
The first stop after the ultrasound was to tell my grandma. My parents already knew I was pregnant.
MY DEAR GIRL... IS THIS YOUR BABY?
I WANTED TO WAIT UNTIL THE ULTRASOUND TO TELL YOU.
AMAZING! AMAZING!!
DON'T SKIP ROPE NOW!
I'd recorded the heartbeat so she could hear it.
BOM BOM
BOM BOM

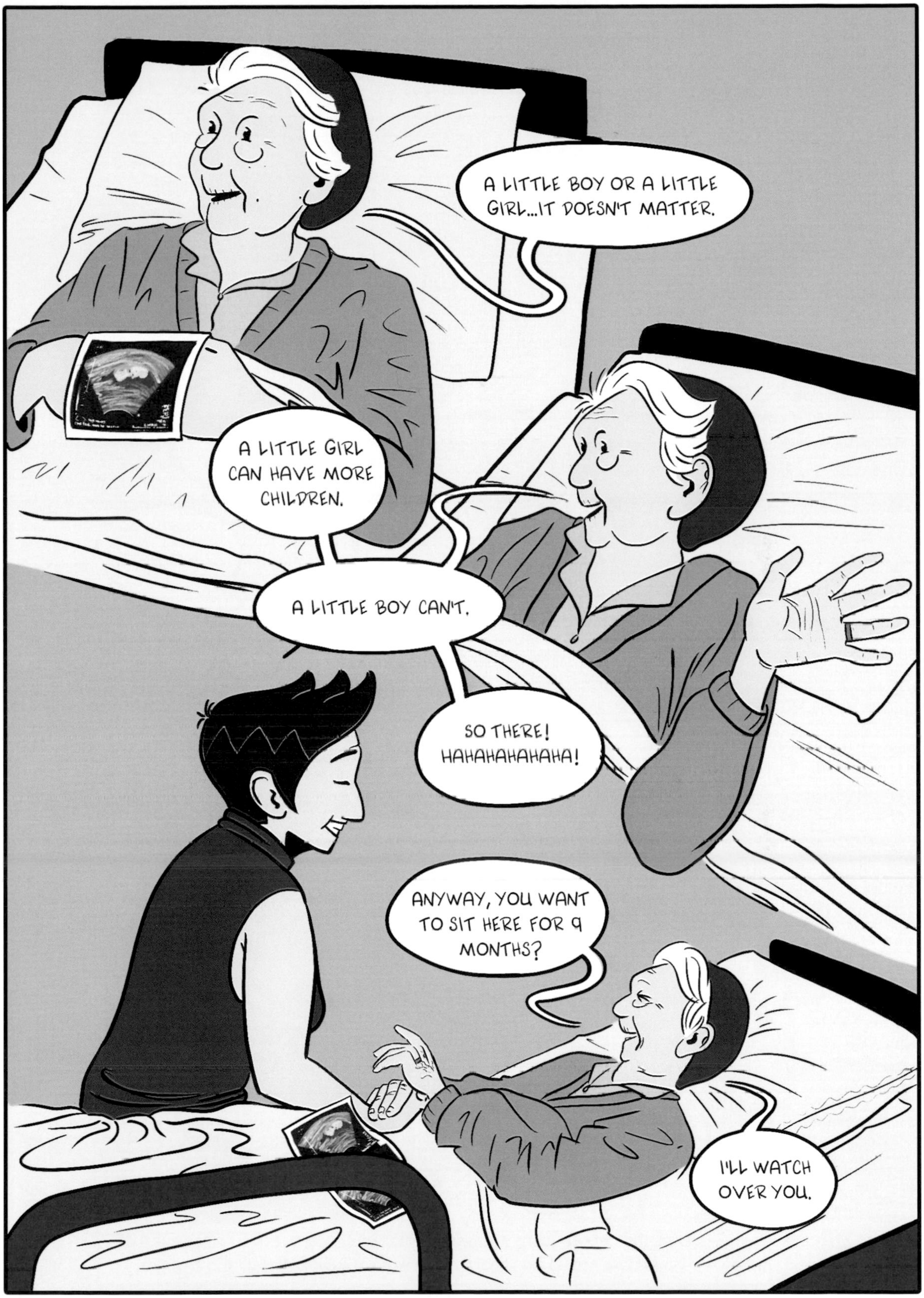
A LITTLE BOY OR A LITTLE GIRL...IT DOESN'T MATTER.
A LITTLE GIRL CAN HAVE MORE CHILDREN.
A LITTLE BOY CAN'T.
SO THERE! HAHAHAHAHAHA!
ANYWAY, YOU WANT TO SIT HERE FOR 9 MONTHS?
I'LL WATCH OVER YOU.

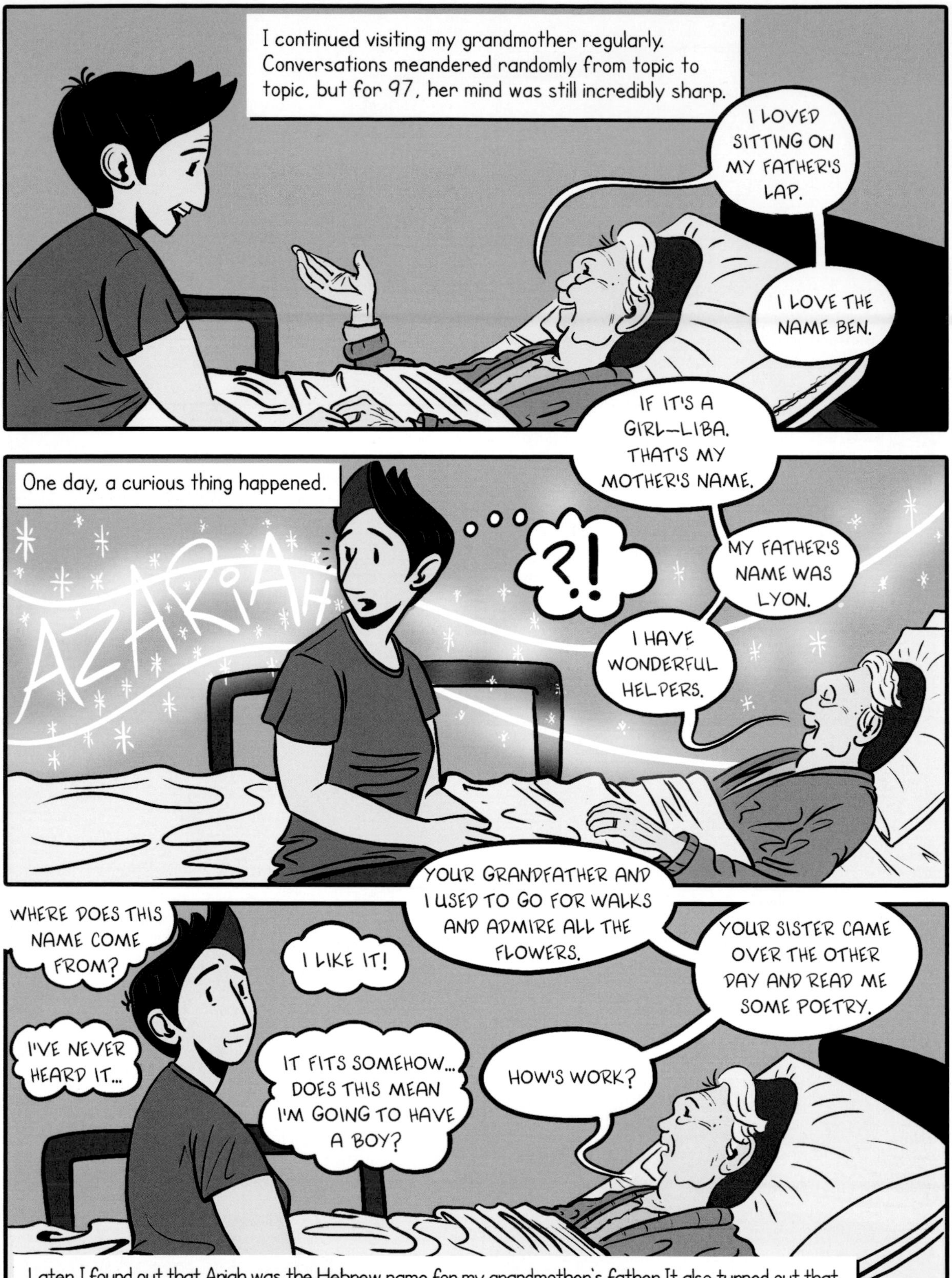
I continued visiting my grandmother regularly. Conversations meandered randomly from topic to topic, but for 97, her mind was still incredibly sharp.
I LOVED SITTING ON MY FATHER'S LAP.
I LOVE THE NAME BEN.
IF IT'S A GIRL—LIBA. THAT'S MY MOTHER'S NAME.
One day, a curious thing happened.
AZARiAH
?!
MY FATHER'S NAME WAS LYON.
I HAVE WONDERFUL HELPERS.
WHERE DOES THIS NAME COME FROM?
I LIKE IT!
YOUR GRANDFATHER AND I USED TO GO FOR WALKS AND ADMIRE ALL THE FLOWERS.
YOUR SISTER CAME OVER THE OTHER DAY AND READ ME SOME POETRY.
I'VE NEVER HEARD IT...
IT FITS SOMEHOW... DOES THIS MEAN I'M GOING TO HAVE A BOY?
HOW'S WORK?
Later, I found out that Ariah was the Hebrew name for my grandmother's father. It also turned out that, had I been a boy, my mother would have named me Ezra. Azariah was like a conflation of the 2 names.

Because my "advanced maternal age" meant I was at a higher risk of having issues with the baby's health, I decided to undergo fetal genetic testing to make sure the baby was OK. I had 3 options for testing.

The SIPS test is not the most accurate test, but it was free and would raise any flags. It was a 3-part test that was spaced out over several weeks.

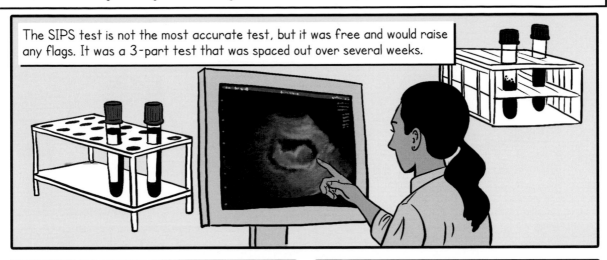

The NIPT claims to be 99% accurate, but costs several hundred dollars—unless you get flagged for a potential issue, in which case it's covered by the provincial Medical Services Plan.

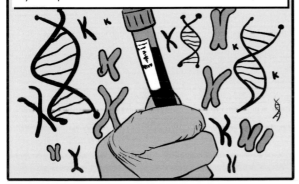

An amnio is supposed to be 100% conclusive. There was noooo way I was getting that huge needle inserted into my abdomen, coming within centimetres of my baby, and possibly causing a miscarriage.

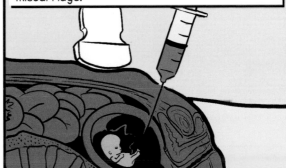

I opted for the SIPS test.

THESE ARE THE REQUISITION FORMS.

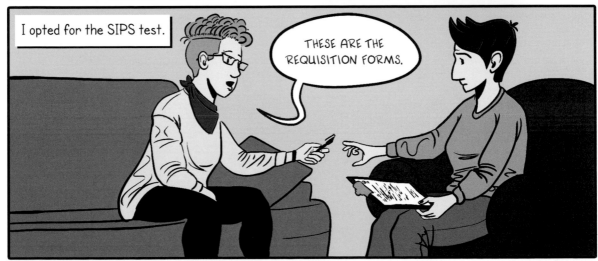

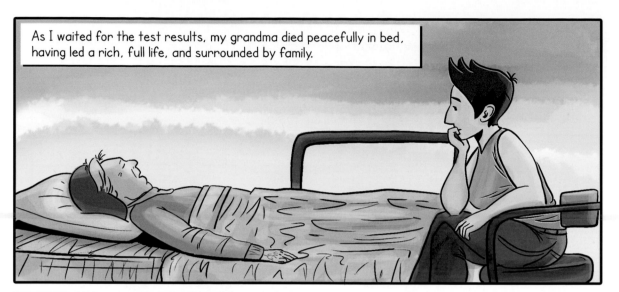

As I waited for the test results, my grandma died peacefully in bed, having led a rich, full life, and surrounded by family.

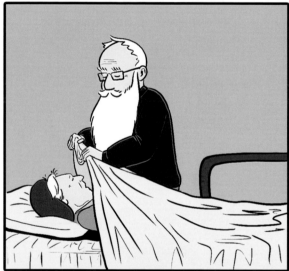

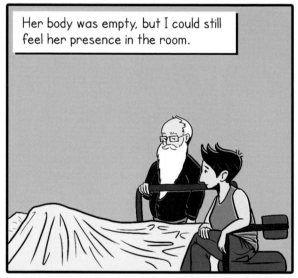

Her body was empty, but I could still feel her presence in the room.

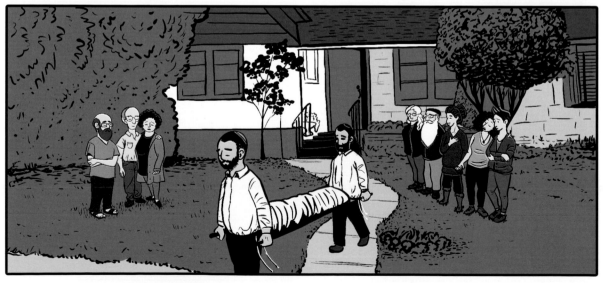

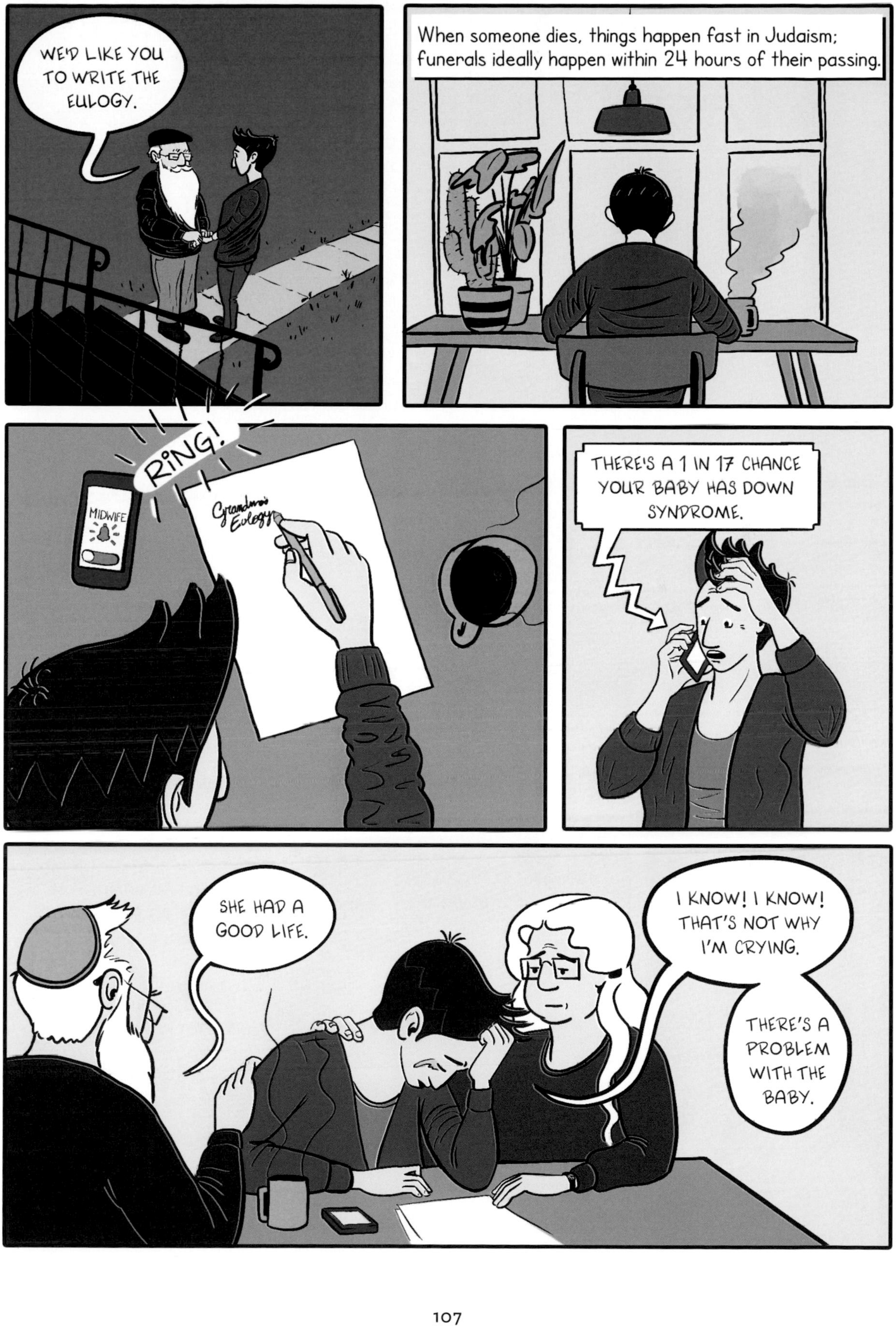
WE'D LIKE YOU TO WRITE THE EULOGY.
When someone dies, things happen fast in Judaism; funerals ideally happen within 24 hours of their passing.
RING!
MIDWIFE
Grandma's Eulogy
THERE'S A 1 IN 17 CHANCE YOUR BABY HAS DOWN SYNDROME.
SHE HAD A GOOD LIFE.
I KNOW! I KNOW! THAT'S NOT WHY I'M CRYING.
THERE'S A PROBLEM WITH THE BABY.

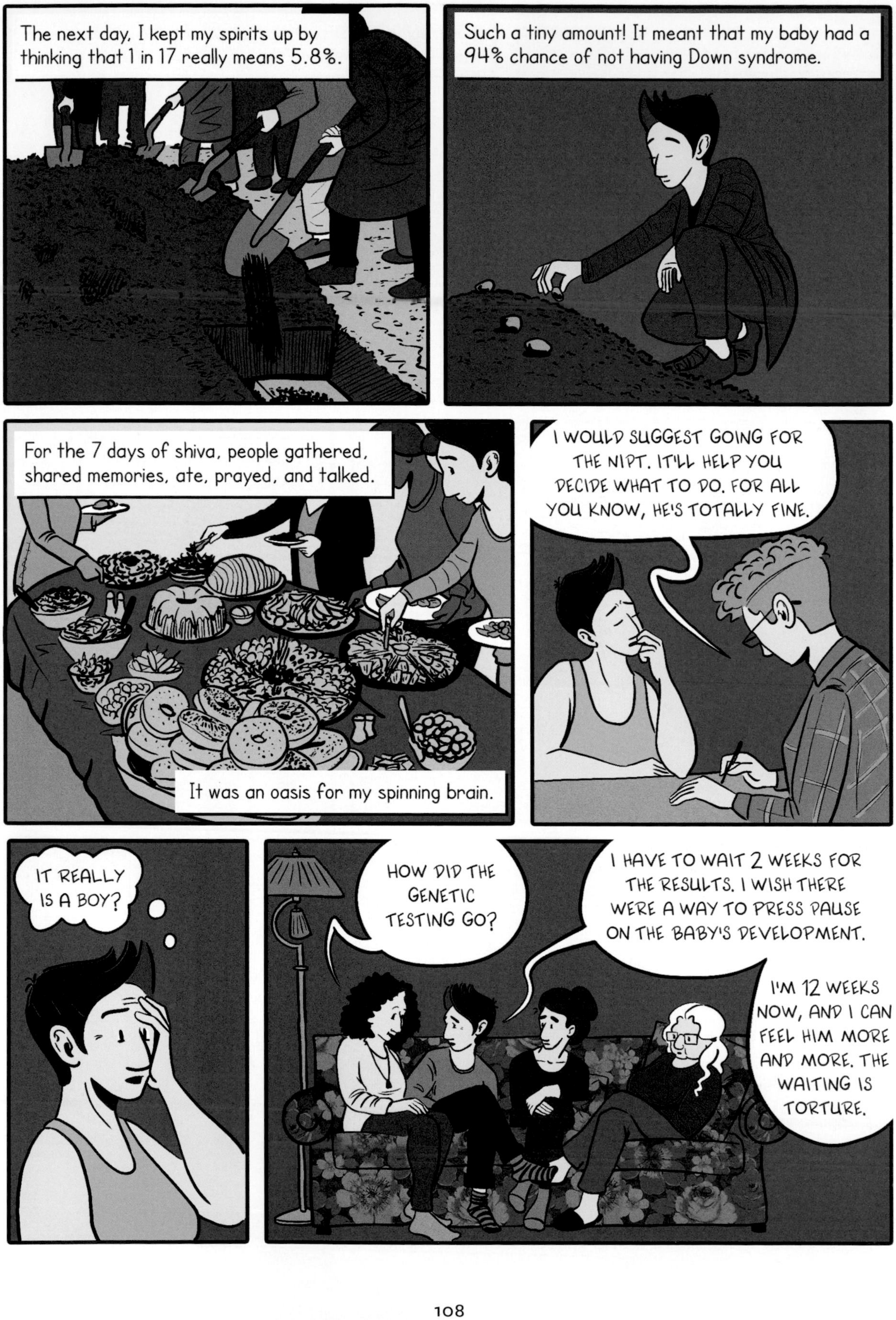

The next day, I kept my spirits up by thinking that 1 in 17 really means 5.8%.
Such a tiny amount! It meant that my baby had a 94% chance of not having Down syndrome.
For the 7 days of shiva, people gathered, shared memories, ate, prayed, and talked.
It was an oasis for my spinning brain.
I WOULD SUGGEST GOING FOR THE NIPT. IT'LL HELP YOU DECIDE WHAT TO DO. FOR ALL YOU KNOW, HE'S TOTALLY FINE.
IT REALLY IS A BOY?
HOW DID THE GENETIC TESTING GO?
I HAVE TO WAIT 2 WEEKS FOR THE RESULTS. I WISH THERE WERE A WAY TO PRESS PAUSE ON THE BABY'S DEVELOPMENT.
I'M 12 WEEKS NOW, AND I CAN FEEL HIM MORE AND MORE. THE WAITING IS TORTURE.

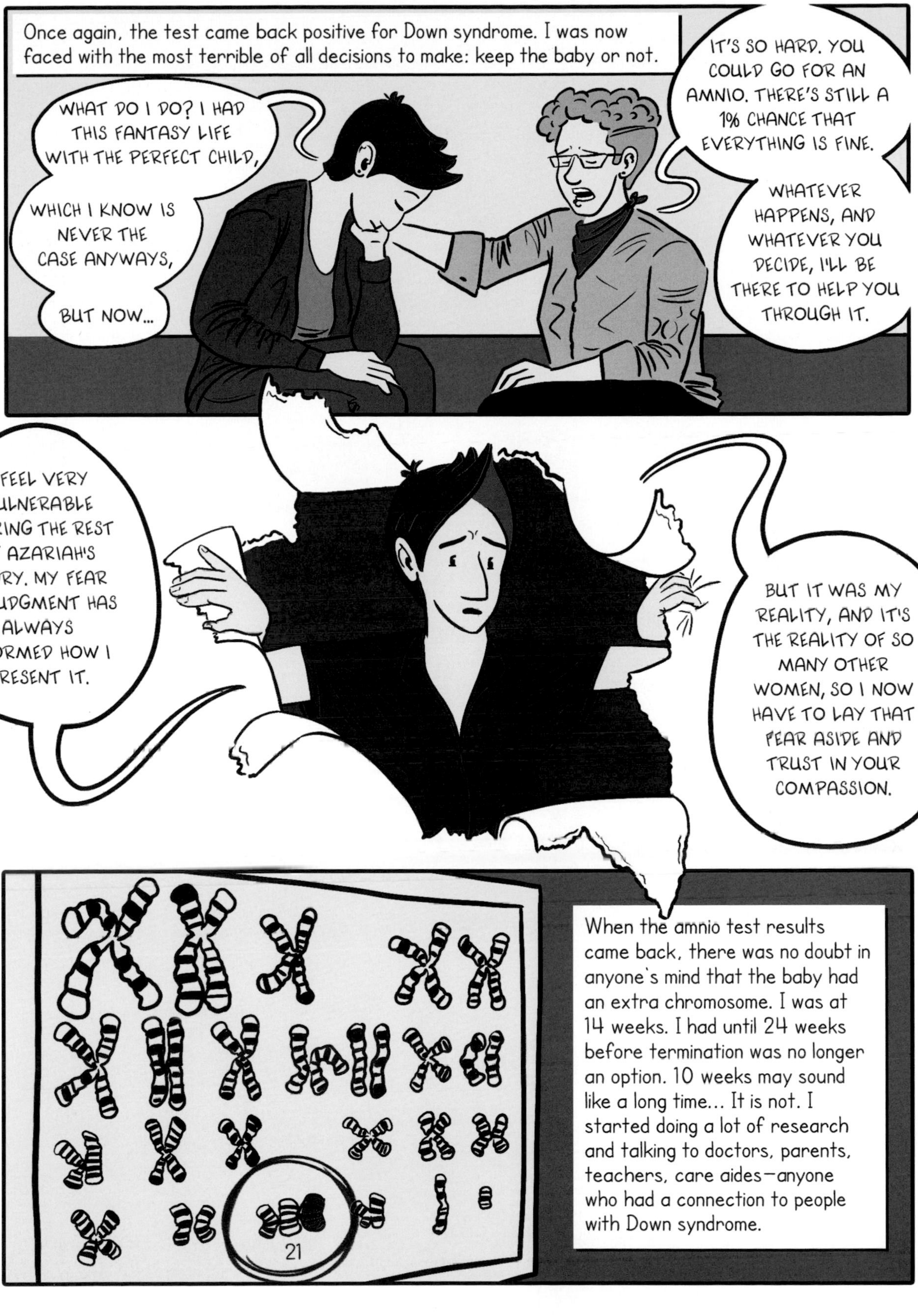

Once again, the test came back positive for Down syndrome. I was now faced with the most terrible of all decisions to make: keep the baby or not.
WHAT DO I DO? I HAD THIS FANTASY LIFE WITH THE PERFECT CHILD,
WHICH I KNOW IS NEVER THE CASE ANYWAYS,
BUT NOW...
IT'S SO HARD. YOU COULD GO FOR AN AMNIO. THERE'S STILL A 1% CHANCE THAT EVERYTHING IS FINE.
WHATEVER HAPPENS, AND WHATEVER YOU DECIDE, I'LL BE THERE TO HELP YOU THROUGH IT.
I FEEL VERY VULNERABLE SHARING THE REST OF AZARIAH'S STORY. MY FEAR OF JUDGMENT HAS ALWAYS INFORMED HOW I PRESENT IT.
BUT IT WAS MY REALITY, AND IT'S THE REALITY OF SO MANY OTHER WOMEN, SO I NOW HAVE TO LAY THAT FEAR ASIDE AND TRUST IN YOUR COMPASSION.
21
When the amnio test results came back, there was no doubt in anyone's mind that the baby had an extra chromosome. I was at 14 weeks. I had until 24 weeks before termination was no longer an option. 10 weeks may sound like a long time... It is not. I started doing a lot of research and talking to doctors, parents, teachers, care aides—anyone who had a connection to people with Down syndrome.

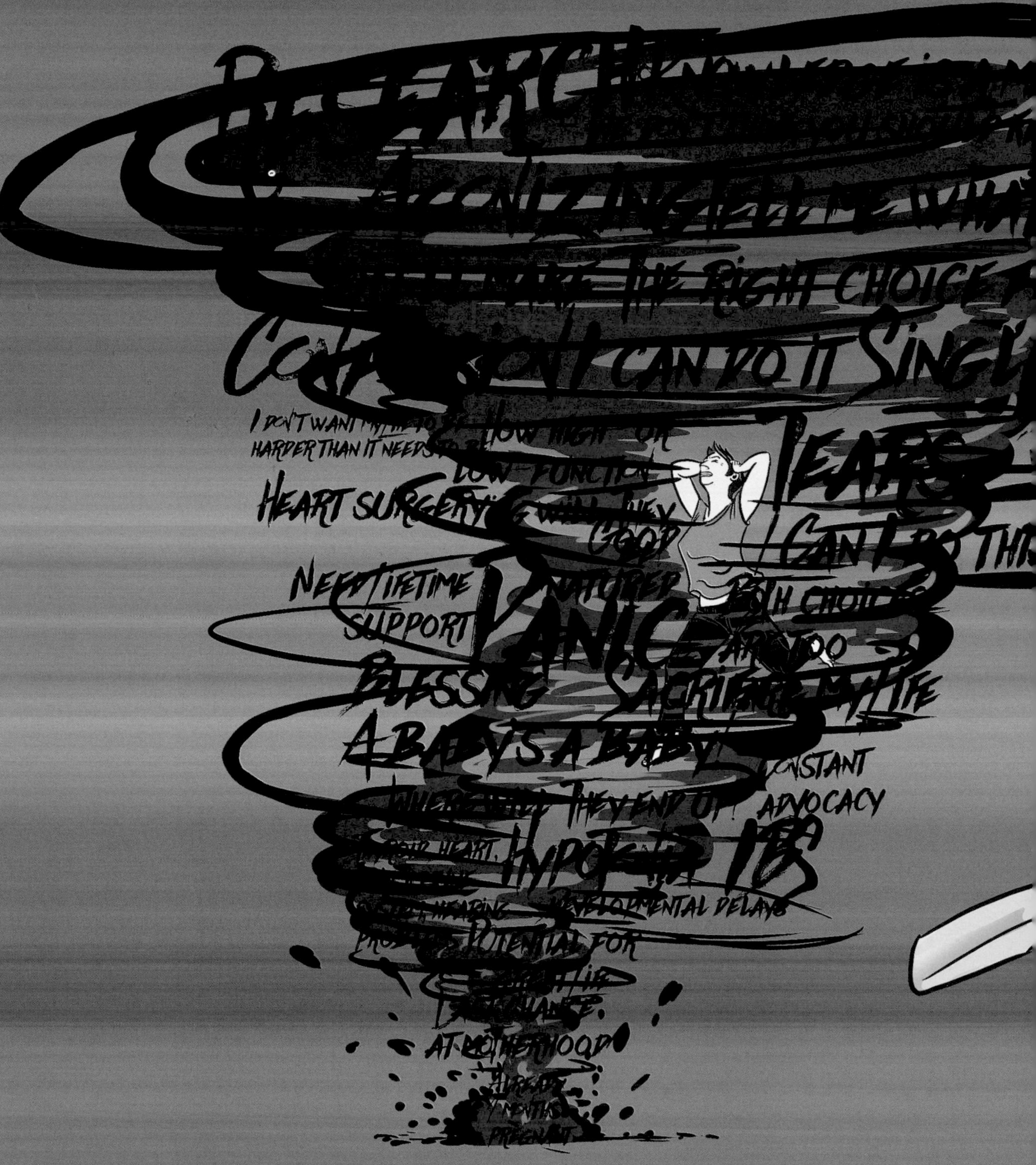
RESEARCH
TELL ME WHAT
MAKE THE RIGHT CHOICE
CAN DO IT SINGL
I DON'T WANT
HARDER THAN IT NEEDS
HOW HIGH OR
LOW FUNCTION
HEART SURGERY
GOOD
TEARS
NEED LIFETIME SUPPORT
PANIC
ARE TOO
BLESSING
A BABY'S A BABY
ADVOCACY
THEY END UP
DEVELOPMENTAL DELAYS
POTENTIAL FOR
AT MOTHERHOOD
PREGNANT

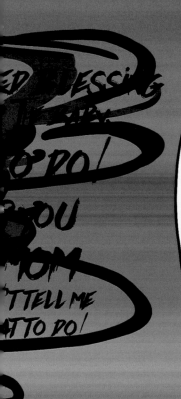

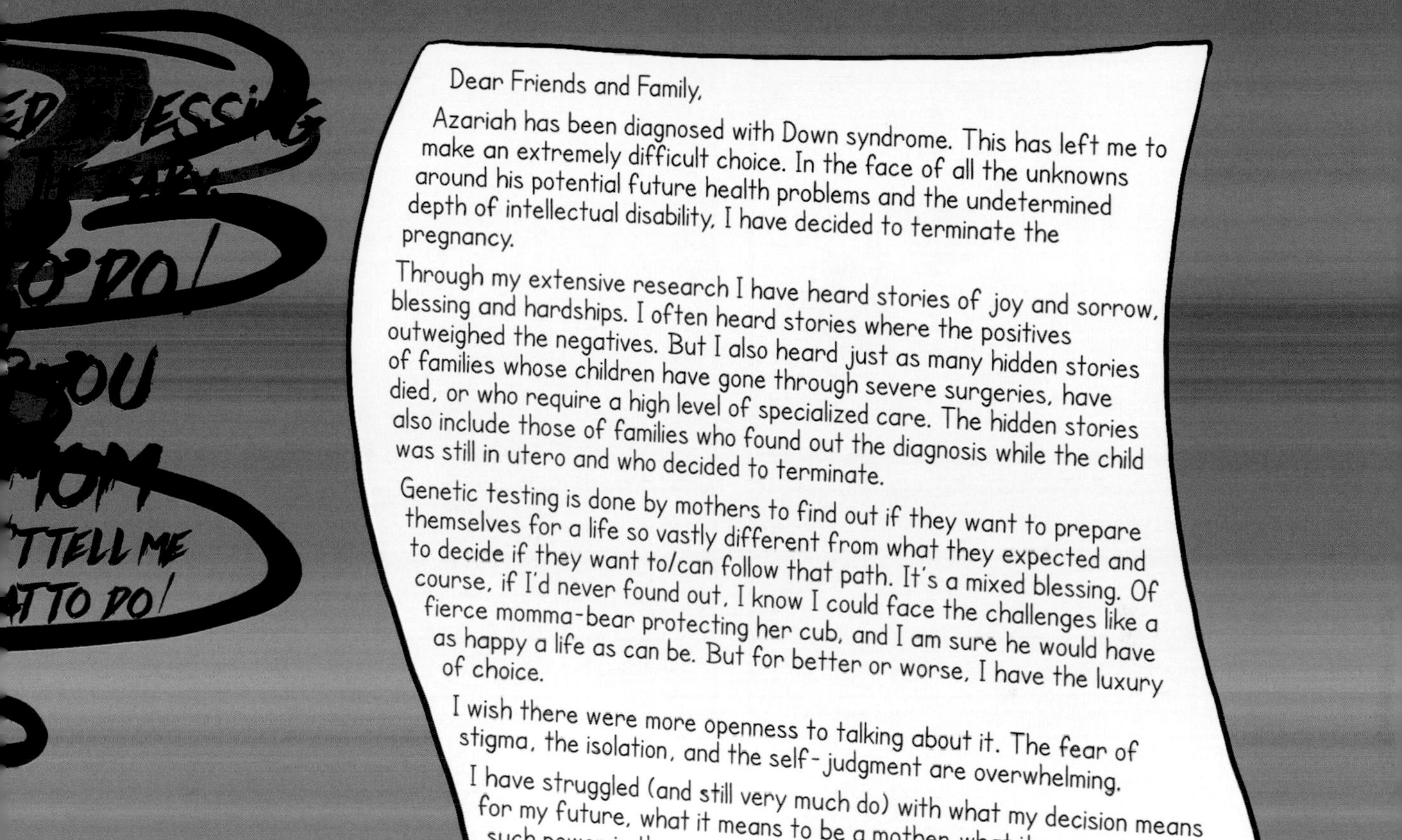

Dear Friends and Family,

Azariah has been diagnosed with Down syndrome. This has left me to make an extremely difficult choice. In the face of all the unknowns around his potential future health problems and the undetermined depth of intellectual disability, I have decided to terminate the pregnancy.

Through my extensive research I have heard stories of joy and sorrow, blessing and hardships. I often heard stories where the positives outweighed the negatives. But I also heard just as many hidden stories of families whose children have gone through severe surgeries, have died, or who require a high level of specialized care. The hidden stories also include those of families who found out the diagnosis while the child was still in utero and who decided to terminate.

Genetic testing is done by mothers to find out if they want to prepare themselves for a life so vastly different from what they expected and to decide if they want to/can follow that path. It's a mixed blessing. Of course, if I'd never found out, I know I could face the challenges like a fierce momma-bear protecting her cub, and I am sure he would have as happy a life as can be. But for better or worse, I have the luxury of choice.

I wish there were more openness to talking about it. The fear of stigma, the isolation, and the self-judgment are overwhelming.

I have struggled (and still very much do) with what my decision means for my future, what it means to be a mother, what it means to have such power in the giving and taking of life, what it means as a physically and intellectually able person to consciously choose to permanently and intimately accept or not accept a person with disability into my life, whether my decision is an act of selfishness and where the line is between selflessness and dangerous self-abnegation. I have flip-flopped on my decision and desires more times than I can count. All paths feel impossible and hard.

Not all of you will agree with my choice, but, although this decision doesn't lessen the grief, or offer relief, it is what is right for me. Know that in the short time Azariah will have been in my life, so much life has been lived, lessons have been learned, and grace allowed.

I feel truly blessed with the community I have around me and find solace and strength in the kindness and support you've offered me in the last year. I will continue the journey towards motherhood.

Myriam

Despite having sent that letter, doubts still plagued me. One more thing happened the day before the first phase of the termination that helped me confirm my decision.

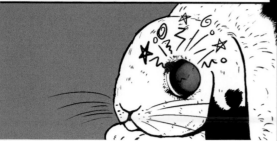

Sherbert had now been on meds for 6 months and her health had not improved. I finally agreed to her surgery.

Unfortunately, my timing was terrible. Sherbert's surgery ended up being scheduled for the day before I had to go into the hospital.

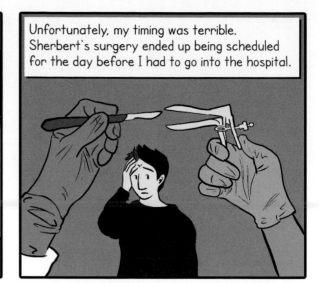

It wasn't easy leaving her at the vet's.

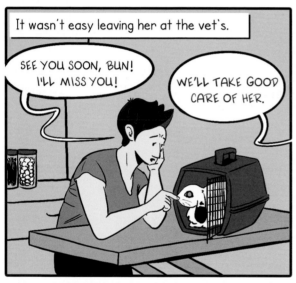

SEE YOU SOON, BUN! I'LL MISS YOU!

WE'LL TAKE GOOD CARE OF HER.

Hours later,

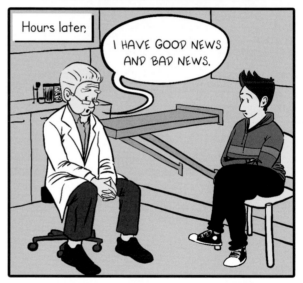

I HAVE GOOD NEWS AND BAD NEWS.

It turned out that although the eye removal had gone perfectly, the abscess had gone deep into the inner ear. When they removed it and flushed the ear, the inner ear nerve got damaged, leaving Sherbert with vestibular disease. In other words, she had a serious head tilt, uncontrollable dizziness, rolling due to loss of balance, and nystagmus (involuntary rapid eye movements) in her one good eye.

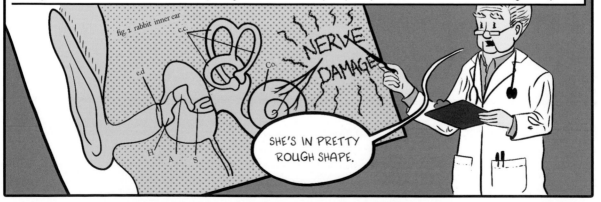

fig. 2 rabbit inner ear

NERVE DAMAGE

SHE'S IN PRETTY ROUGH SHAPE.

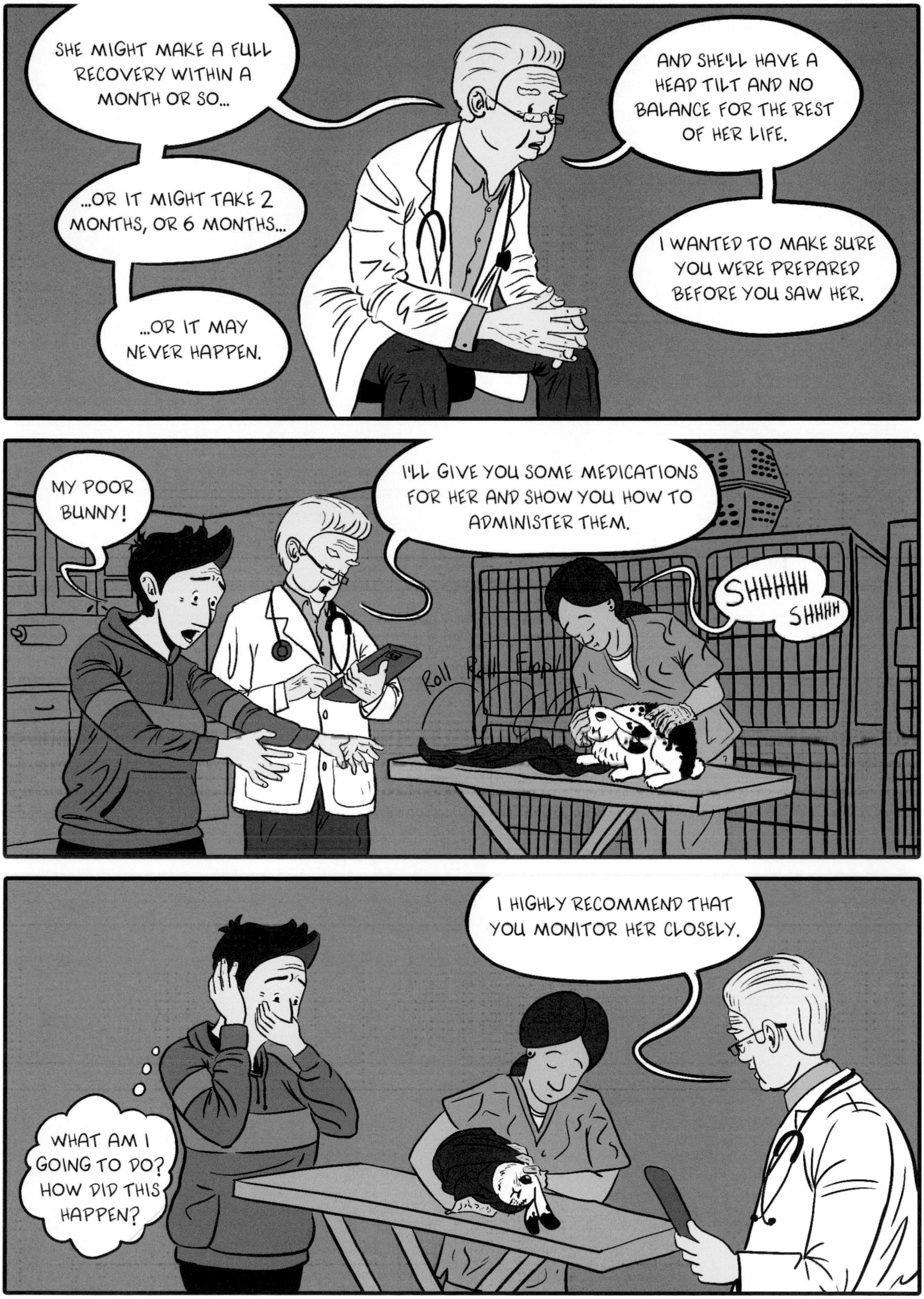
SHE MIGHT MAKE A FULL RECOVERY WITHIN A MONTH OR SO...
...OR IT MIGHT TAKE 2 MONTHS, OR 6 MONTHS...
...OR IT MAY NEVER HAPPEN.
AND SHE'LL HAVE A HEAD TILT AND NO BALANCE FOR THE REST OF HER LIFE.
I WANTED TO MAKE SURE YOU WERE PREPARED BEFORE YOU SAW HER.
MY POOR BUNNY!
I'LL GIVE YOU SOME MEDICATIONS FOR HER AND SHOW YOU HOW TO ADMINISTER THEM.
Roll Roll Flop!
SHHHHH
SHHHH
I HIGHLY RECOMMEND THAT YOU MONITOR HER CLOSELY.
WHAT AM I GOING TO DO? HOW DID THIS HAPPEN?

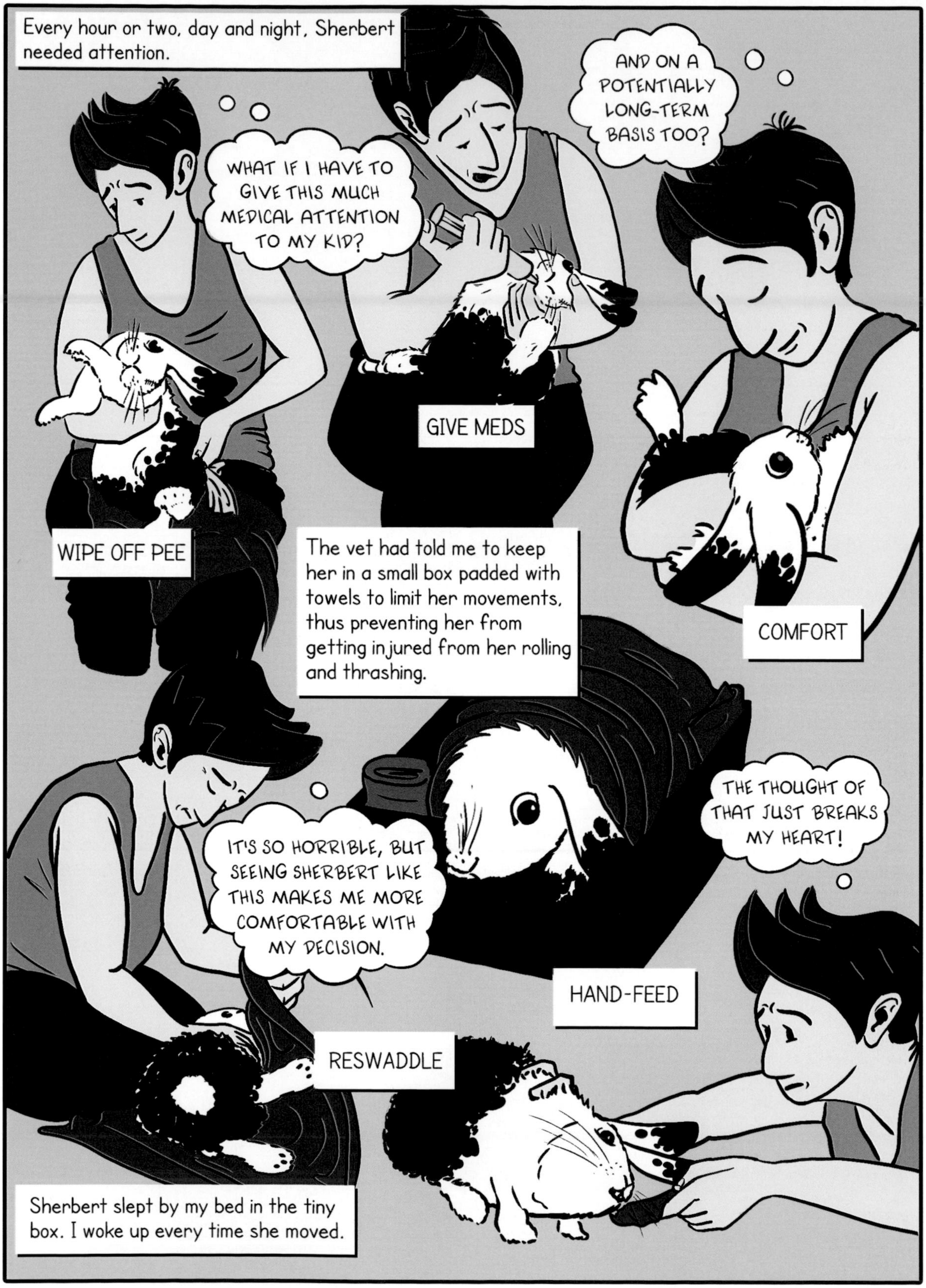
Every hour or two, day and night, Sherbert needed attention.
WHAT IF I HAVE TO GIVE THIS MUCH MEDICAL ATTENTION TO MY KID?
AND ON A POTENTIALLY LONG-TERM BASIS TOO?
WIPE OFF PEE
GIVE MEDS
COMFORT
The vet had told me to keep her in a small box padded with towels to limit her movements, thus preventing her from getting injured from her rolling and thrashing.
IT'S SO HORRIBLE, BUT SEEING SHERBERT LIKE THIS MAKES ME MORE COMFORTABLE WITH MY DECISION.
THE THOUGHT OF THAT JUST BREAKS MY HEART!
HAND-FEED
RESWADDLE
Sherbert slept by my bed in the tiny box. I woke up every time she moved.

By dawn I was exhausted. After considering going to the hospital alone in a taxi, I got a friend to drive me there.

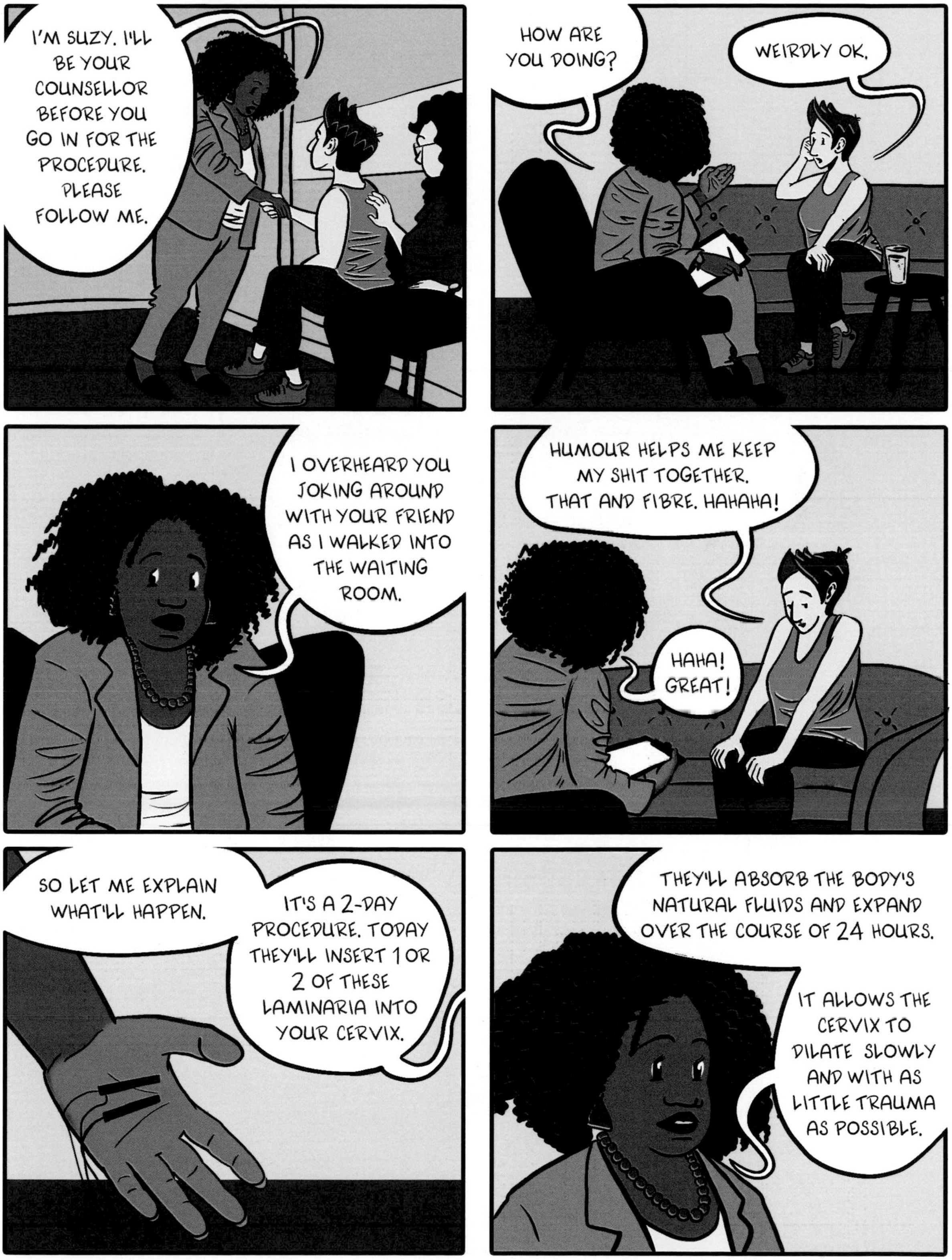

I'M SUZY. I'LL BE YOUR COUNSELLOR BEFORE YOU GO IN FOR THE PROCEDURE. PLEASE FOLLOW ME.
HOW ARE YOU DOING?
WEIRDLY OK.
I OVERHEARD YOU JOKING AROUND WITH YOUR FRIEND AS I WALKED INTO THE WAITING ROOM.
HUMOUR HELPS ME KEEP MY SHIT TOGETHER. THAT AND FIBRE. HAHAHA!
HAHA! GREAT!
SO LET ME EXPLAIN WHAT'LL HAPPEN.
IT'S A 2-DAY PROCEDURE. TODAY THEY'LL INSERT 1 OR 2 OF THESE LAMINARIA INTO YOUR CERVIX.
THEY'LL ABSORB THE BODY'S NATURAL FLUIDS AND EXPAND OVER THE COURSE OF 24 HOURS.
IT ALLOWS THE CERVIX TO DILATE SLOWLY AND WITH AS LITTLE TRAUMA AS POSSIBLE.

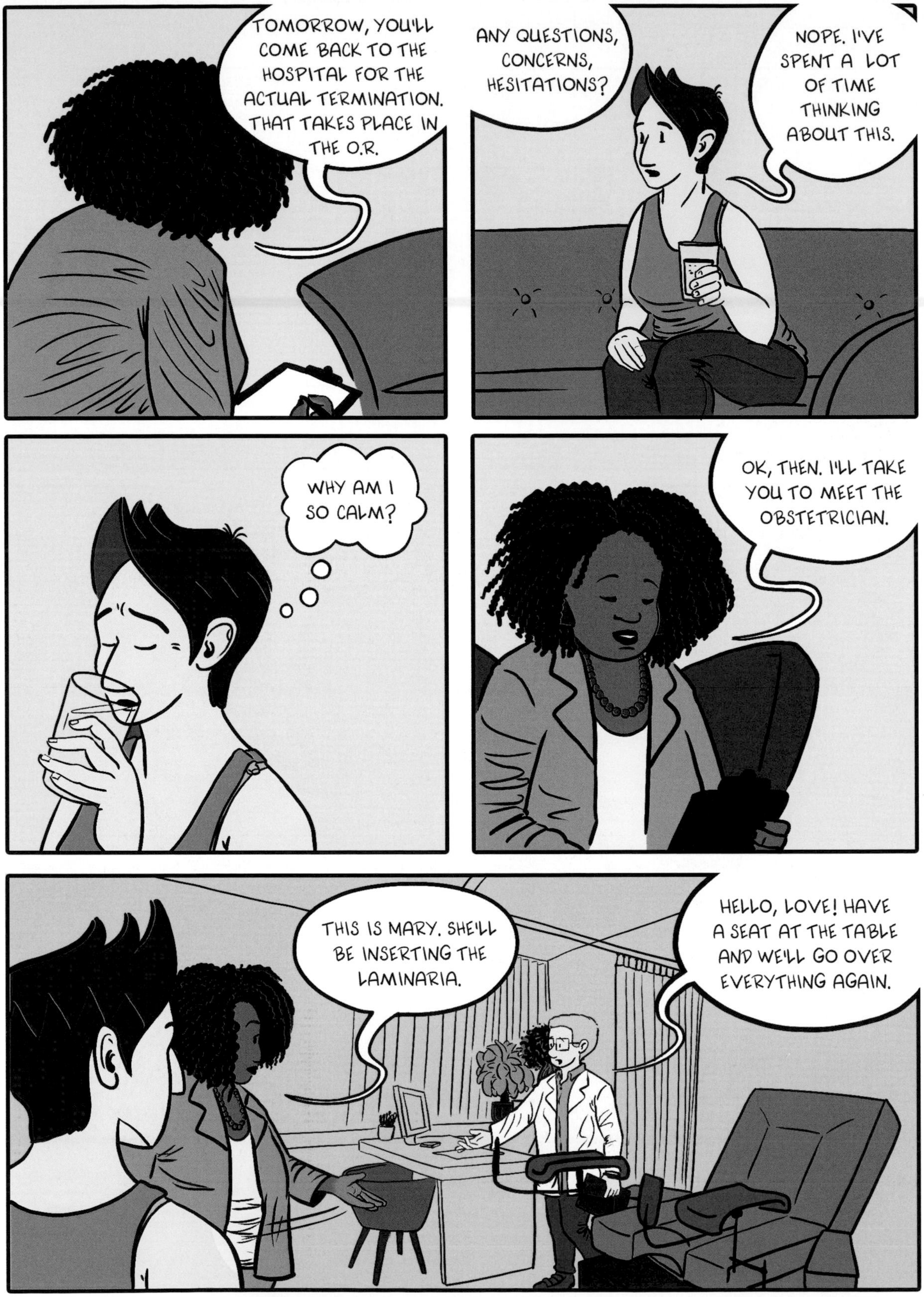
TOMORROW, YOU'LL COME BACK TO THE HOSPITAL FOR THE ACTUAL TERMINATION. THAT TAKES PLACE IN THE O.R.
ANY QUESTIONS, CONCERNS, HESITATIONS?
NOPE. I'VE SPENT A LOT OF TIME THINKING ABOUT THIS.
WHY AM I SO CALM?
OK, THEN. I'LL TAKE YOU TO MEET THE OBSTETRICIAN.
THIS IS MARY. SHE'LL BE INSERTING THE LAMINARIA.
HELLO, LOVE! HAVE A SEAT AT THE TABLE AND WE'LL GO OVER EVERYTHING AGAIN.

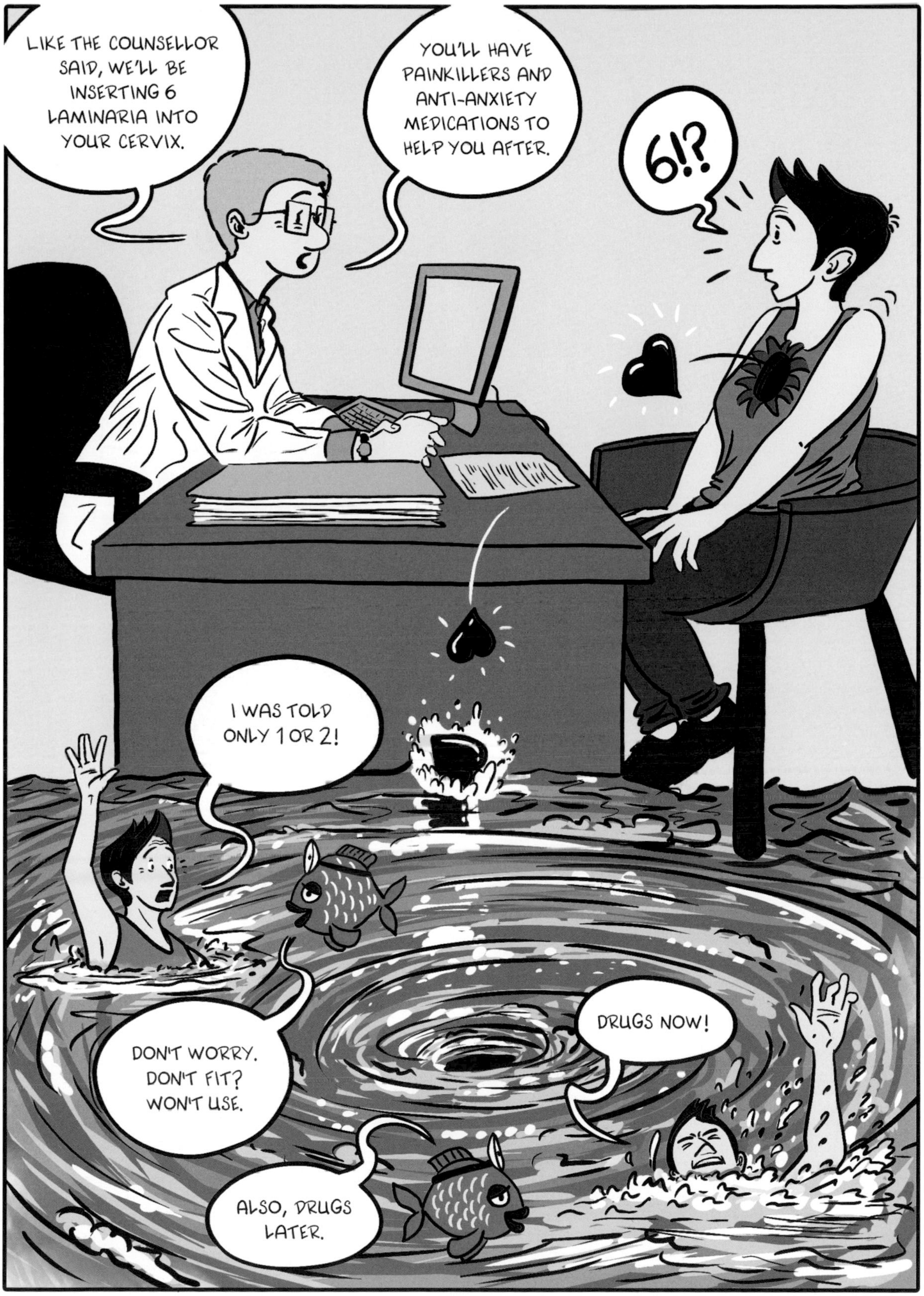
LIKE THE COUNSELLOR SAID, WE'LL BE INSERTING 6 LAMINARIA INTO YOUR CERVIX.
YOU'LL HAVE PAINKILLERS AND ANTI-ANXIETY MEDICATIONS TO HELP YOU AFTER.
6!?
I WAS TOLD ONLY 1 OR 2!
DON'T WORRY. DON'T FIT? WON'T USE.
DRUGS NOW!
ALSO, DRUGS LATER.

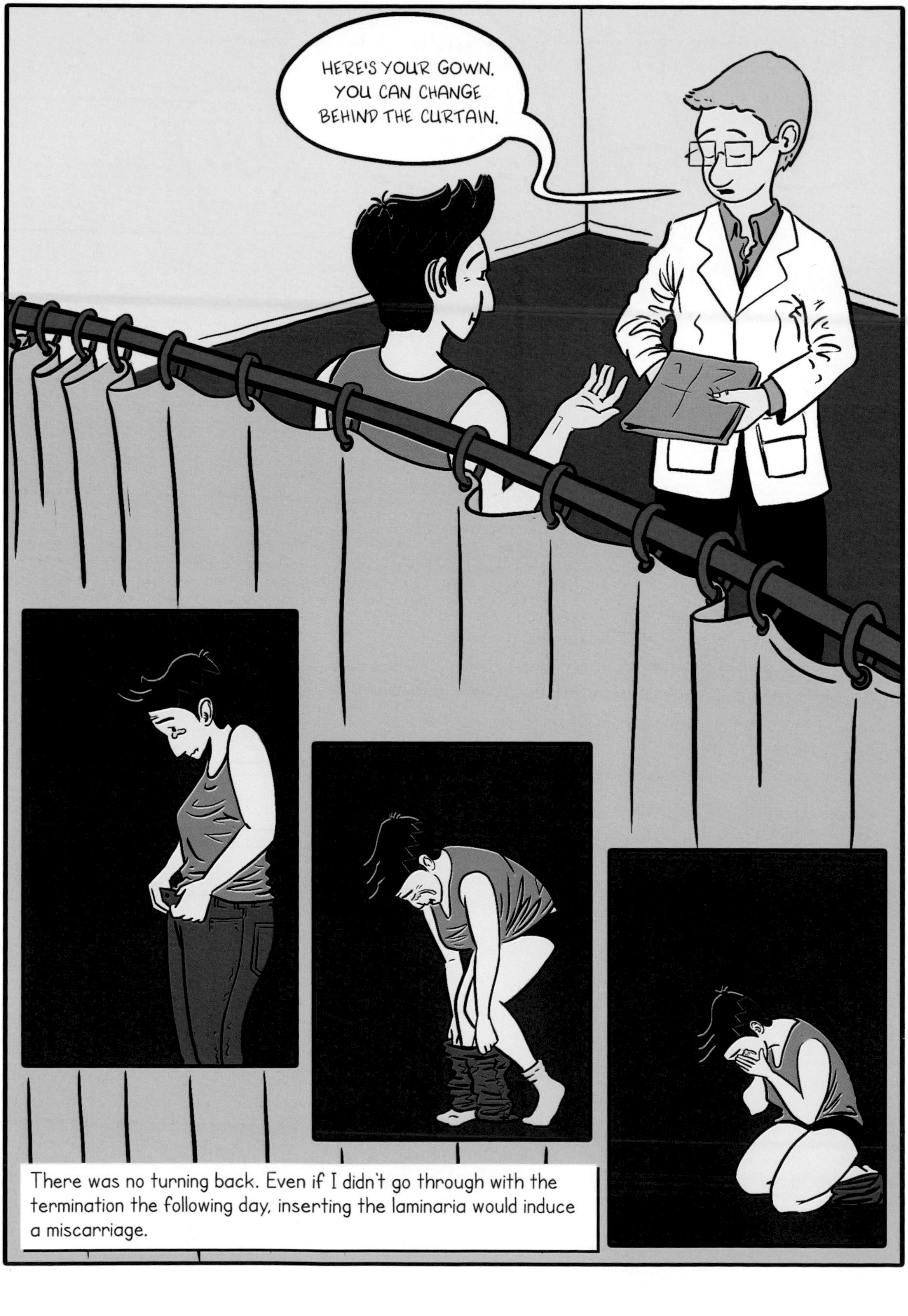
HERE'S YOUR GOWN. YOU CAN CHANGE BEHIND THE CURTAIN.
There was no turning back. Even if I didn't go through with the termination the following day, inserting the laminaria would induce a miscarriage.

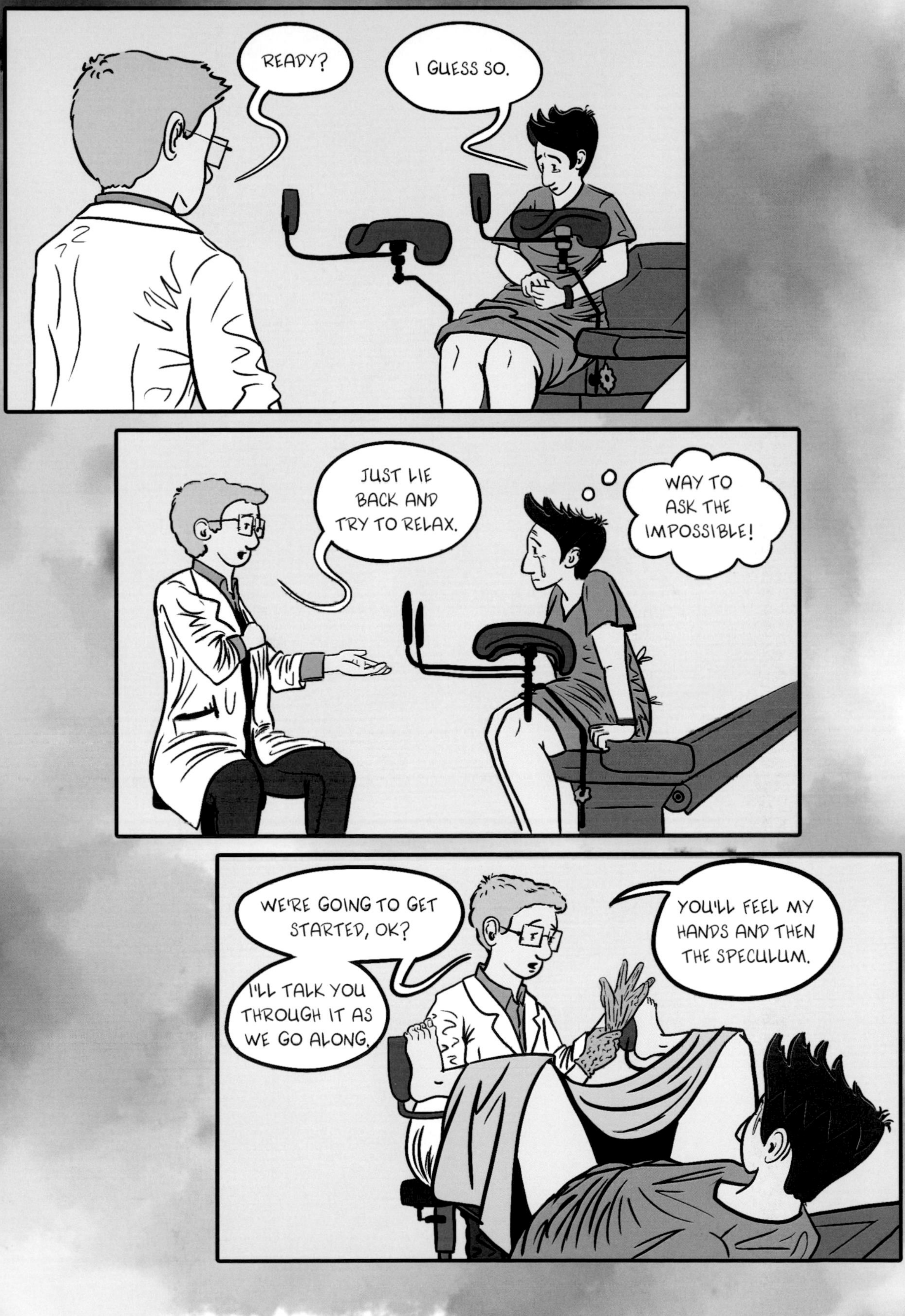
READY?
I GUESS SO.
JUST LIE BACK AND TRY TO RELAX.
WAY TO ASK THE IMPOSSIBLE!
WE'RE GOING TO GET STARTED, OK?
I'LL TALK YOU THROUGH IT AS WE GO ALONG.
YOU'LL FEEL MY HANDS AND THEN THE SPECULUM.

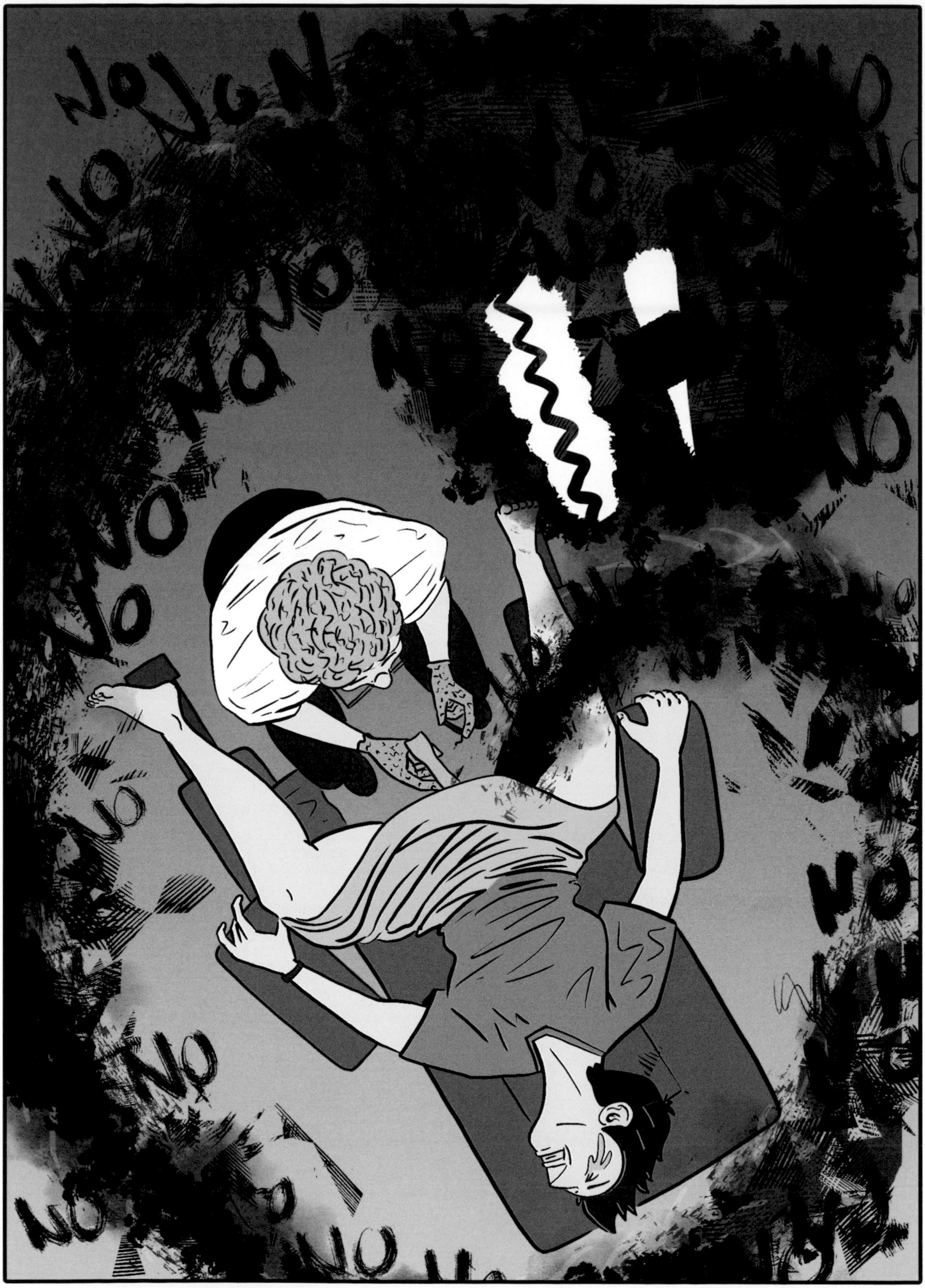
NO NO NO NO NO NO NO NO NO NO NO NO NO NO NO NO

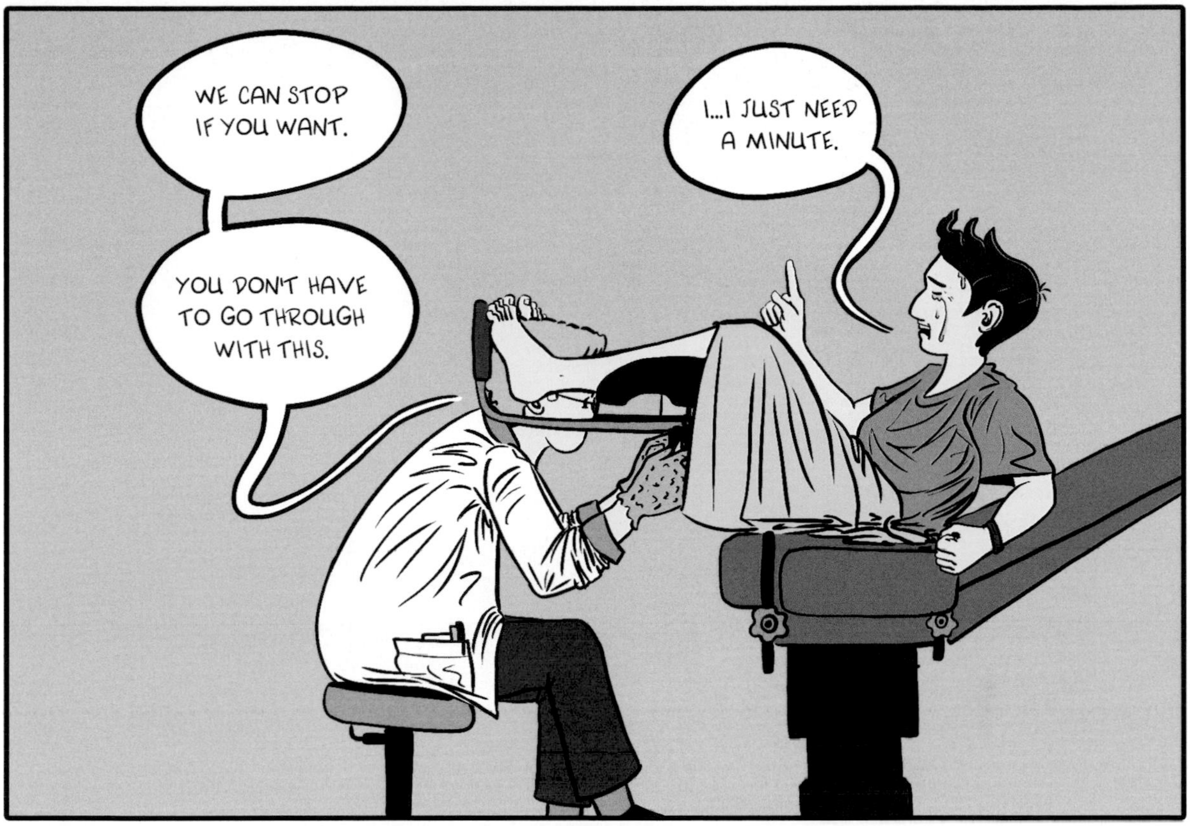
WE CAN STOP IF YOU WANT.
YOU DON'T HAVE TO GO THROUGH WITH THIS.
I...I JUST NEED A MINUTE.

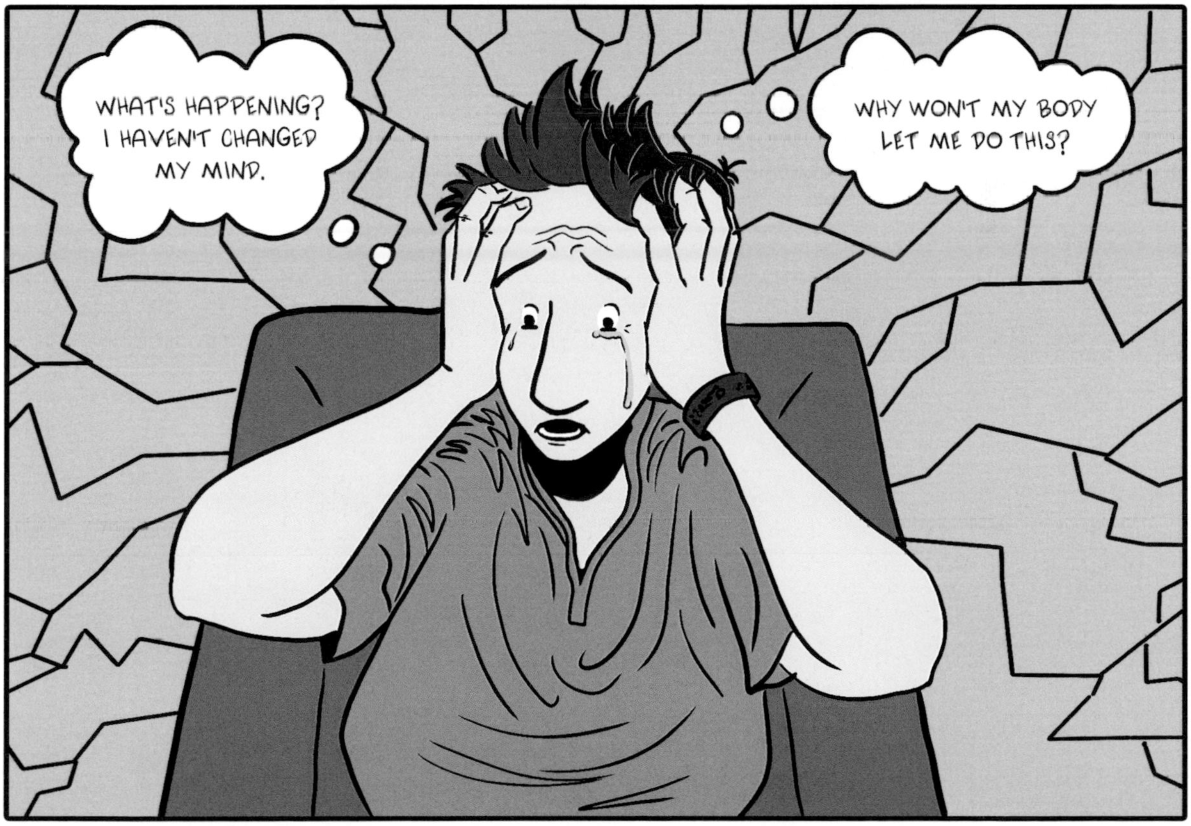
WHAT'S HAPPENING? I HAVEN'T CHANGED MY MIND.
WHY WON'T MY BODY LET ME DO THIS?

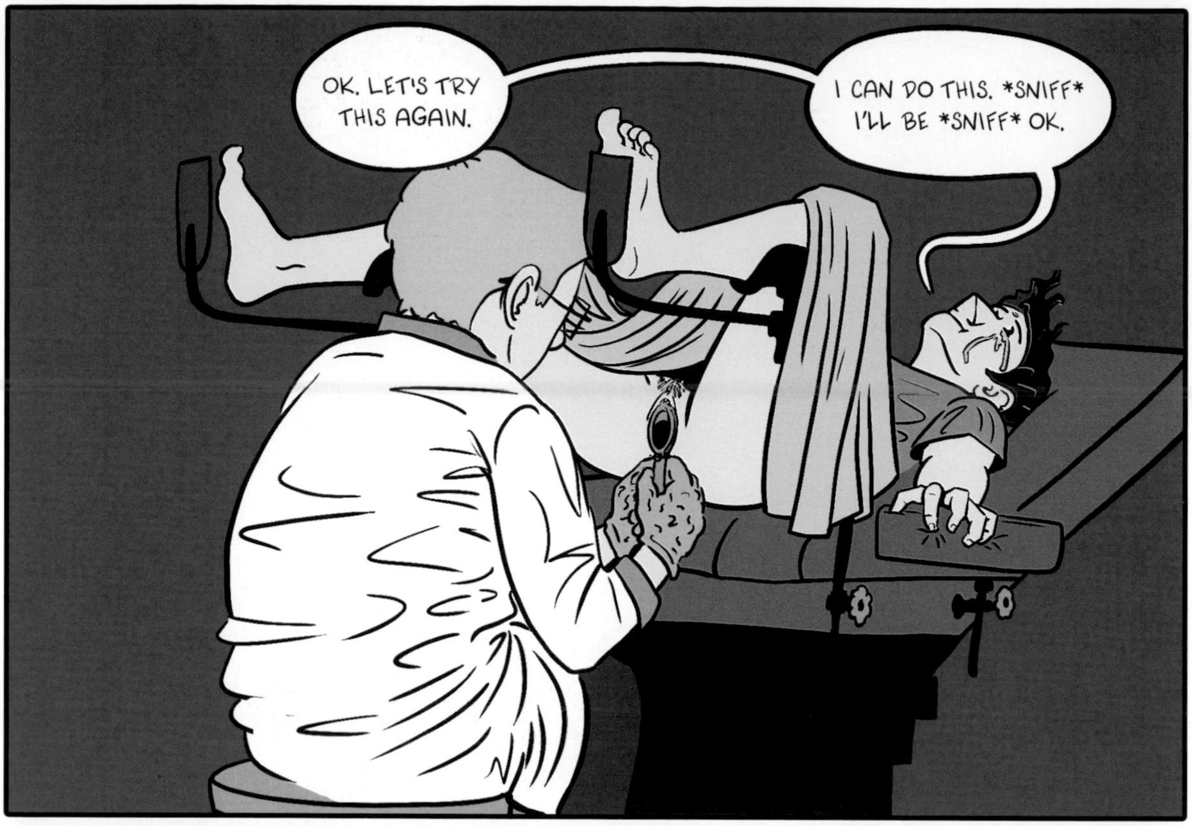
OK. LET'S TRY THIS AGAIN.
I CAN DO THIS. *SNIFF* I'LL BE *SNIFF* OK.

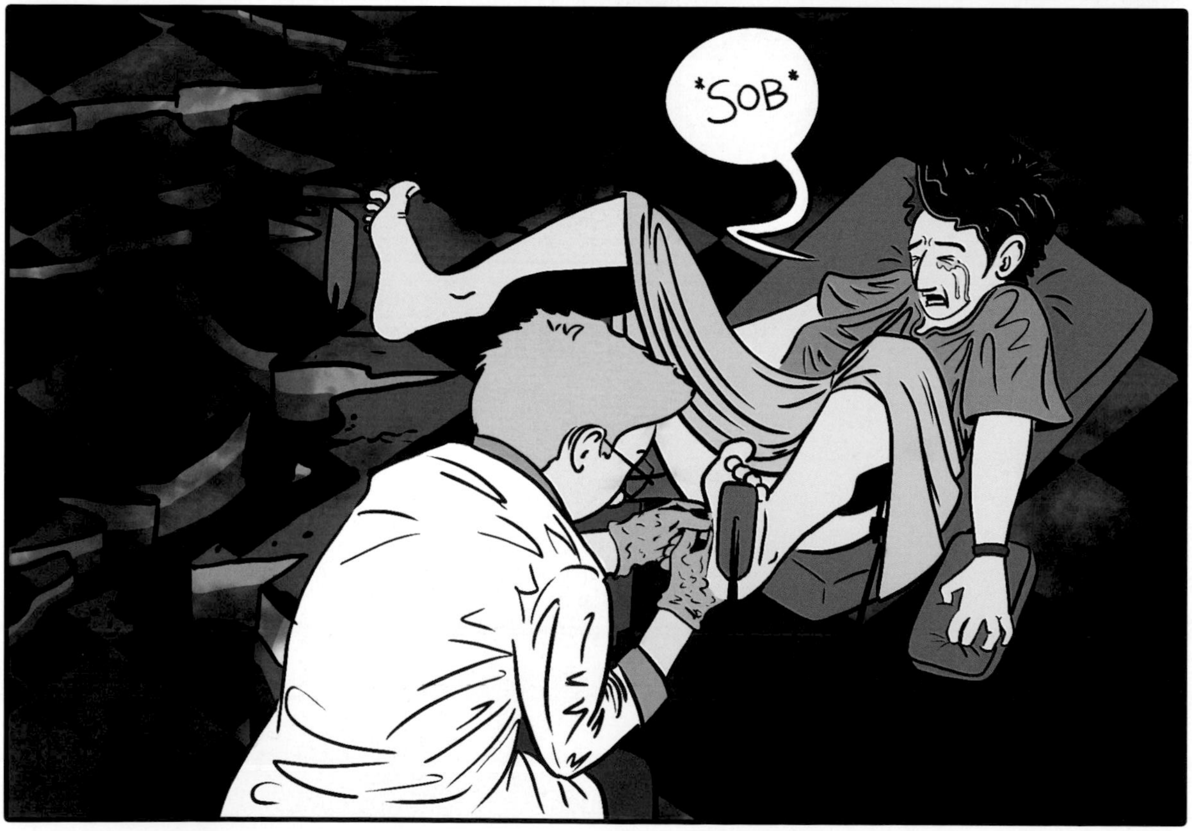
SOB

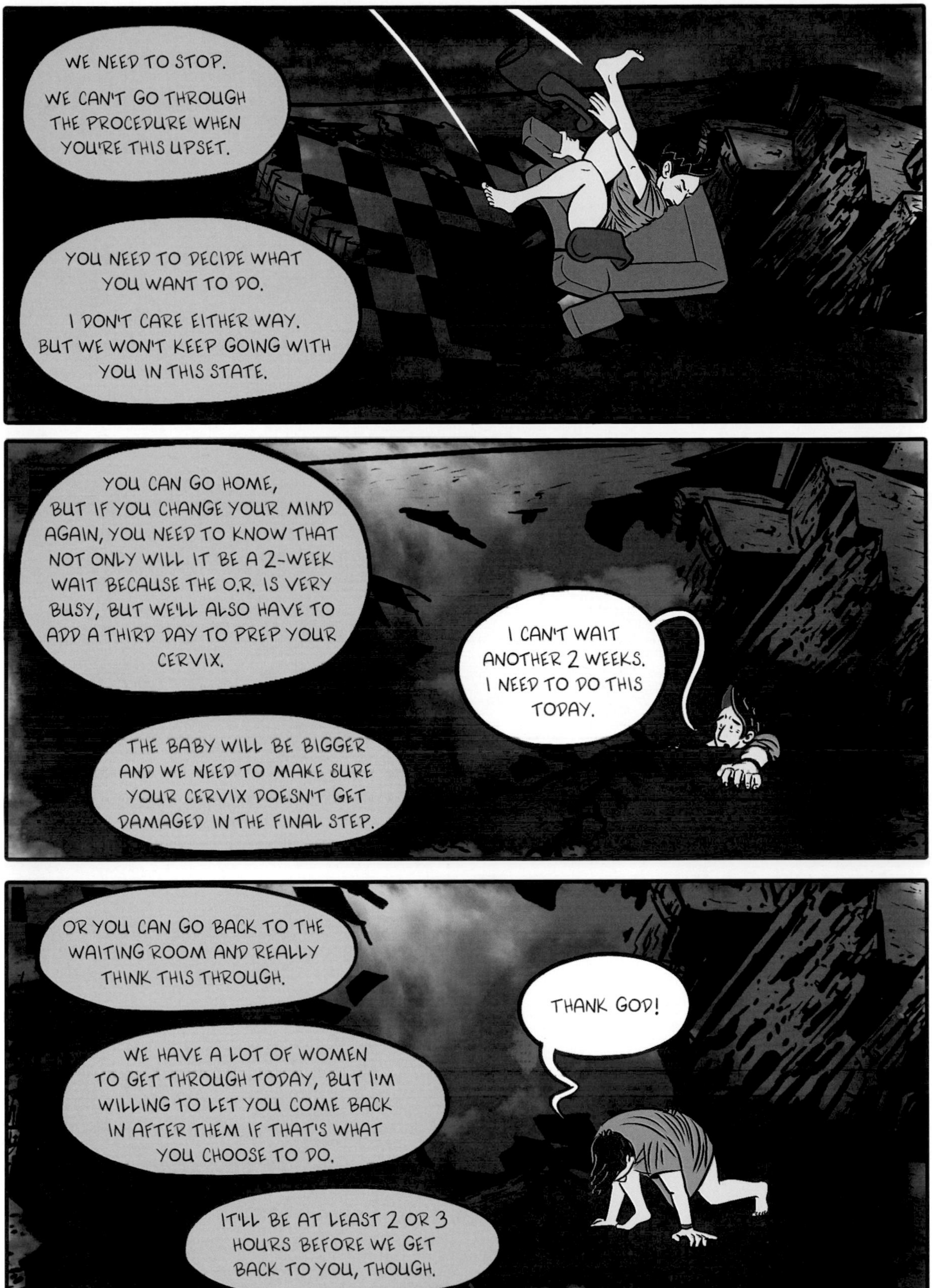
WE NEED TO STOP.
WE CAN'T GO THROUGH THE PROCEDURE WHEN YOU'RE THIS UPSET.
YOU NEED TO DECIDE WHAT YOU WANT TO DO.
I DON'T CARE EITHER WAY. BUT WE WON'T KEEP GOING WITH YOU IN THIS STATE.
YOU CAN GO HOME, BUT IF YOU CHANGE YOUR MIND AGAIN, YOU NEED TO KNOW THAT NOT ONLY WILL IT BE A 2-WEEK WAIT BECAUSE THE O.R. IS VERY BUSY, BUT WE'LL ALSO HAVE TO ADD A THIRD DAY TO PREP YOUR CERVIX.
THE BABY WILL BE BIGGER AND WE NEED TO MAKE SURE YOUR CERVIX DOESN'T GET DAMAGED IN THE FINAL STEP.
I CAN'T WAIT ANOTHER 2 WEEKS. I NEED TO DO THIS TODAY.
OR YOU CAN GO BACK TO THE WAITING ROOM AND REALLY THINK THIS THROUGH.
THANK GOD!
WE HAVE A LOT OF WOMEN TO GET THROUGH TODAY, BUT I'M WILLING TO LET YOU COME BACK IN AFTER THEM IF THAT'S WHAT YOU CHOOSE TO DO.
IT'LL BE AT LEAST 2 OR 3 HOURS BEFORE WE GET BACK TO YOU, THOUGH.

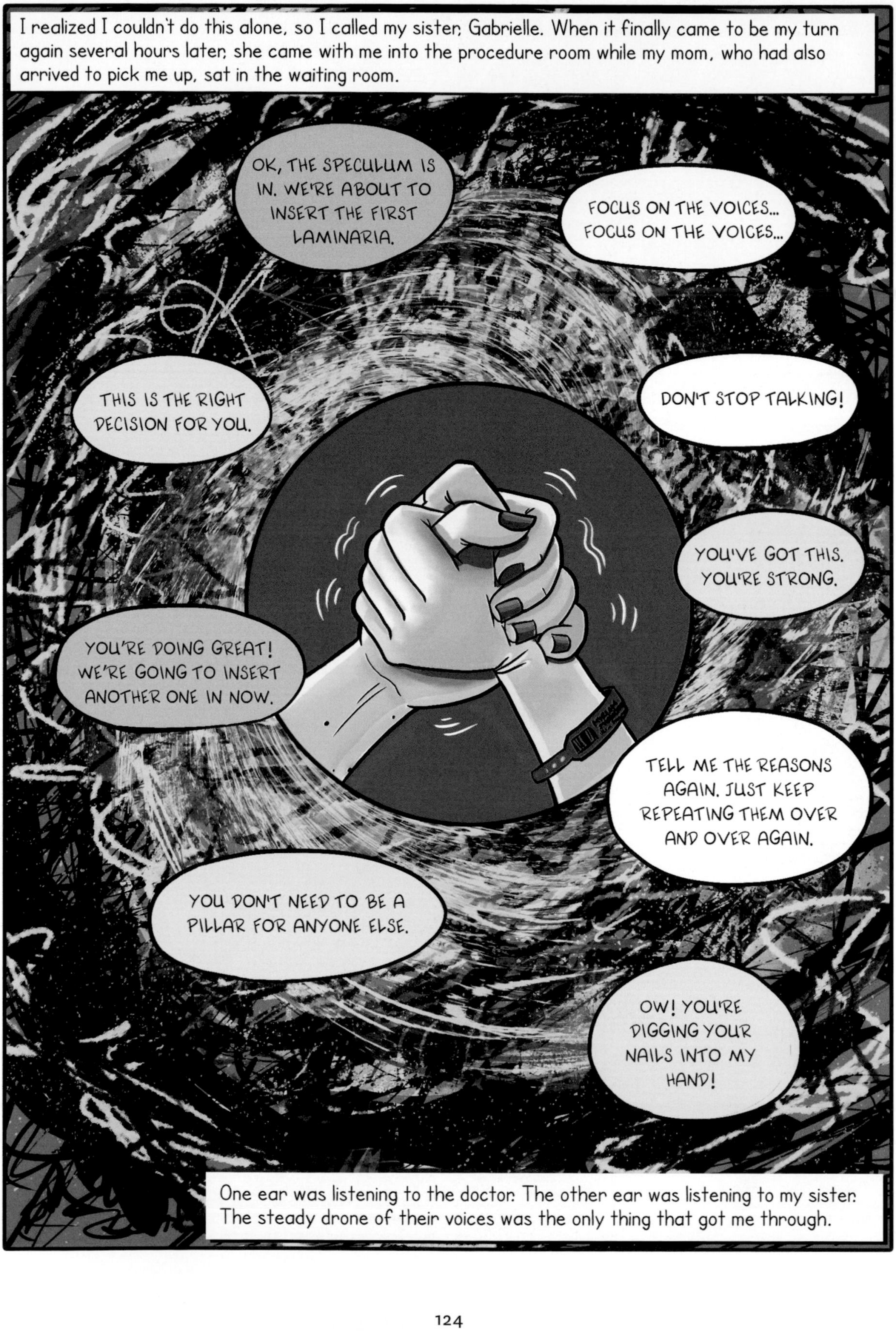
I realized I couldn't do this alone, so I called my sister, Gabrielle. When it finally came to be my turn again several hours later, she came with me into the procedure room while my mom, who had also arrived to pick me up, sat in the waiting room.
OK, THE SPECULUM IS IN. WE'RE ABOUT TO INSERT THE FIRST LAMINARIA.
FOCUS ON THE VOICES... FOCUS ON THE VOICES...
THIS IS THE RIGHT DECISION FOR YOU.
DON'T STOP TALKING!
YOU'VE GOT THIS. YOU'RE STRONG.
YOU'RE DOING GREAT! WE'RE GOING TO INSERT ANOTHER ONE IN NOW.
TELL ME THE REASONS AGAIN. JUST KEEP REPEATING THEM OVER AND OVER AGAIN.
YOU DON'T NEED TO BE A PILLAR FOR ANYONE ELSE.
OW! YOU'RE DIGGING YOUR NAILS INTO MY HAND!
One ear was listening to the doctor. The other ear was listening to my sister. The steady drone of their voices was the only thing that got me through.

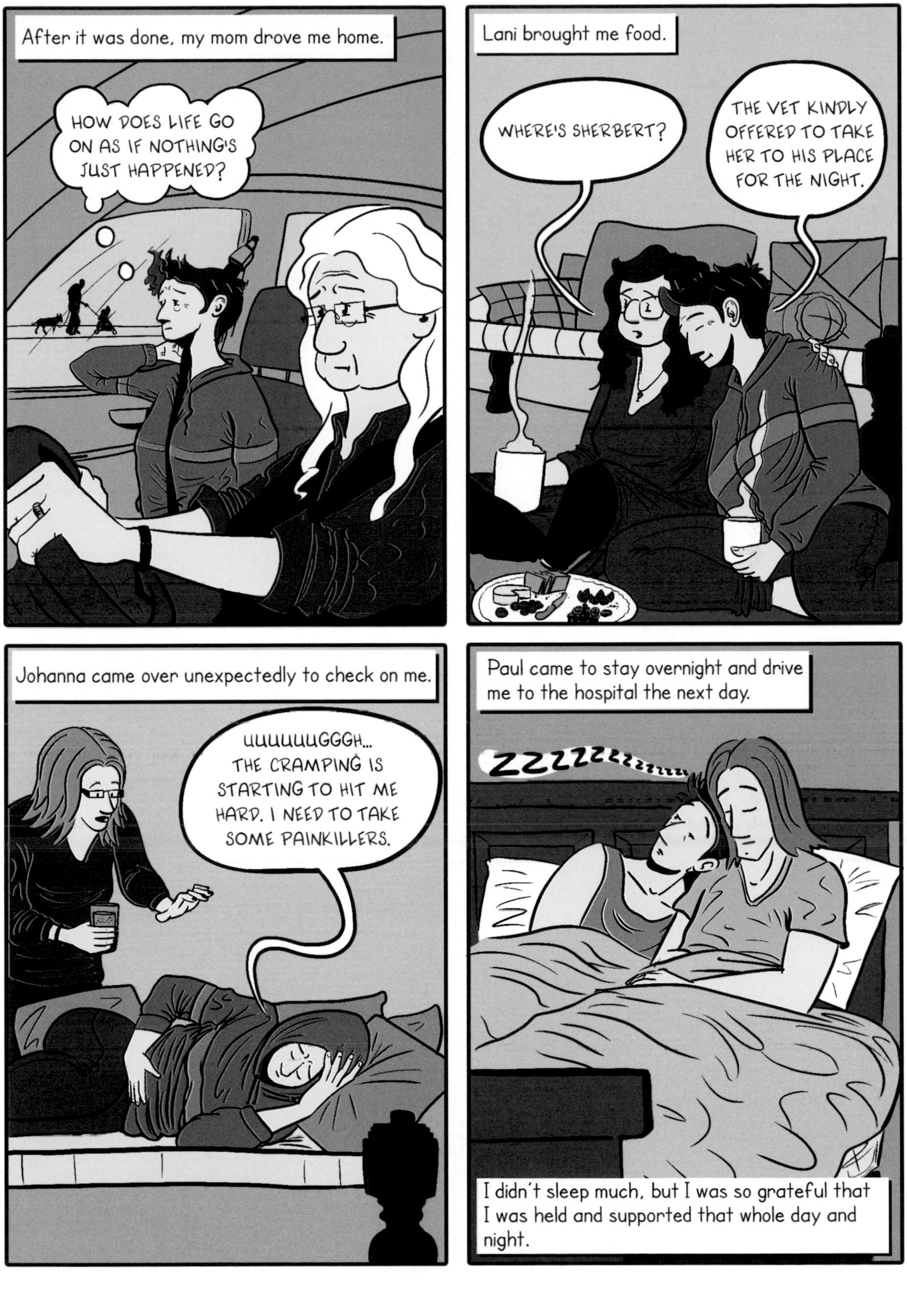
After it was done, my mom drove me home.
HOW DOES LIFE GO ON AS IF NOTHING'S JUST HAPPENED?
Lani brought me food.
WHERE'S SHERBERT?
THE VET KINDLY OFFERED TO TAKE HER TO HIS PLACE FOR THE NIGHT.
Johanna came over unexpectedly to check on me.
UUUUUUGGGH... THE CRAMPING IS STARTING TO HIT ME HARD. I NEED TO TAKE SOME PAINKILLERS.
Paul came to stay overnight and drive me to the hospital the next day.
ZZZZZzzzzzz
I didn't sleep much, but I was so grateful that I was held and supported that whole day and night.

At the hospital, Paul and my midwife did a good job of distracting me. Perhaps too good a job.

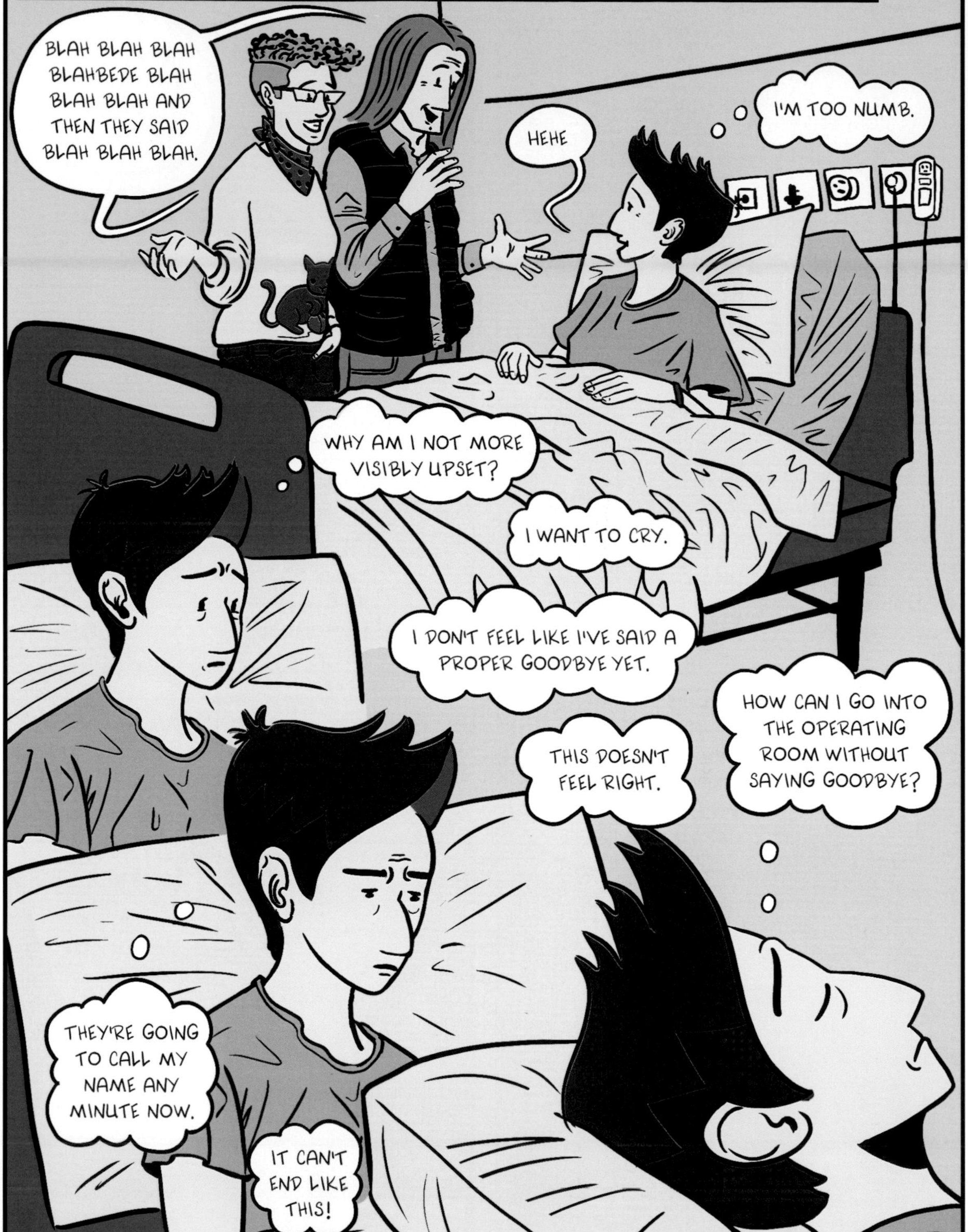
BLAH BLAH BLAH BLAHBEDE BLAH BLAH BLAH AND THEN THEY SAID BLAH BLAH BLAH.
HEHE
I'M TOO NUMB.
WHY AM I NOT MORE VISIBLY UPSET?
I WANT TO CRY.
I DON'T FEEL LIKE I'VE SAID A PROPER GOODBYE YET.
HOW CAN I GO INTO THE OPERATING ROOM WITHOUT SAYING GOODBYE?
THIS DOESN'T FEEL RIGHT.
THEY'RE GOING TO CALL MY NAME ANY MINUTE NOW.
IT CAN'T END LIKE THIS!

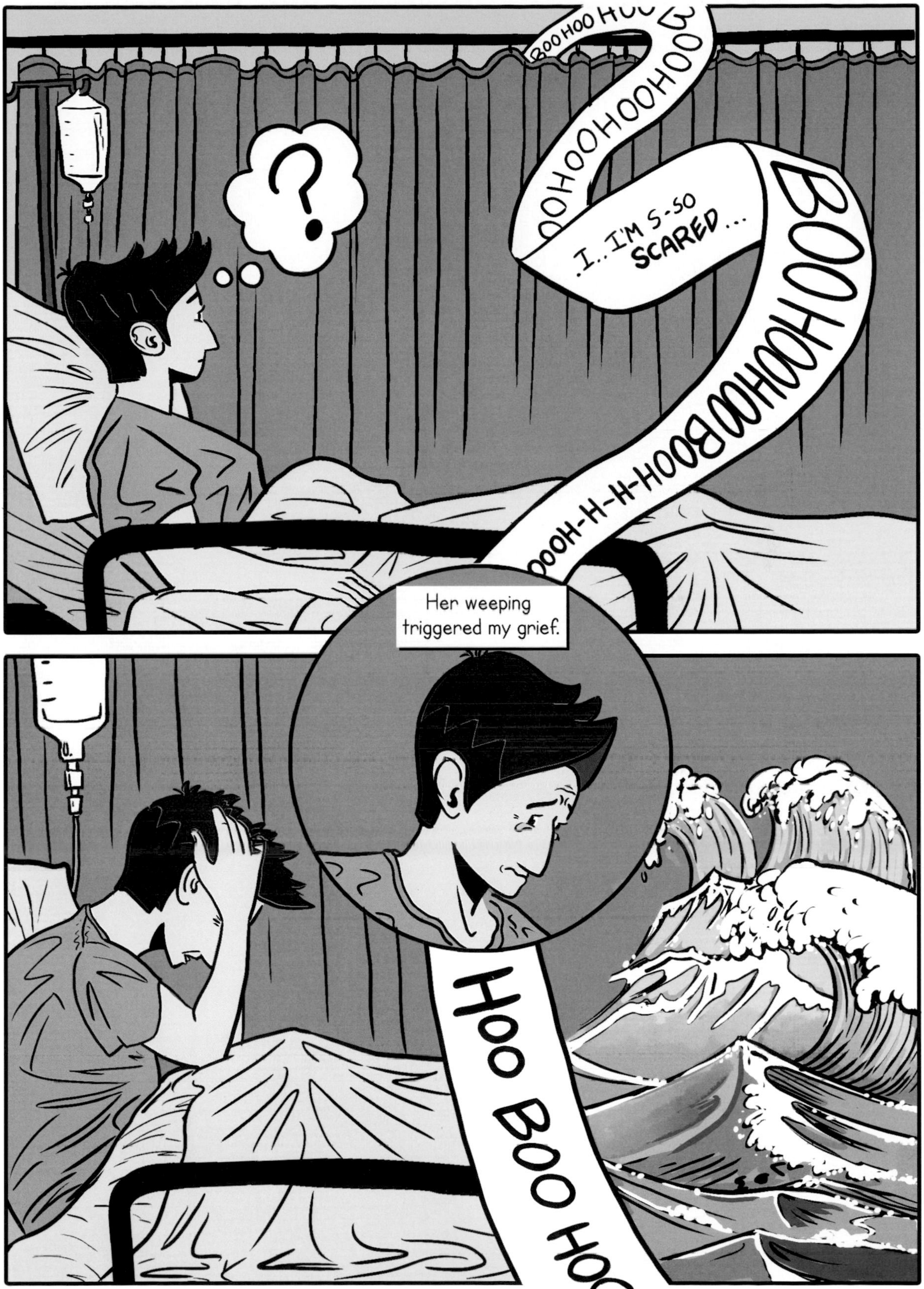
?
BOO HOO HOO
BOOHOOHOOHOO
..I..I'M S-SO SCARED...
BOOHOOHOOBOOH-H-HOOOO
Her weeping triggered my grief.
HOO BOO HOO

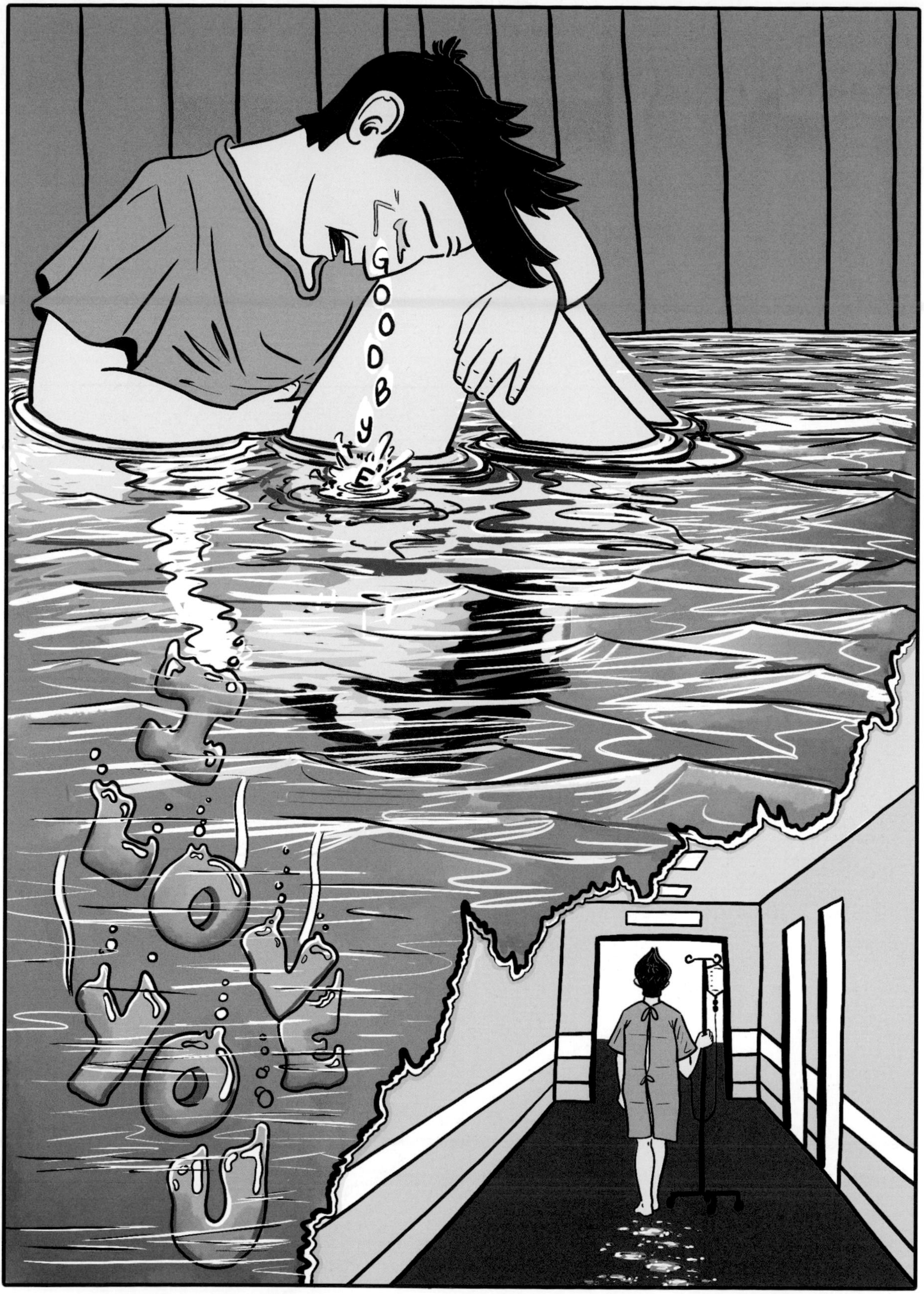
GOODBYE

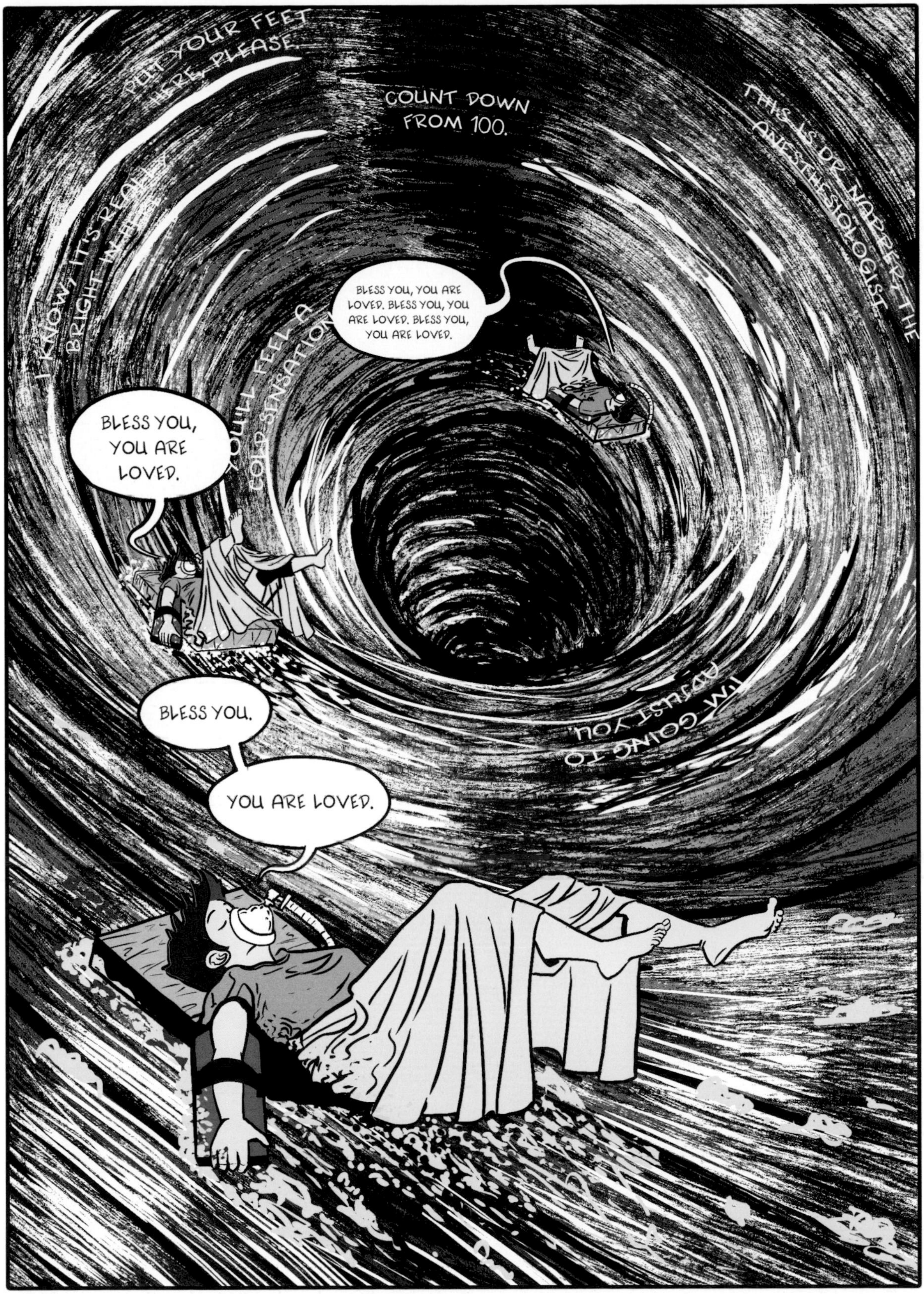
PUT YOUR FEET HERE, PLEASE.
COUNT DOWN FROM 100.
THIS IS DR. NAPPER, THE ANESTHESIOLOGIST.
I KNOW, IT'S REALLY BRIGHT IN
YOU'LL FEEL A COLD SENSATION.
BLESS YOU, YOU ARE LOVED. BLESS YOU, YOU ARE LOVED. BLESS YOU, YOU ARE LOVED.
BLESS YOU, YOU ARE LOVED.
I'M GOING TO ADJUST YOU.
BLESS YOU.
YOU ARE LOVED.

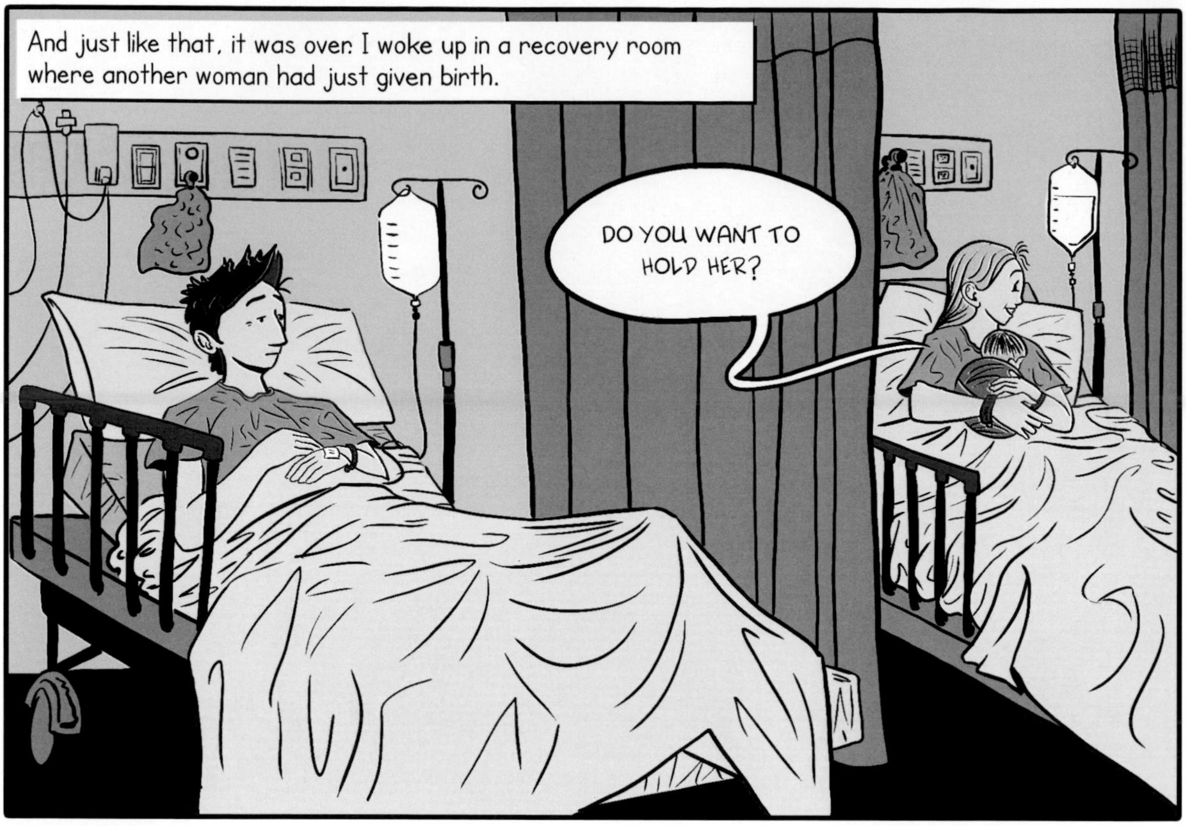
And just like that, it was over. I woke up in a recovery room where another woman had just given birth.
DO YOU WANT TO HOLD HER?

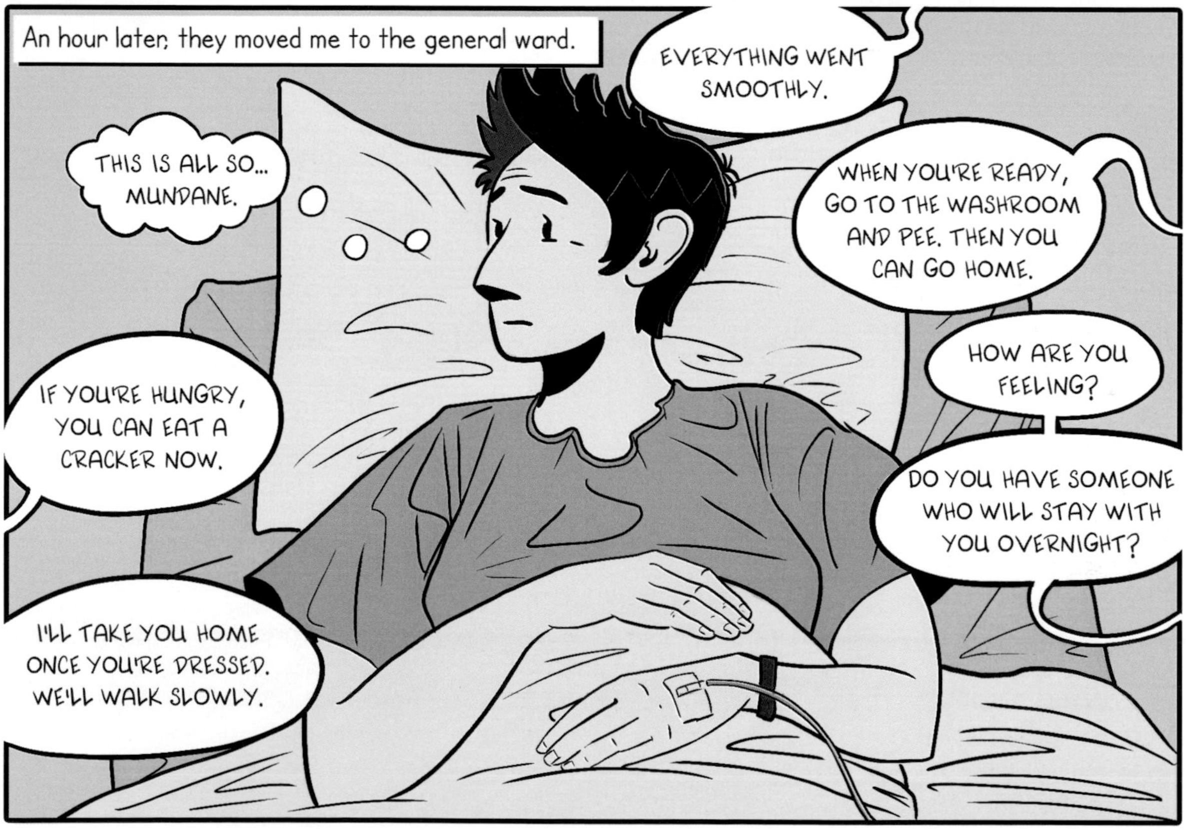
An hour later, they moved me to the general ward.
EVERYTHING WENT SMOOTHLY.
THIS IS ALL SO... MUNDANE.
WHEN YOU'RE READY, GO TO THE WASHROOM AND PEE. THEN YOU CAN GO HOME.
IF YOU'RE HUNGRY, YOU CAN EAT A CRACKER NOW.
HOW ARE YOU FEELING?
DO YOU HAVE SOMEONE WHO WILL STAY WITH YOU OVERNIGHT?
I'LL TAKE YOU HOME ONCE YOU'RE DRESSED. WE'LL WALK SLOWLY.

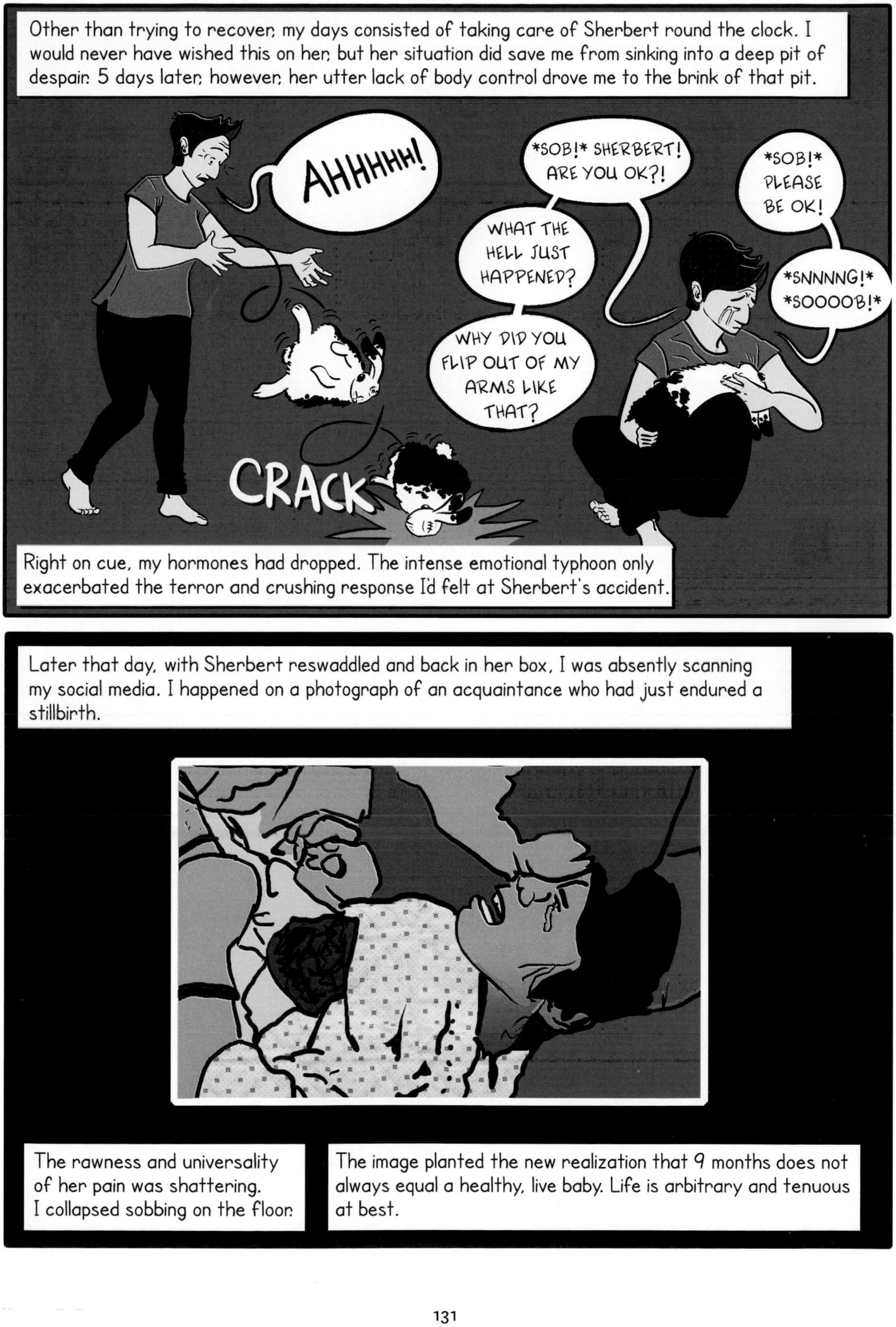
Other than trying to recover, my days consisted of taking care of Sherbert round the clock. I would never have wished this on her, but her situation did save me from sinking into a deep pit of despair. 5 days later, however, her utter lack of body control drove me to the brink of that pit.
AHHHHH!
CRACK
WHAT THE HELL JUST HAPPENED?
WHY DID YOU FLIP OUT OF MY ARMS LIKE THAT?
SOB! SHERBERT! ARE YOU OK?!
SOB! PLEASE BE OK!
SNNNNG! *SOOOOB!*
Right on cue, my hormones had dropped. The intense emotional typhoon only exacerbated the terror and crushing response I'd felt at Sherbert's accident.
Later that day, with Sherbert reswaddled and back in her box, I was absently scanning my social media. I happened on a photograph of an acquaintance who had just endured a stillbirth.
The rawness and universality of her pain was shattering. I collapsed sobbing on the floor.
The image planted the new realization that 9 months does not always equal a healthy, live baby. Life is arbitrary and tenuous at best.

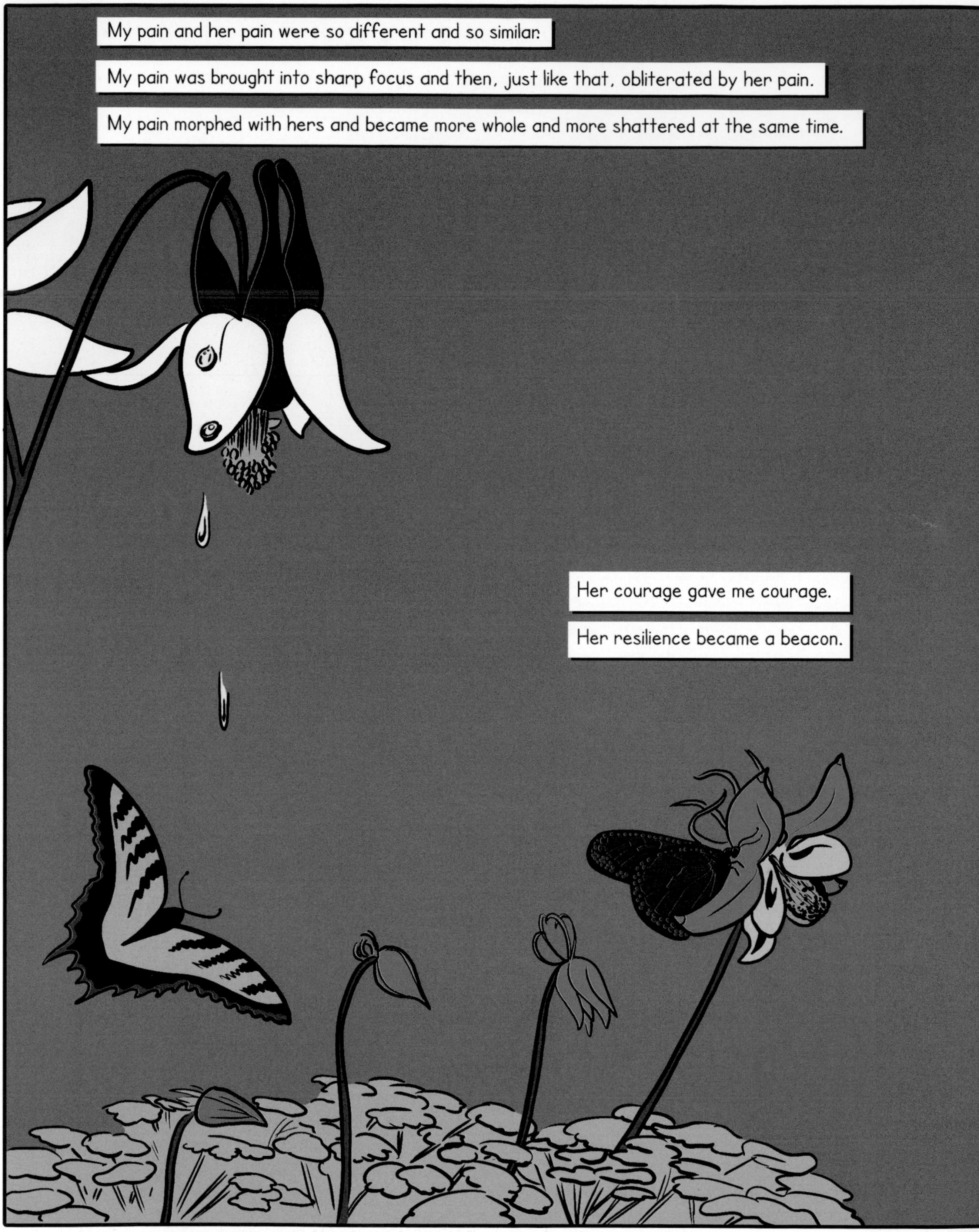
My pain and her pain were so different and so similar.
My pain was brought into sharp focus and then, just like that, obliterated by her pain.
My pain morphed with hers and became more whole and more shattered at the same time.
Her courage gave me courage.
Her resilience became a beacon.

Perhaps all the dragons of our lives are princesses who are only waiting to see us once beautiful and brave. Perhaps everything terrible is in its deepest being something helpless that wants help from us.

So you must not be frightened if a sadness rises up before you larger than any you have ever seen; if a restiveness, like light and cloud shadows, passes over your hands and over all you do. You must think that something is happening with you, that life has not forgotten you, that it holds you in its hand; it will not let you fall. Why do you want to shut out of your life any uneasiness, any miseries, or any depressions? For after all, you do not know what work these conditions are doing inside you.

ˣ-Rainer Maria Rilke

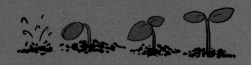

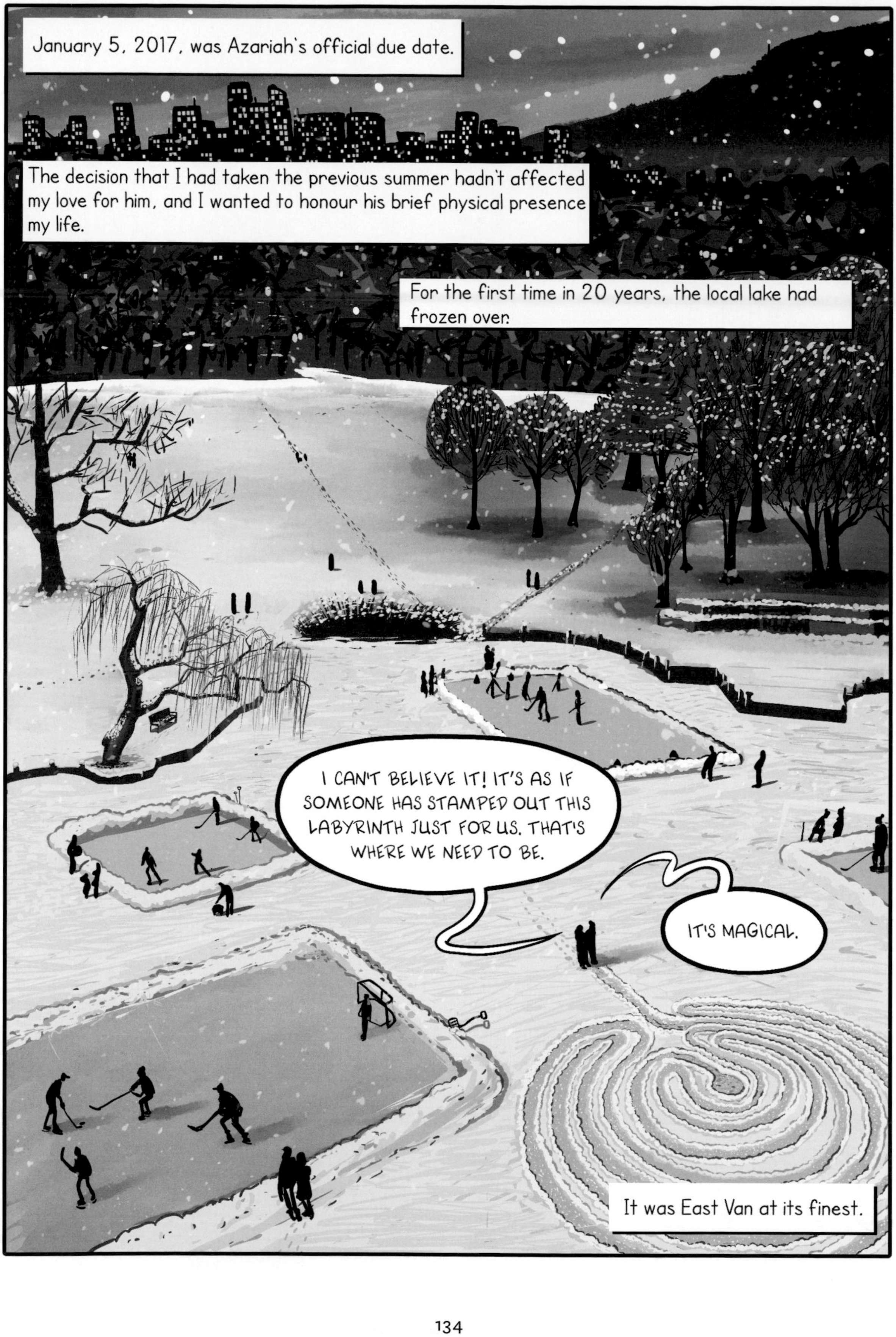
January 5, 2017, was Azariah's official due date.
The decision that I had taken the previous summer hadn't affected my love for him, and I wanted to honour his brief physical presence my life.
For the first time in 20 years, the local lake had frozen over.
I CAN'T BELIEVE IT! IT'S AS IF SOMEONE HAS STAMPED OUT THIS LABYRINTH JUST FOR US. THAT'S WHERE WE NEED TO BE.
IT'S MAGICAL.
It was East Van at its finest.

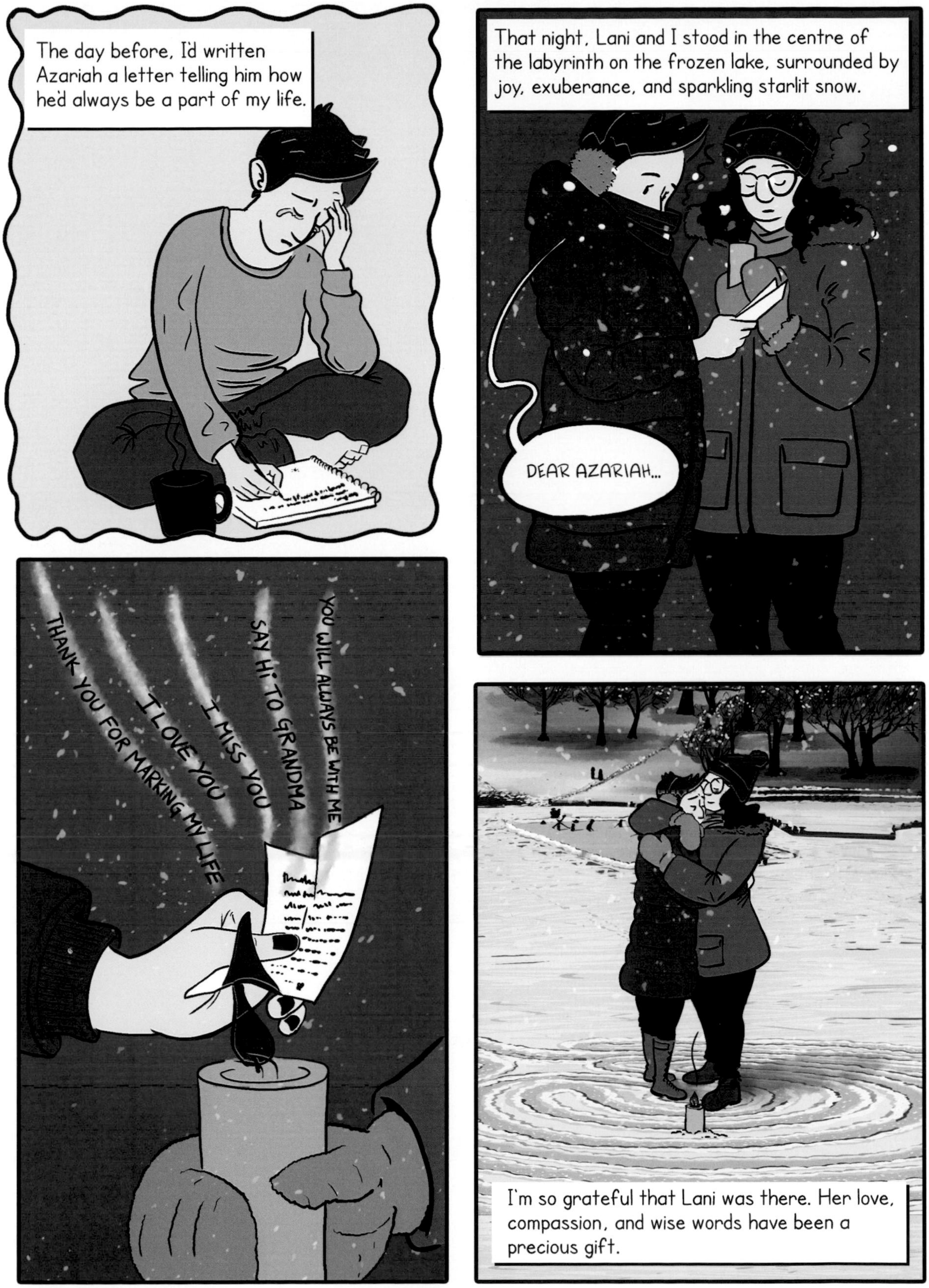

The day before, I'd written Azariah a letter telling him how he'd always be a part of my life.
That night, Lani and I stood in the centre of the labyrinth on the frozen lake, surrounded by joy, exuberance, and sparkling starlit snow.
DEAR AZARIAH...
THANK YOU FOR MARKING MY LIFE
I LOVE YOU
I MISS YOU
SAY HI TO GRANDMA
YOU WILL ALWAYS BE WITH ME
I'm so grateful that Lani was there. Her love, compassion, and wise words have been a precious gift.

YEAR THREE

AUGUST 2016–DECEMBER 2017

Test-Tube Baby

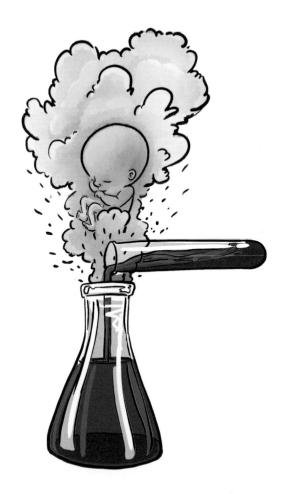

Chapter 4

The Little Eggs That Couldn't

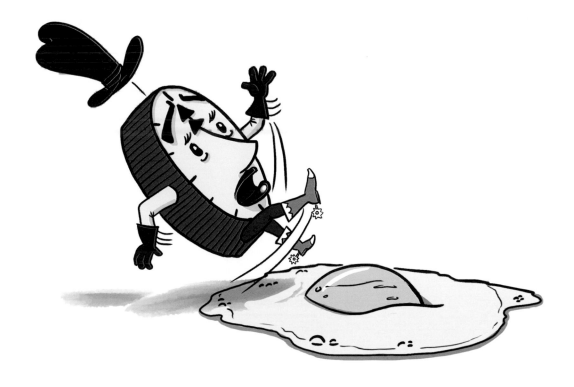

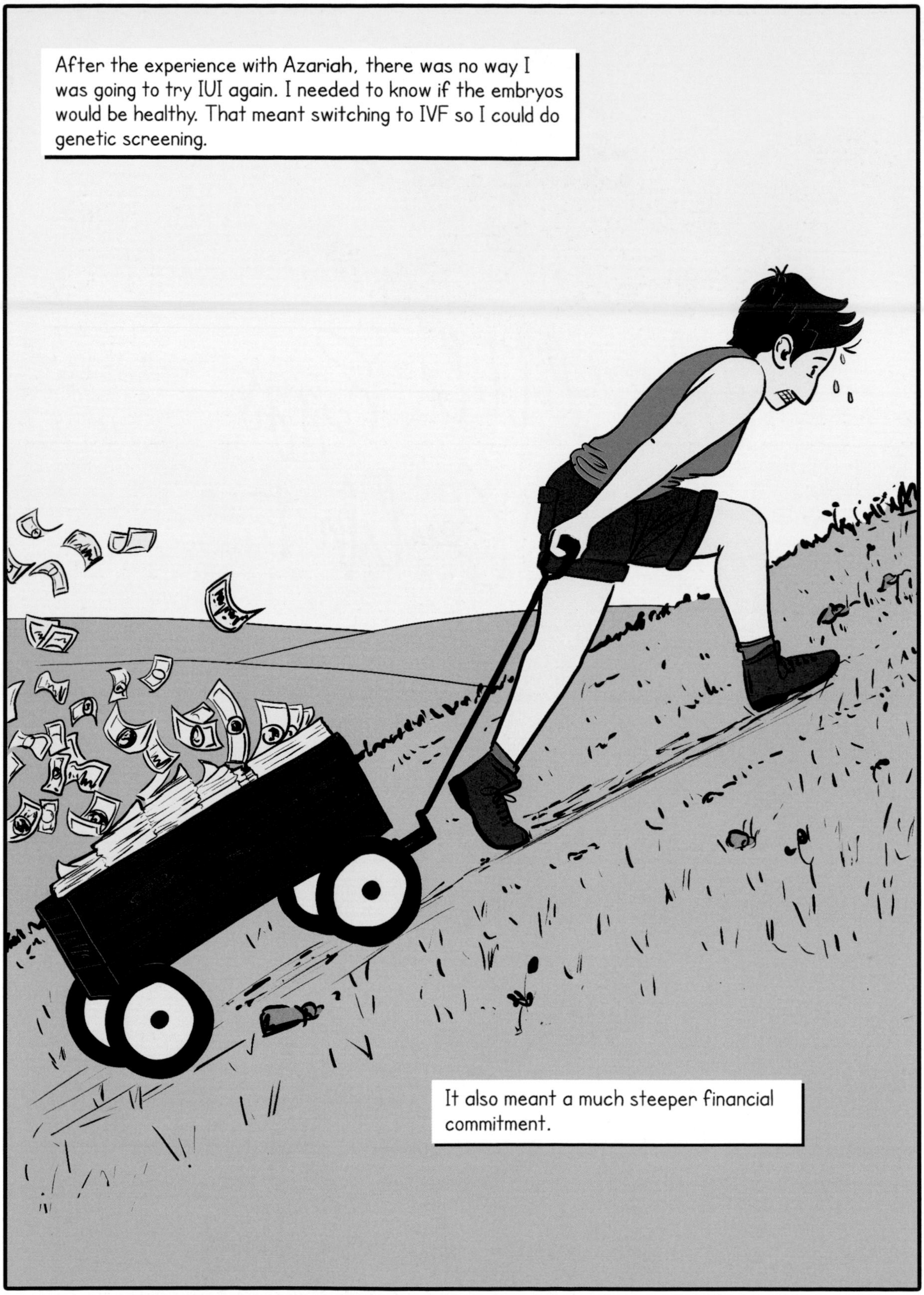
After the experience with Azariah, there was no way I was going to try IUI again. I needed to know if the embryos would be healthy. That meant switching to IVF so I could do genetic screening.
It also meant a much steeper financial commitment.

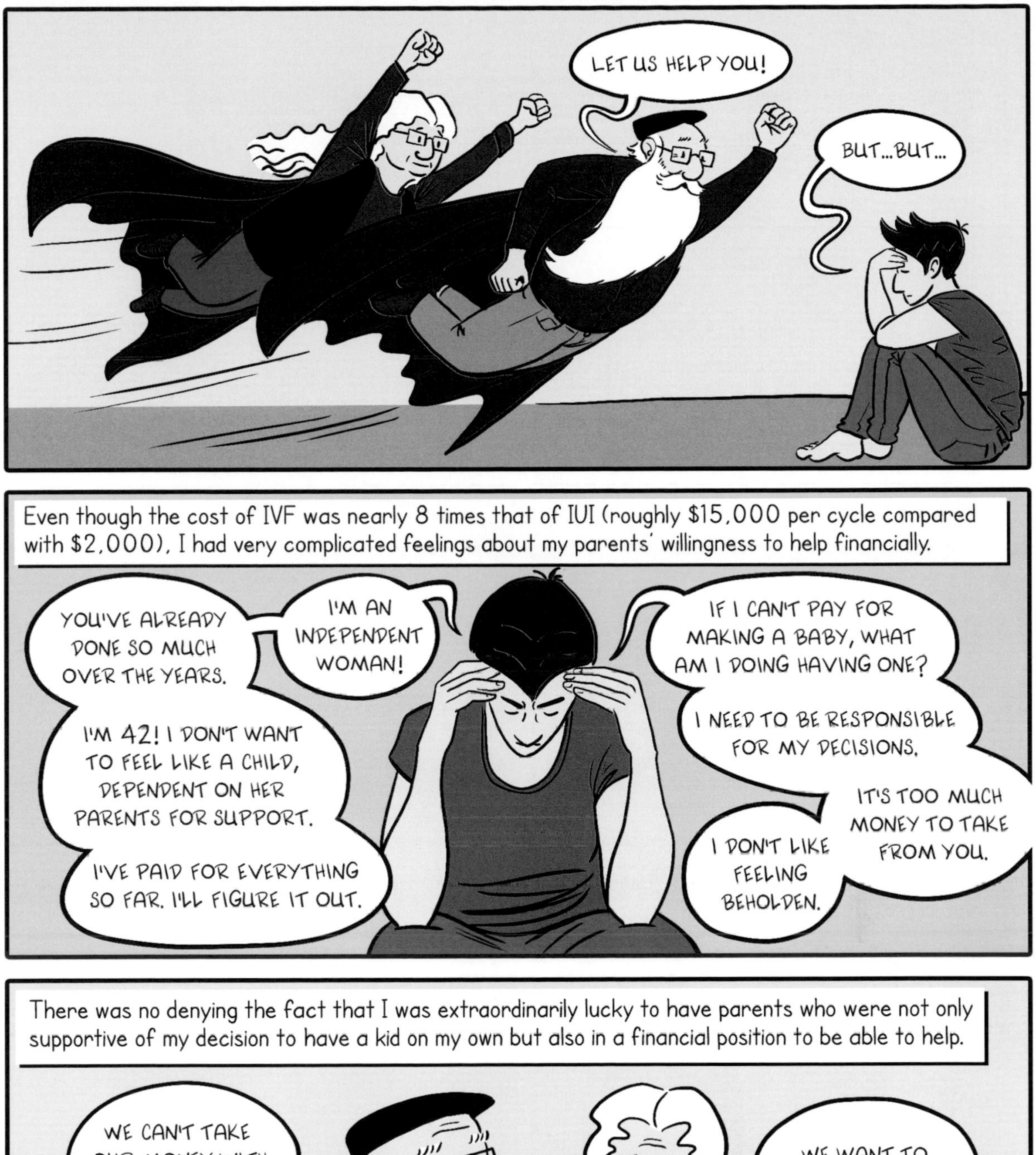
LET US HELP YOU!
BUT...BUT...
Even though the cost of IVF was nearly 8 times that of IUI (roughly $15,000 per cycle compared with $2,000), I had very complicated feelings about my parents' willingness to help financially.
YOU'VE ALREADY DONE SO MUCH OVER THE YEARS.
I'M AN INDEPENDENT WOMAN!
I'M 42! I DON'T WANT TO FEEL LIKE A CHILD, DEPENDENT ON HER PARENTS FOR SUPPORT.
I'VE PAID FOR EVERYTHING SO FAR. I'LL FIGURE IT OUT.
IF I CAN'T PAY FOR MAKING A BABY, WHAT AM I DOING HAVING ONE?
I NEED TO BE RESPONSIBLE FOR MY DECISIONS.
IT'S TOO MUCH MONEY TO TAKE FROM YOU.
I DON'T LIKE FEELING BEHOLDEN.
There was no denying the fact that I was extraordinarily lucky to have parents who were not only supportive of my decision to have a kid on my own but also in a financial position to be able to help.
WE CAN'T TAKE OUR MONEY WITH US WHEN WE DIE.
PLUS, WE WANT GRANDKIDS!
WE WANT TO DO THIS FOR YOU.

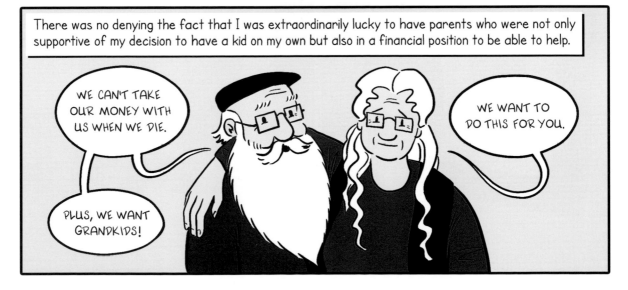

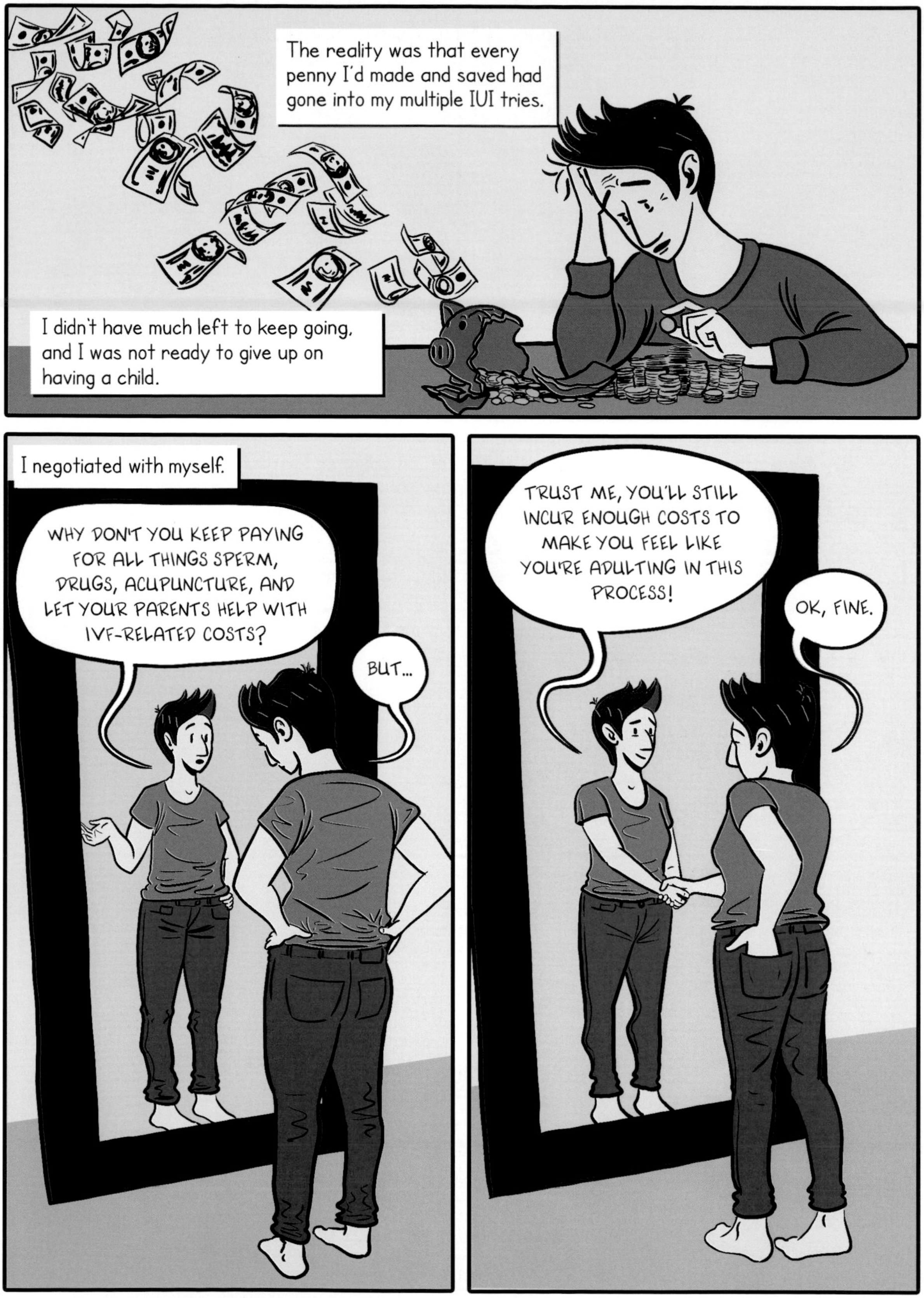
The reality was that every penny I'd made and saved had gone into my multiple IUI tries.
I didn't have much left to keep going, and I was not ready to give up on having a child.
I negotiated with myself.
WHY DON'T YOU KEEP PAYING FOR ALL THINGS SPERM, DRUGS, ACUPUNCTURE, AND LET YOUR PARENTS HELP WITH IVF-RELATED COSTS?
BUT...
TRUST ME, YOU'LL STILL INCUR ENOUGH COSTS TO MAKE YOU FEEL LIKE YOU'RE ADULTING IN THIS PROCESS!
OK, FINE.

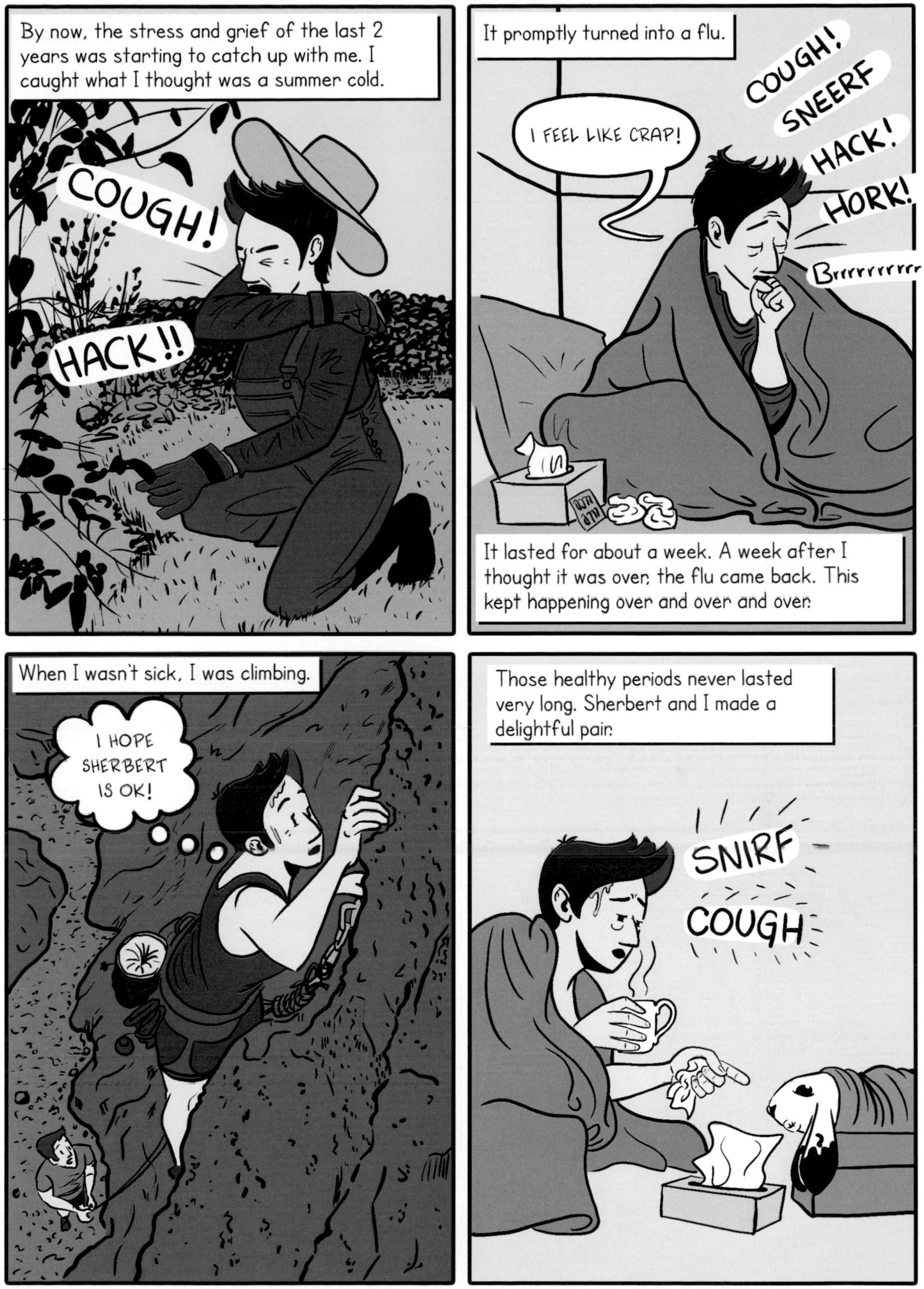
By now, the stress and grief of the last 2 years was starting to catch up with me. I caught what I thought was a summer cold.
COUGH!
HACK!!
It promptly turned into a flu.
I FEEL LIKE CRAP!
COUGH!
SNEERF
HACK!
HORK!
Brrrrrrrrr
It lasted for about a week. A week after I thought it was over, the flu came back. This kept happening over and over and over.
When I wasn't sick, I was climbing.
I HOPE SHERBERT IS OK!
Those healthy periods never lasted very long. Sherbert and I made a delightful pair.
SNIRF
COUGH

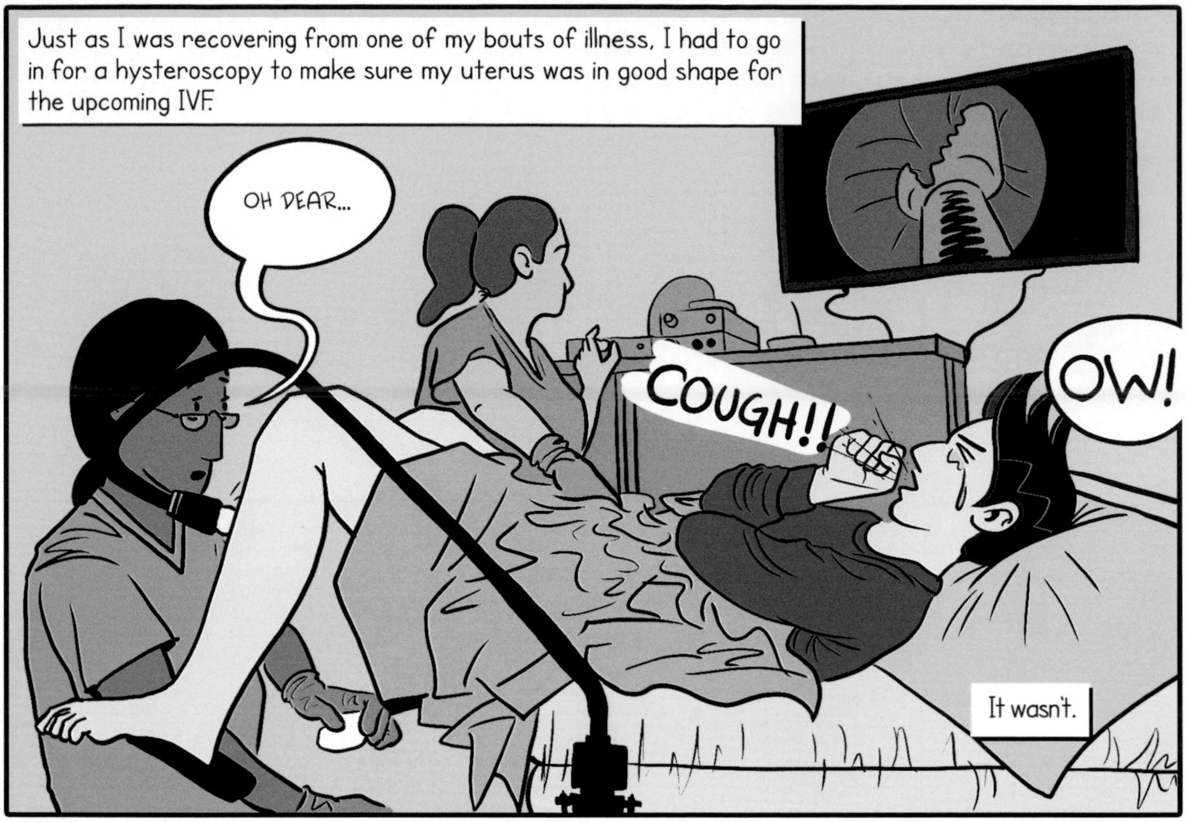
Just as I was recovering from one of my bouts of illness, I had to go in for a hysteroscopy to make sure my uterus was in good shape for the upcoming IVF.
OH DEAR...
COUGH!!
OW!
It wasn't.

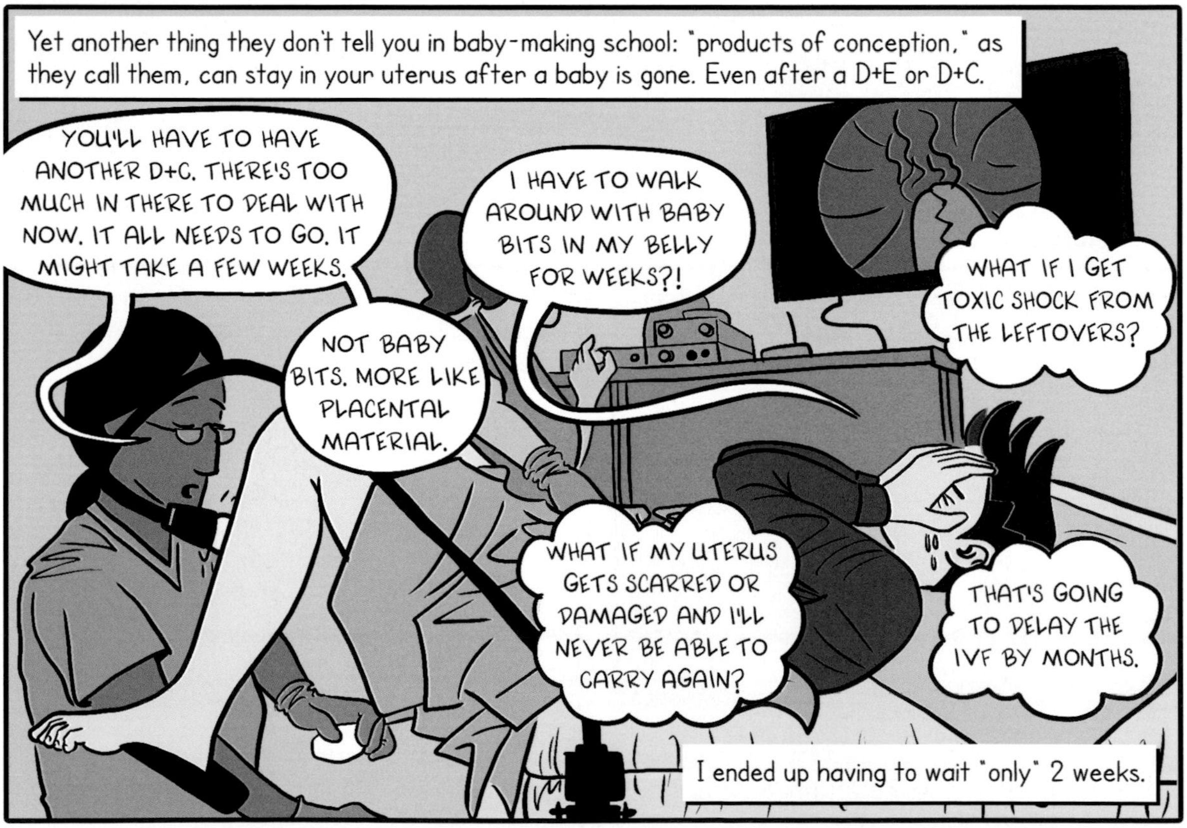
Yet another thing they don't tell you in baby-making school: "products of conception," as they call them, can stay in your uterus after a baby is gone. Even after a D+E or D+C.
YOU'LL HAVE TO HAVE ANOTHER D+C. THERE'S TOO MUCH IN THERE TO DEAL WITH NOW. IT ALL NEEDS TO GO. IT MIGHT TAKE A FEW WEEKS.
I HAVE TO WALK AROUND WITH BABY BITS IN MY BELLY FOR WEEKS?!
NOT BABY BITS. MORE LIKE PLACENTAL MATERIAL.
WHAT IF I GET TOXIC SHOCK FROM THE LEFTOVERS?
WHAT IF MY UTERUS GETS SCARRED OR DAMAGED AND I'LL NEVER BE ABLE TO CARRY AGAIN?
THAT'S GOING TO DELAY THE IVF BY MONTHS.
I ended up having to wait "only" 2 weeks.

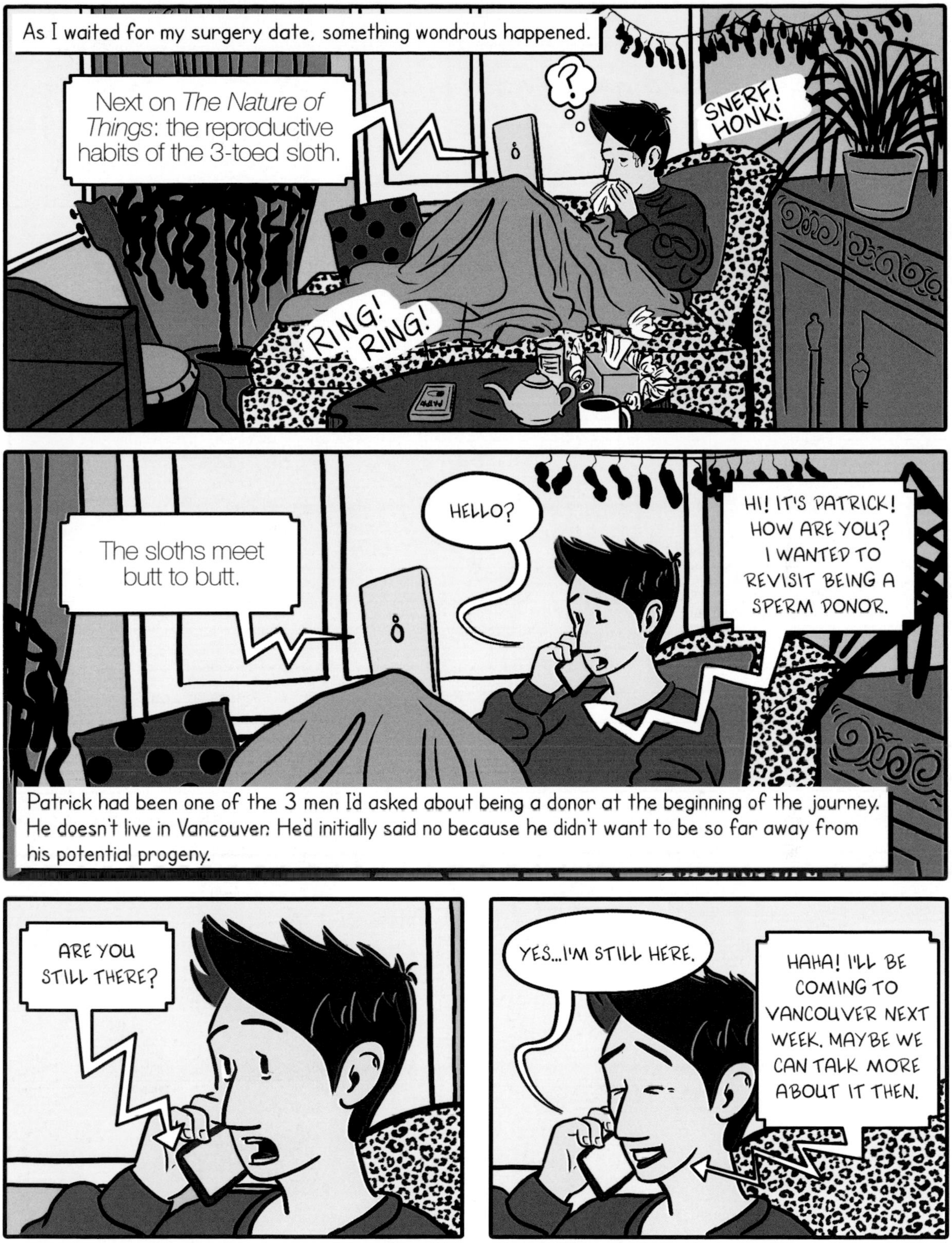
As I waited for my surgery date, something wondrous happened.
Next on *The Nature of Things*: the reproductive habits of the 3-toed sloth.
?
SNERF! HONK!
RING! RING!
HELLO?
The sloths meet butt to butt.
HI! IT'S PATRICK! HOW ARE YOU? I WANTED TO REVISIT BEING A SPERM DONOR.
Patrick had been one of the 3 men I'd asked about being a donor at the beginning of the journey. He doesn't live in Vancouver. He'd initially said no because he didn't want to be so far away from his potential progeny.
ARE YOU STILL THERE?
YES...I'M STILL HERE.
HAHA! I'LL BE COMING TO VANCOUVER NEXT WEEK. MAYBE WE CAN TALK MORE ABOUT IT THEN.

The phone call happened to coincide with my running out of anonymous donor sperm. I had been debating whether to buy more of the same or to choose a new donor. Patrick had been high on my list of known donors, so this presented an intriguing possibility.

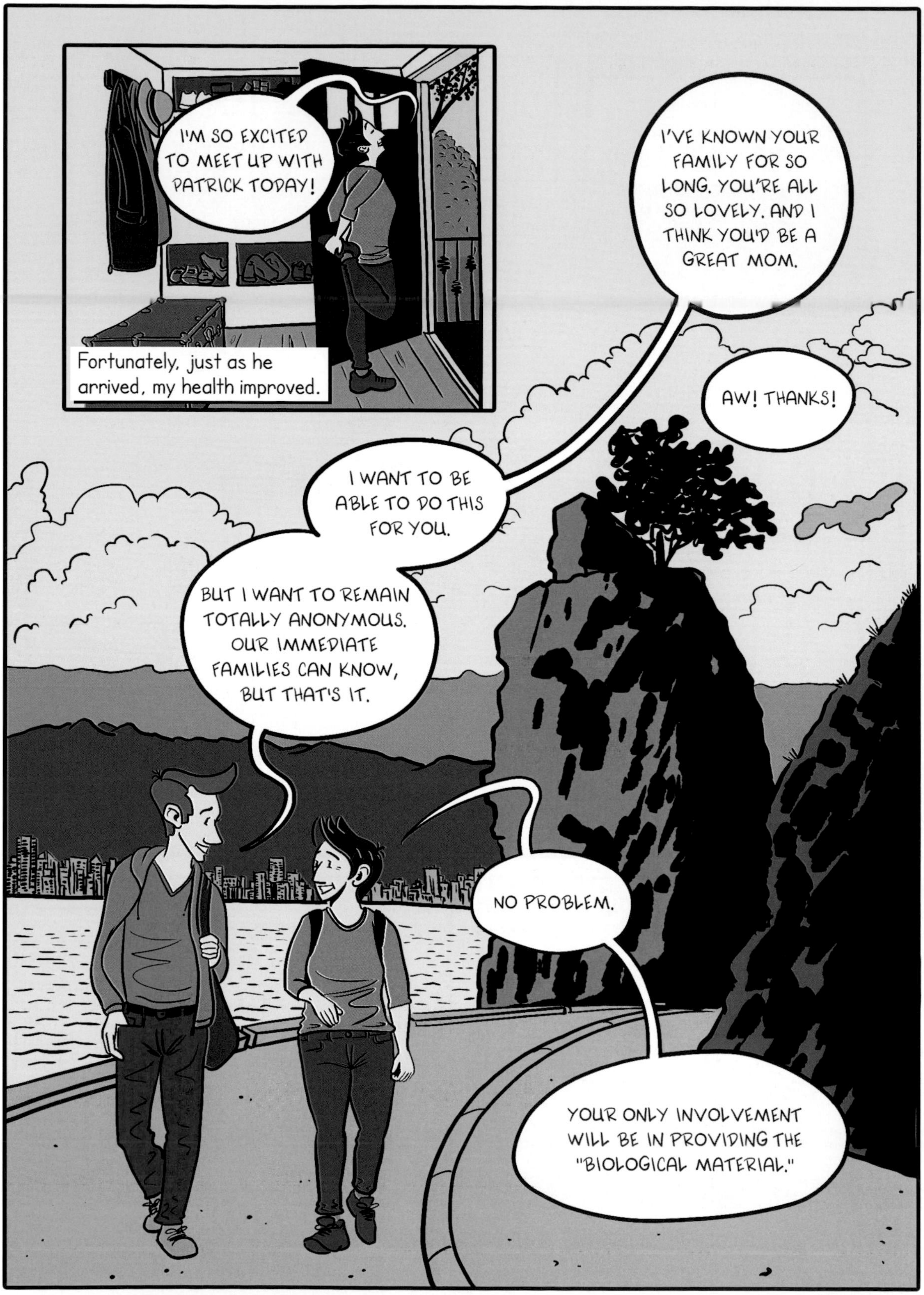
I'M SO EXCITED TO MEET UP WITH PATRICK TODAY!
Fortunately, just as he arrived, my health improved.
I'VE KNOWN YOUR FAMILY FOR SO LONG. YOU'RE ALL SO LOVELY. AND I THINK YOU'D BE A GREAT MOM.
AW! THANKS!
I WANT TO BE ABLE TO DO THIS FOR YOU.
BUT I WANT TO REMAIN TOTALLY ANONYMOUS. OUR IMMEDIATE FAMILIES CAN KNOW, BUT THAT'S IT.
NO PROBLEM.
YOUR ONLY INVOLVEMENT WILL BE IN PROVIDING THE "BIOLOGICAL MATERIAL."

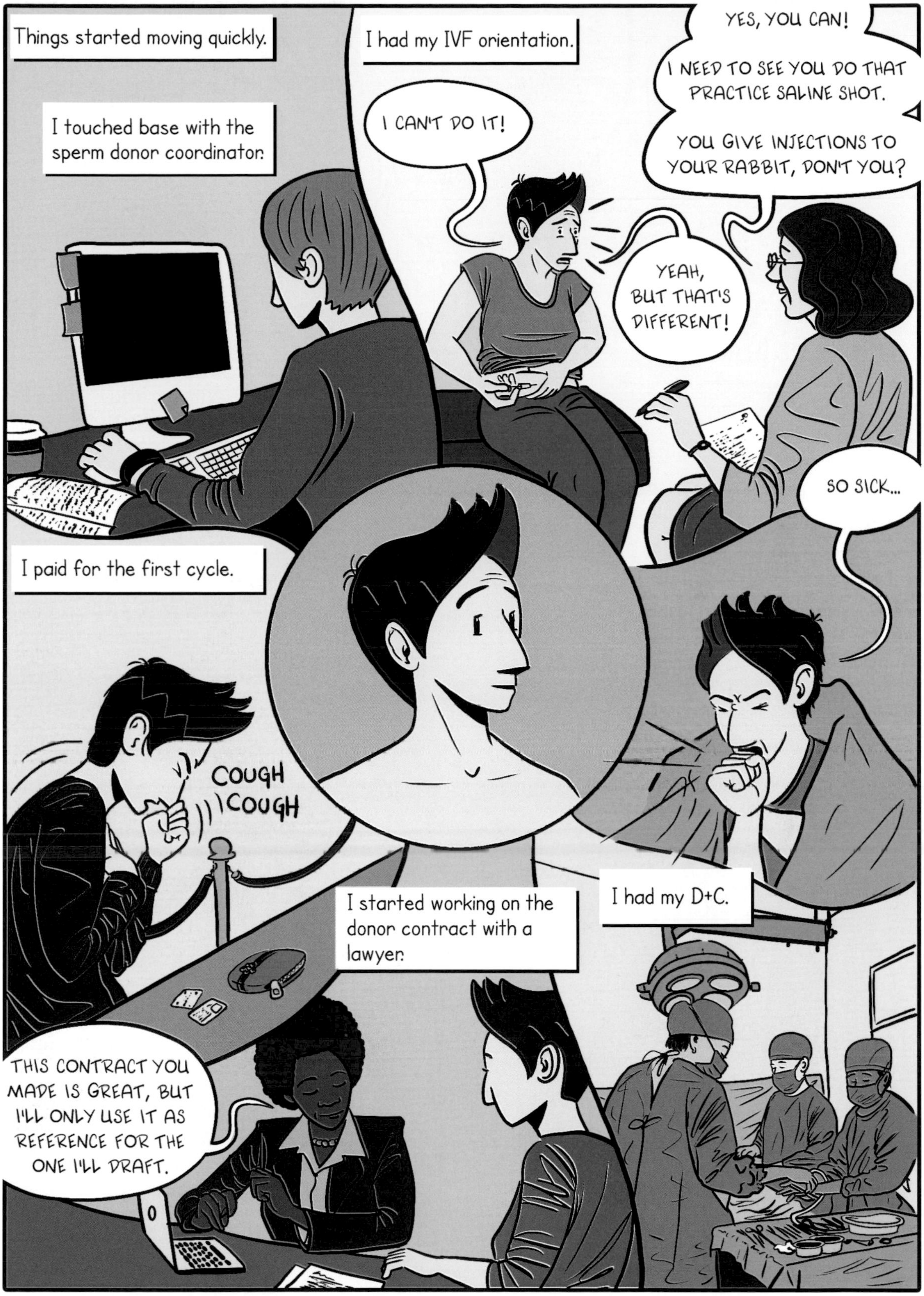

Things started moving quickly.
I touched base with the sperm donor coordinator.
I had my IVF orientation.
I CAN'T DO IT!
YES, YOU CAN!
I NEED TO SEE YOU DO THAT PRACTICE SALINE SHOT.
YOU GIVE INJECTIONS TO YOUR RABBIT, DON'T YOU?
YEAH, BUT THAT'S DIFFERENT!
I paid for the first cycle.
COUGH COUGH
SO SICK...
I started working on the donor contract with a lawyer.
THIS CONTRACT YOU MADE IS GREAT, BUT I'LL ONLY USE IT AS REFERENCE FOR THE ONE I'LL DRAFT.
I had my D+C.

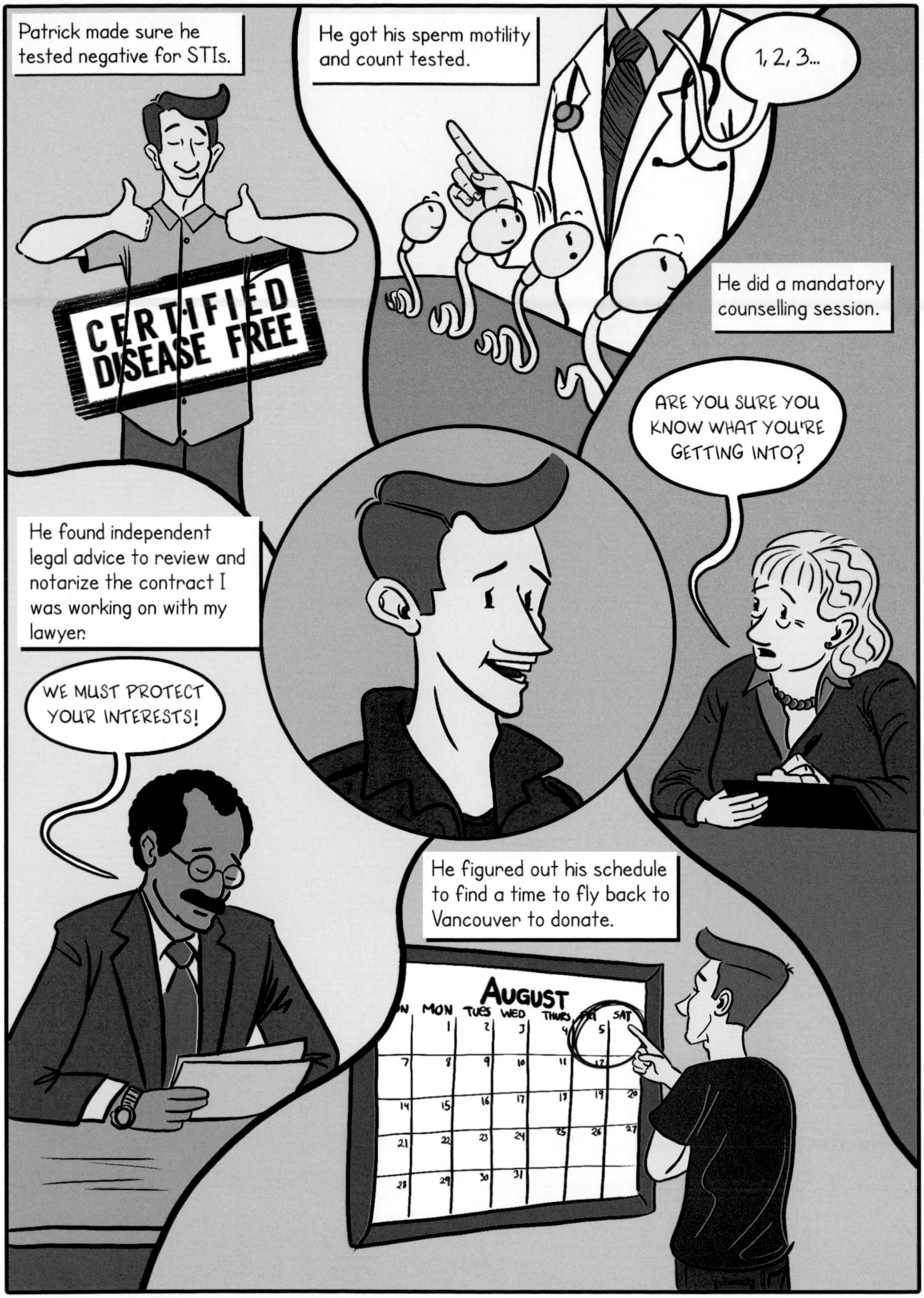
Patrick made sure he tested negative for STIs.
CERTIFIED DISEASE FREE
He got his sperm motility and count tested.
1, 2, 3...
He did a mandatory counselling session.
ARE YOU SURE YOU KNOW WHAT YOU'RE GETTING INTO?
He found independent legal advice to review and notarize the contract I was working on with my lawyer.
WE MUST PROTECT YOUR INTERESTS!
He figured out his schedule to find a time to fly back to Vancouver to donate.
AUGUST

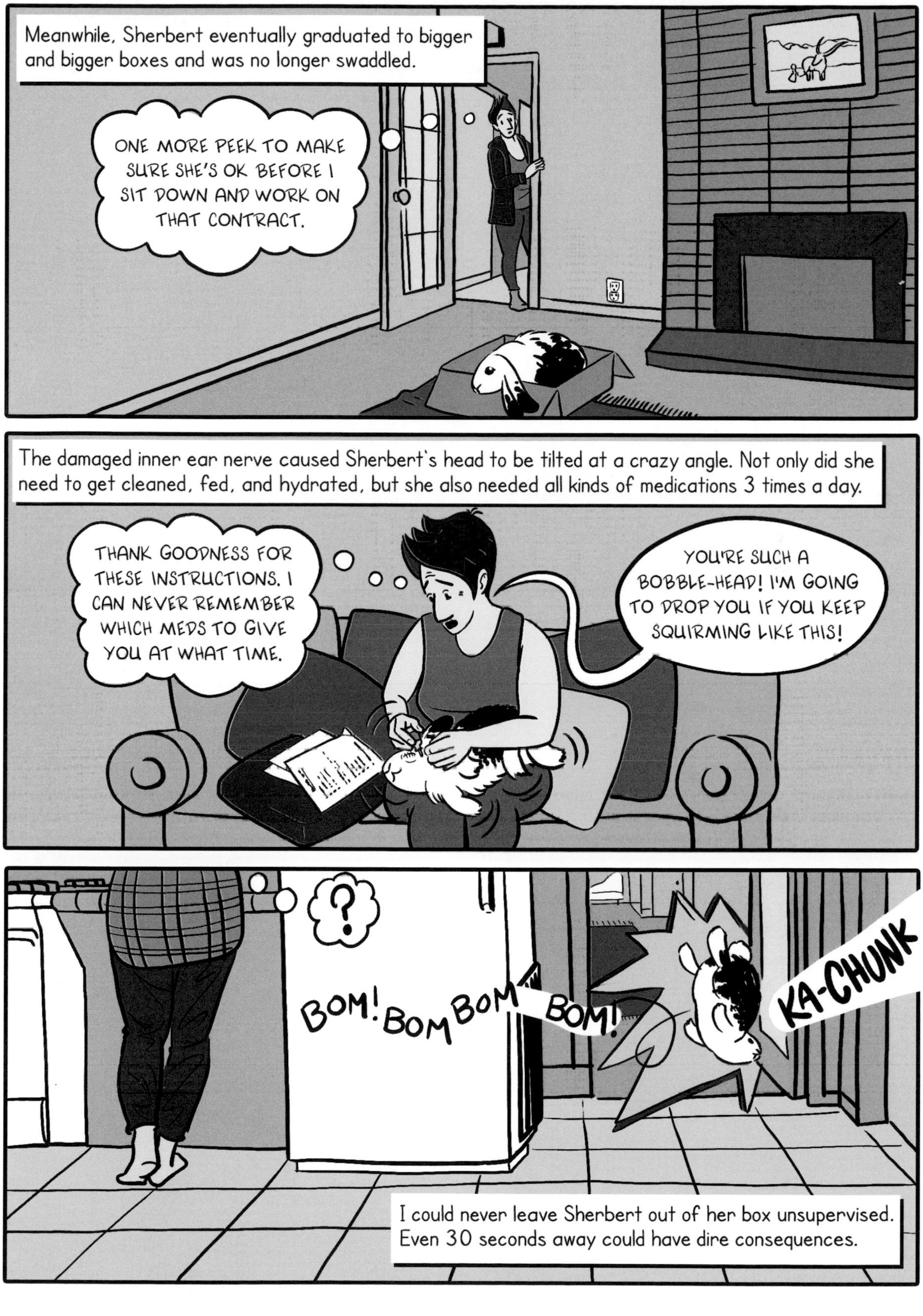

Meanwhile, Sherbert eventually graduated to bigger and bigger boxes and was no longer swaddled.
ONE MORE PEEK TO MAKE SURE SHE'S OK BEFORE I SIT DOWN AND WORK ON THAT CONTRACT.
The damaged inner ear nerve caused Sherbert's head to be tilted at a crazy angle. Not only did she need to get cleaned, fed, and hydrated, but she also needed all kinds of medications 3 times a day.
THANK GOODNESS FOR THESE INSTRUCTIONS. I CAN NEVER REMEMBER WHICH MEDS TO GIVE YOU AT WHAT TIME.
YOU'RE SUCH A BOBBLE-HEAD! I'M GOING TO DROP YOU IF YOU KEEP SQUIRMING LIKE THIS!
?
BOM! BOM BOM BOM!
KA-CHUNK
I could never leave Sherbert out of her box unsupervised. Even 30 seconds away could have dire consequences.

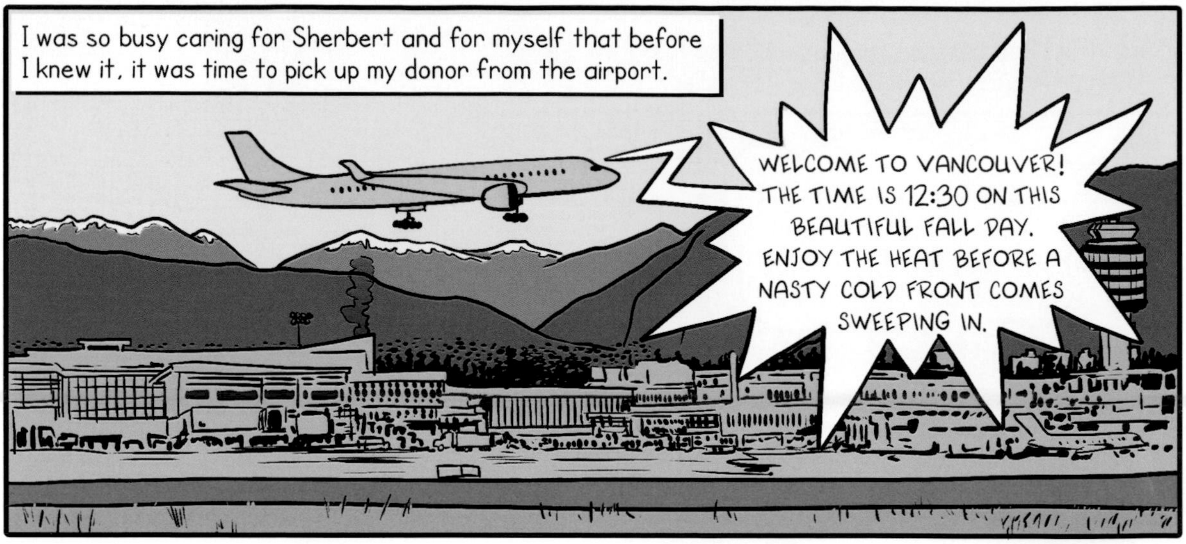
I was so busy caring for Sherbert and for myself that before I knew it, it was time to pick up my donor from the airport.
WELCOME TO VANCOUVER! THE TIME IS 12:30 ON THIS BEAUTIFUL FALL DAY. ENJOY THE HEAT BEFORE A NASTY COLD FRONT COMES SWEEPING IN.

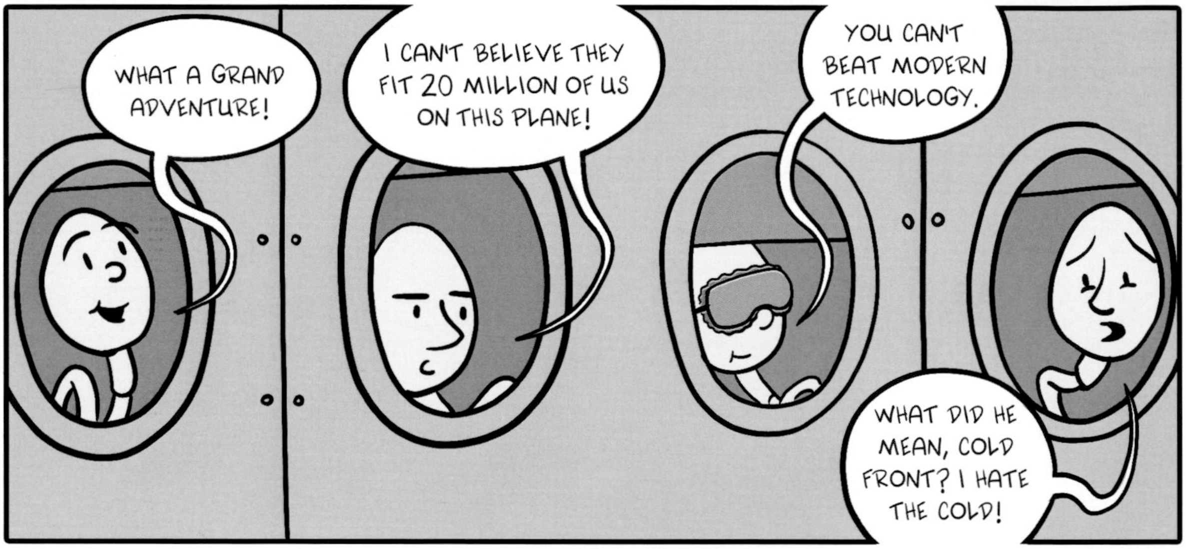
WHAT A GRAND ADVENTURE!
I CAN'T BELIEVE THEY FIT 20 MILLION OF US ON THIS PLANE!
YOU CAN'T BEAT MODERN TECHNOLOGY.
WHAT DID HE MEAN, COLD FRONT? I HATE THE COLD!

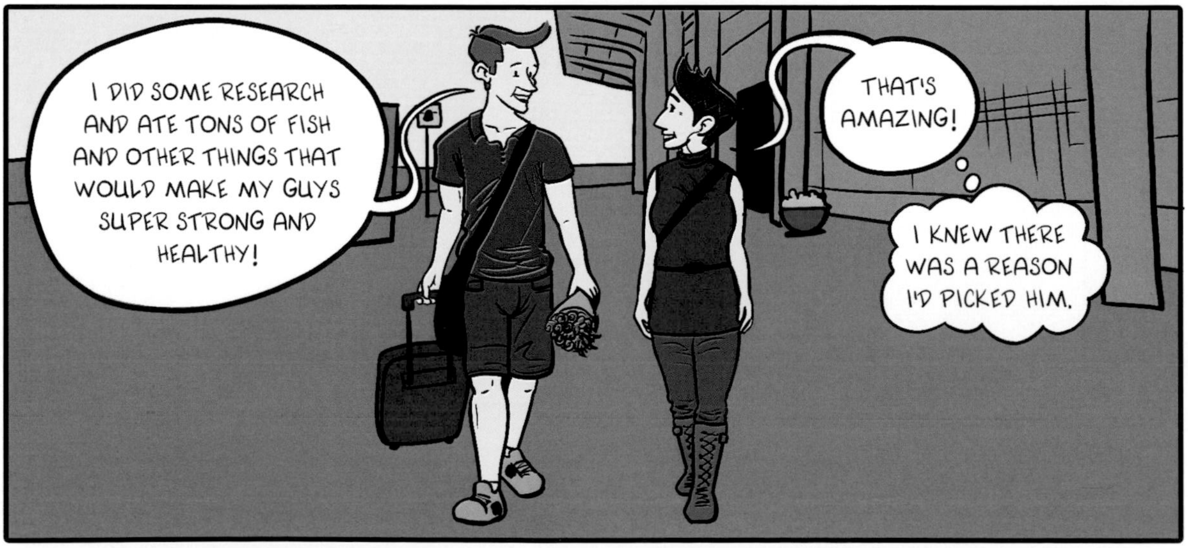
I DID SOME RESEARCH AND ATE TONS OF FISH AND OTHER THINGS THAT WOULD MAKE MY GUYS SUPER STRONG AND HEALTHY!
THAT'S AMAZING!
I KNEW THERE WAS A REASON I'D PICKED HIM.

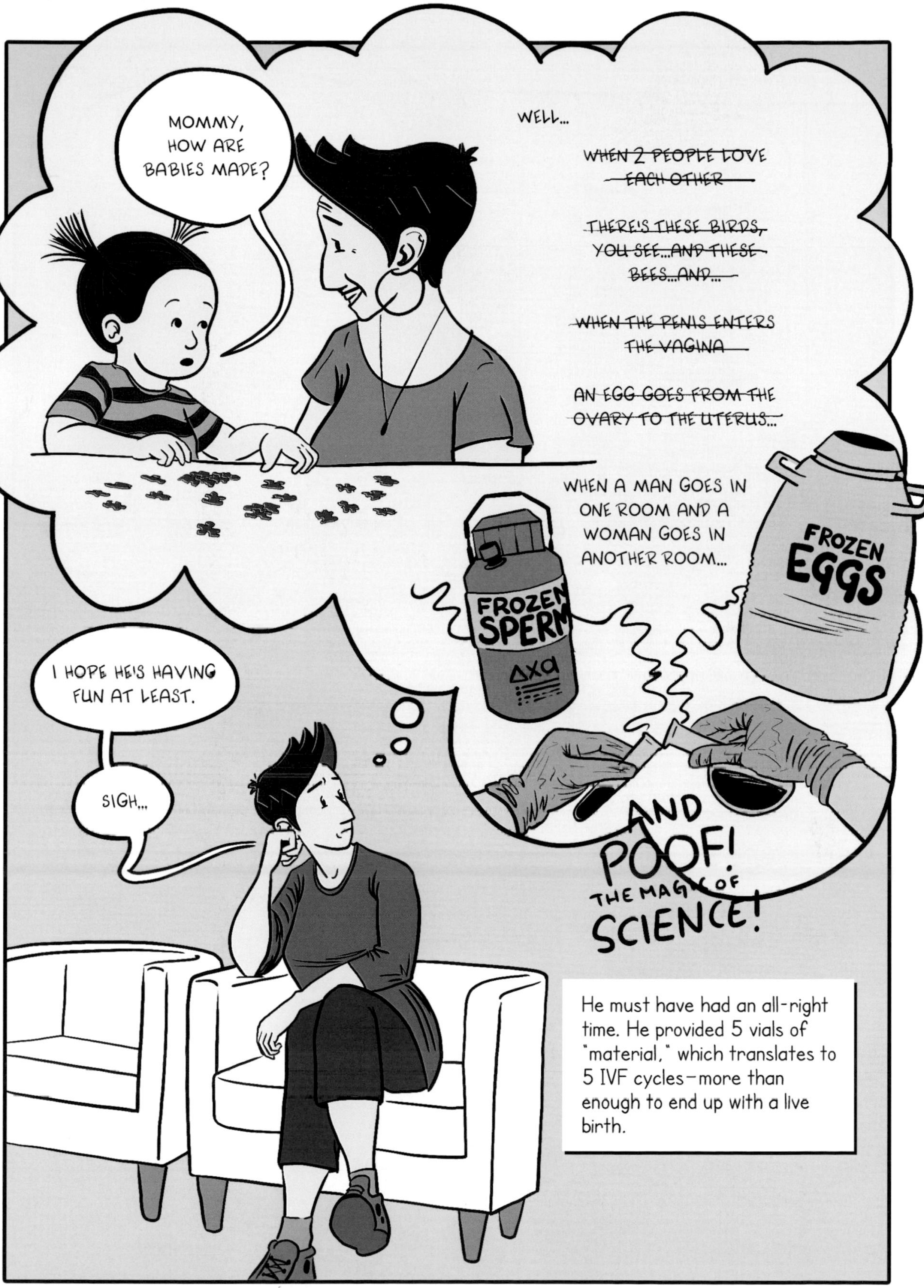
MOMMY, HOW ARE BABIES MADE?
WELL...
WHEN 2 PEOPLE LOVE EACH OTHER
THERE'S THESE BIRDS, YOU SEE...AND THESE BEES...AND...
WHEN THE PENIS ENTERS THE VAGINA
AN EGG GOES FROM THE OVARY TO THE UTERUS...
WHEN A MAN GOES IN ONE ROOM AND A WOMAN GOES IN ANOTHER ROOM...
FROZEN EGGS
FROZEN SPERM
AND POOF! THE MAGIC OF SCIENCE!
I HOPE HE'S HAVING FUN AT LEAST.
SIGH...
He must have had an all-right time. He provided 5 vials of "material," which translates to 5 IVF cycles—more than enough to end up with a live birth.

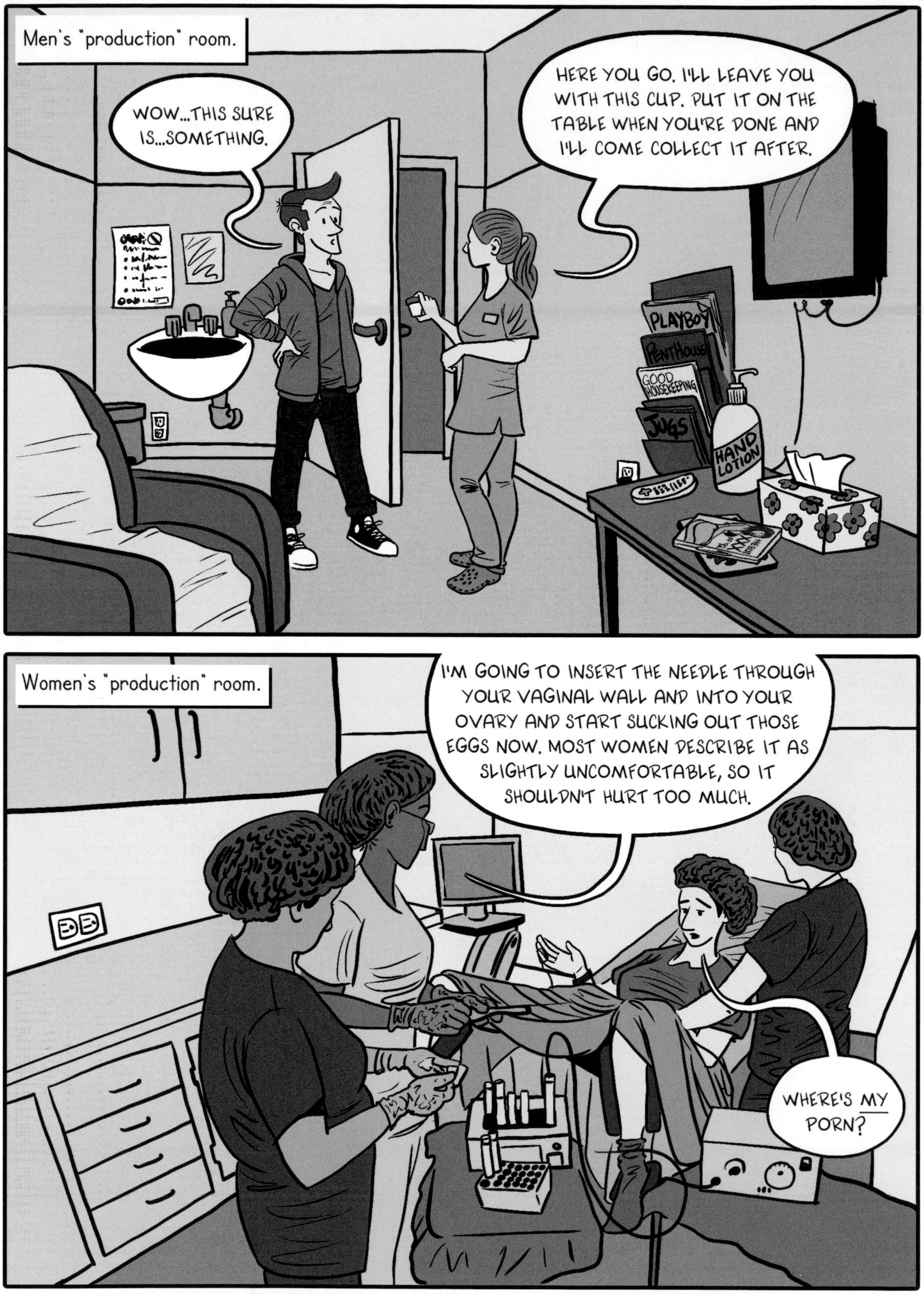
Men's "production" room.
WOW...THIS SURE IS...SOMETHING.
HERE YOU GO. I'LL LEAVE YOU WITH THIS CUP. PUT IT ON THE TABLE WHEN YOU'RE DONE AND I'LL COME COLLECT IT AFTER.
PLAYBOY
PENTHOUSE
GOOD HOUSEKEEPING
JUGS
HAND LOTION
Women's "production" room.
I'M GOING TO INSERT THE NEEDLE THROUGH YOUR VAGINAL WALL AND INTO YOUR OVARY AND START SUCKING OUT THOSE EGGS NOW. MOST WOMEN DESCRIBE IT AS SLIGHTLY UNCOMFORTABLE, SO IT SHOULDN'T HURT TOO MUCH.
WHERE'S MY PORN?

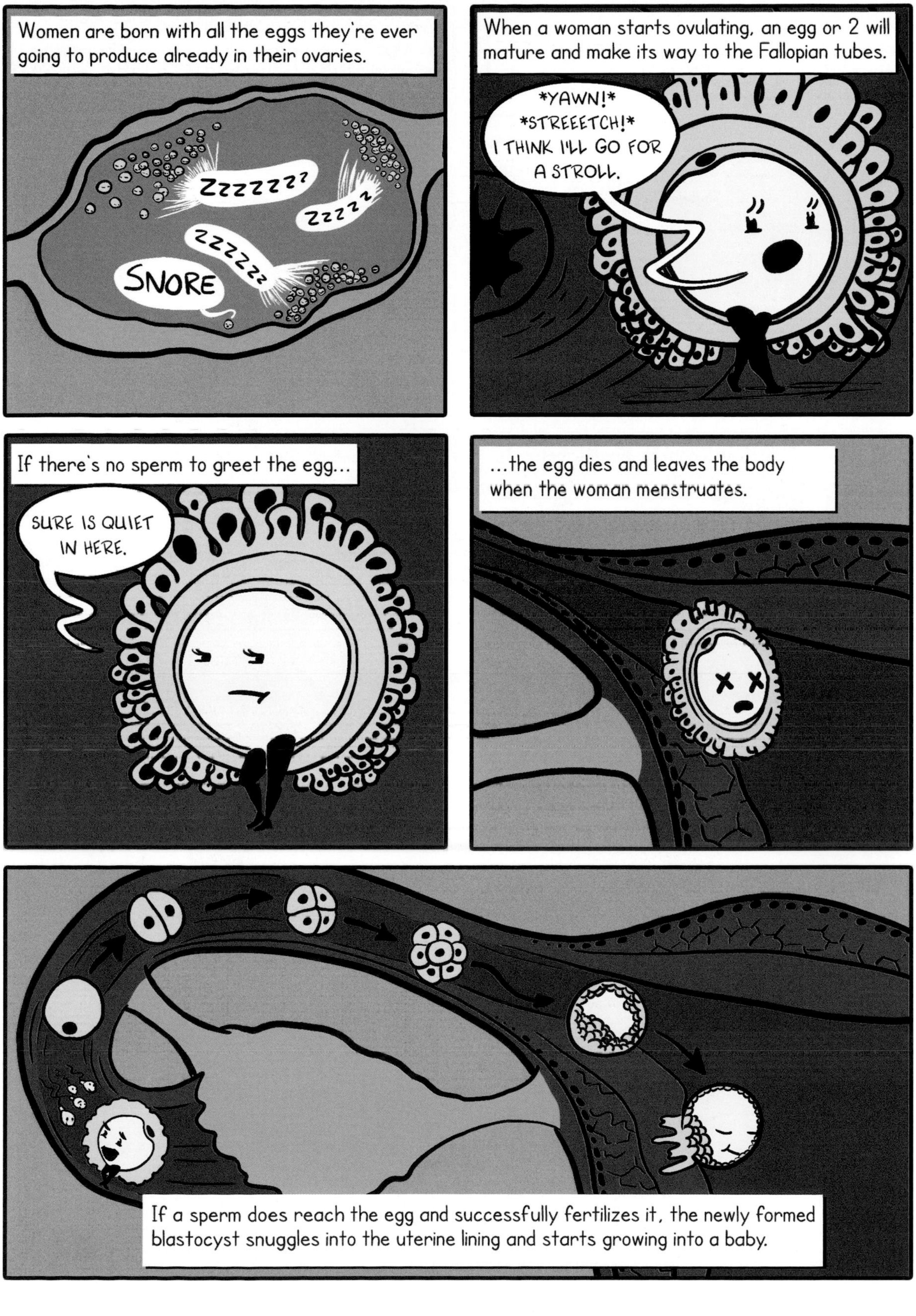

Women are born with all the eggs they're ever going to produce already in their ovaries.
Zzzzzzz
Zzzzz
Zzzzzzz
SNORE
When a woman starts ovulating, an egg or 2 will mature and make its way to the Fallopian tubes.
YAWN! *STREEETCH!* I THINK I'LL GO FOR A STROLL.
If there's no sperm to greet the egg...
SURE IS QUIET IN HERE.
...the egg dies and leaves the body when the woman menstruates.
If a sperm does reach the egg and successfully fertilizes it, the newly formed blastocyst snuggles into the uterine lining and starts growing into a baby.

During an IVF cycle, drugs, injected daily into the belly, are used to force as many egg follicles as possible to mature simultaneously and grow at relatively the same rate.

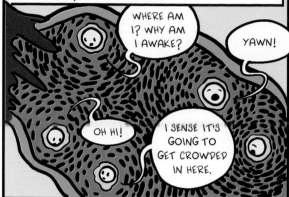

WHERE AM I? WHY AM I AWAKE?

YAWN!

OH HI!

I SENSE IT'S GOING TO GET CROWDED IN HERE.

Over 2 weeks, it's a delicate balancing act of growing follicles without over- or under-growing them, while also ensuring that your body doesn't release them spontaneously.

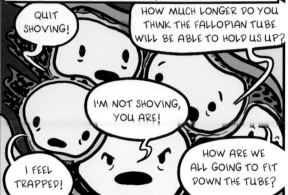

QUIT SHOVING!

HOW MUCH LONGER DO YOU THINK THE FALLOPIAN TUBE WILL BE ABLE TO HOLD US UP?

I'M NOT SHOVING, YOU ARE!

I FEEL TRAPPED!

HOW ARE WE ALL GOING TO FIT DOWN THE TUBE?

Sometimes, one ovary produces more follicles than the other.

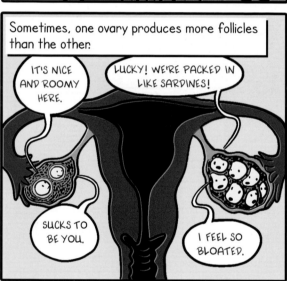

IT'S NICE AND ROOMY HERE.

LUCKY! WE'RE PACKED IN LIKE SARDINES!

SUCKS TO BE YOU.

I FEEL SO BLOATED.

Near the end of the 2 weeks, the follicles are checked via ultrasound to see if they're big enough.

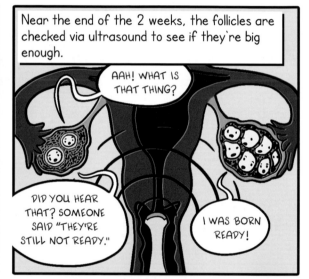

AAH! WHAT IS THAT THING?

DID YOU HEAR THAT? SOMEONE SAID "THEY'RE STILL NOT READY."

I WAS BORN READY!

I bruise easily at the best of times.

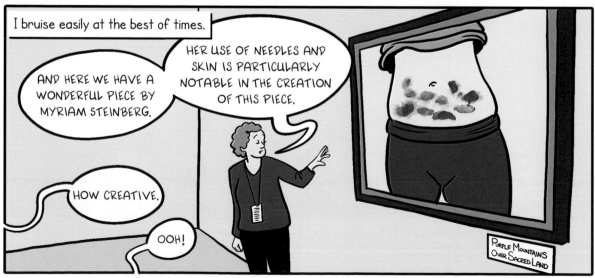

AND HERE WE HAVE A WONDERFUL PIECE BY MYRIAM STEINBERG.

HER USE OF NEEDLES AND SKIN IS PARTICULARLY NOTABLE IN THE CREATION OF THIS PIECE.

HOW CREATIVE.

OOH!

PURPLE MOUNTAINS OVER SACRED LAND

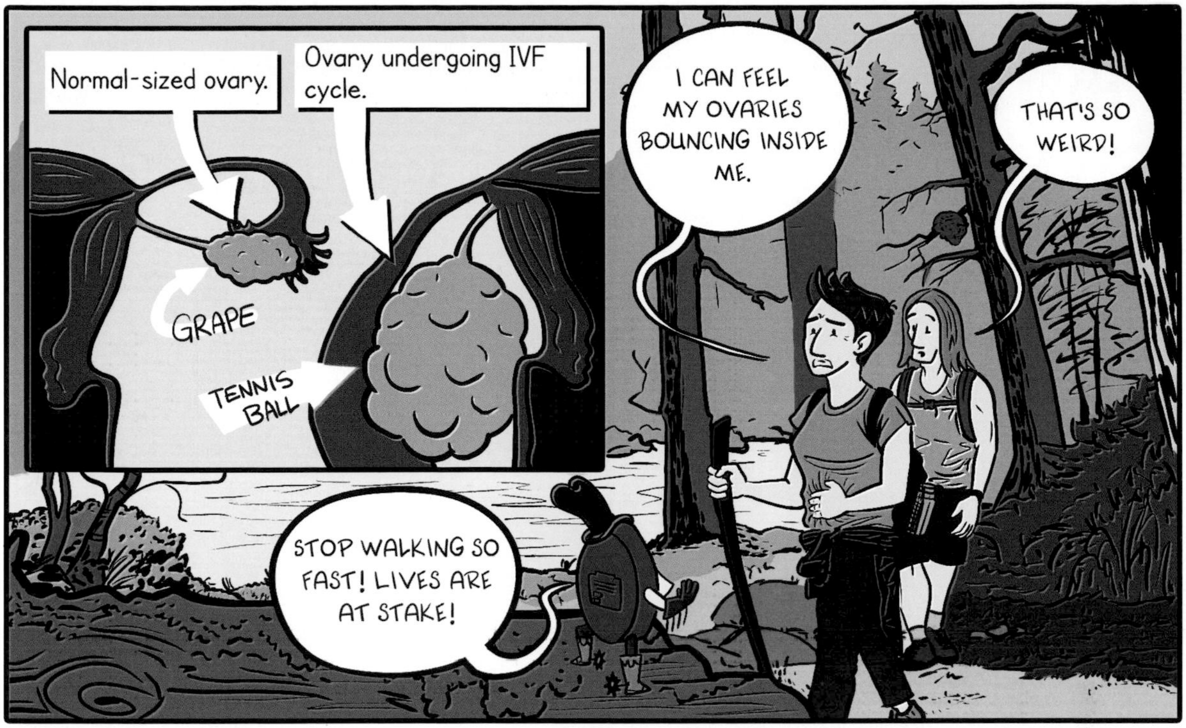
Normal-sized ovary.
Ovary undergoing IVF cycle.
GRAPE
TENNIS BALL
I CAN FEEL MY OVARIES BOUNCING INSIDE ME.
THAT'S SO WEIRD!
STOP WALKING SO FAST! LIVES ARE AT STAKE!

I lived in fear that one wrong move would cause my ovaries to collapse due to their weight and get tangled up in the Fallopian tube, necessitating a trip to the hospital and the loss of the ovary.

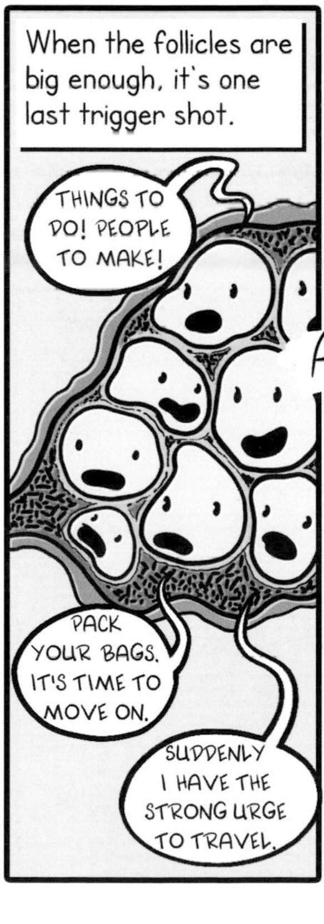
When the follicles are big enough, it's one last trigger shot.
THINGS TO DO! PEOPLE TO MAKE!
PACK YOUR BAGS. IT'S TIME TO MOVE ON.
SUDDENLY I HAVE THE STRONG URGE TO TRAVEL.

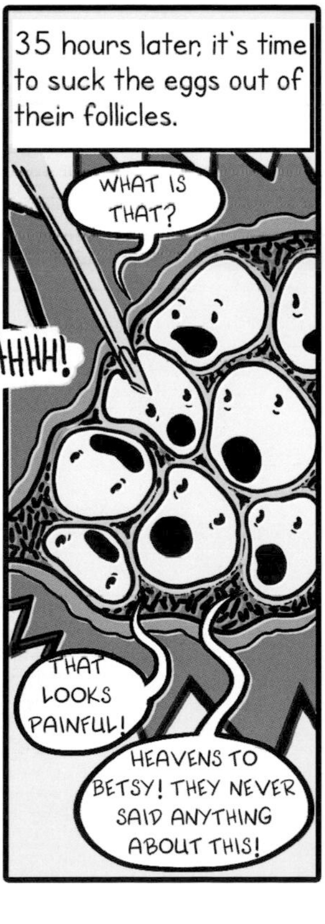
35 hours later, it's time to suck the eggs out of their follicles.
WHAT IS THAT?
AHHH!
THAT LOOKS PAINFUL!
HEAVENS TO BETSY! THEY NEVER SAID ANYTHING ABOUT THIS!

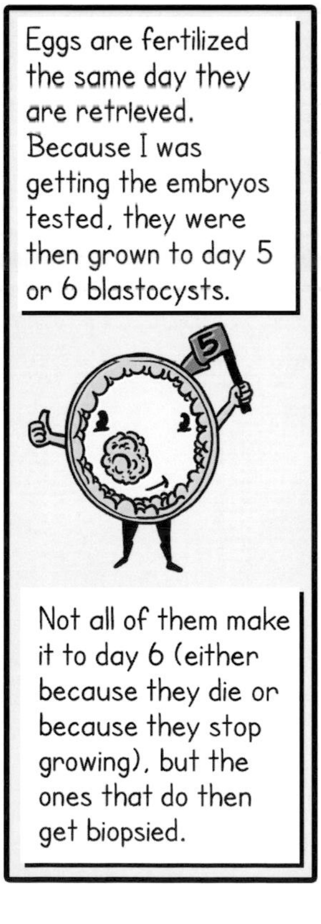
Eggs are fertilized the same day they are retrieved. Because I was getting the embryos tested, they were then grown to day 5 or 6 blastocysts.
5
Not all of them make it to day 6 (either because they die or because they stop growing), but the ones that do then get biopsied.

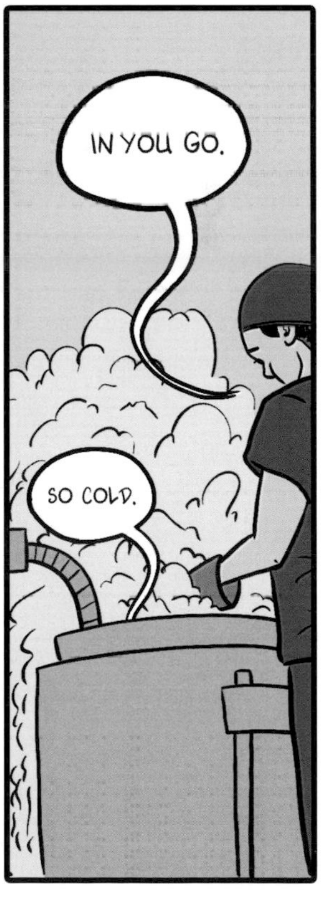
IN YOU GO.
SO COLD.

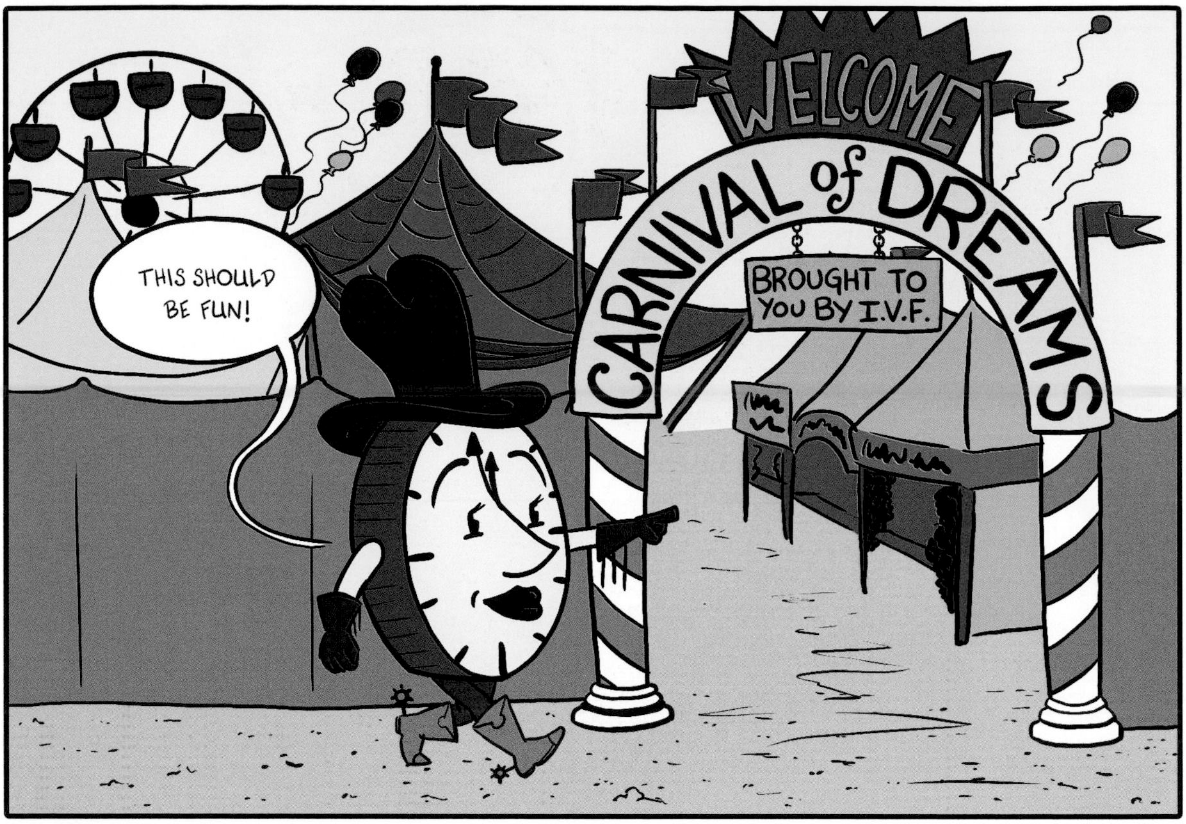
WELCOME
CARNIVAL of DREAMS
BROUGHT TO YOU BY I.V.F.
THIS SHOULD BE FUN!

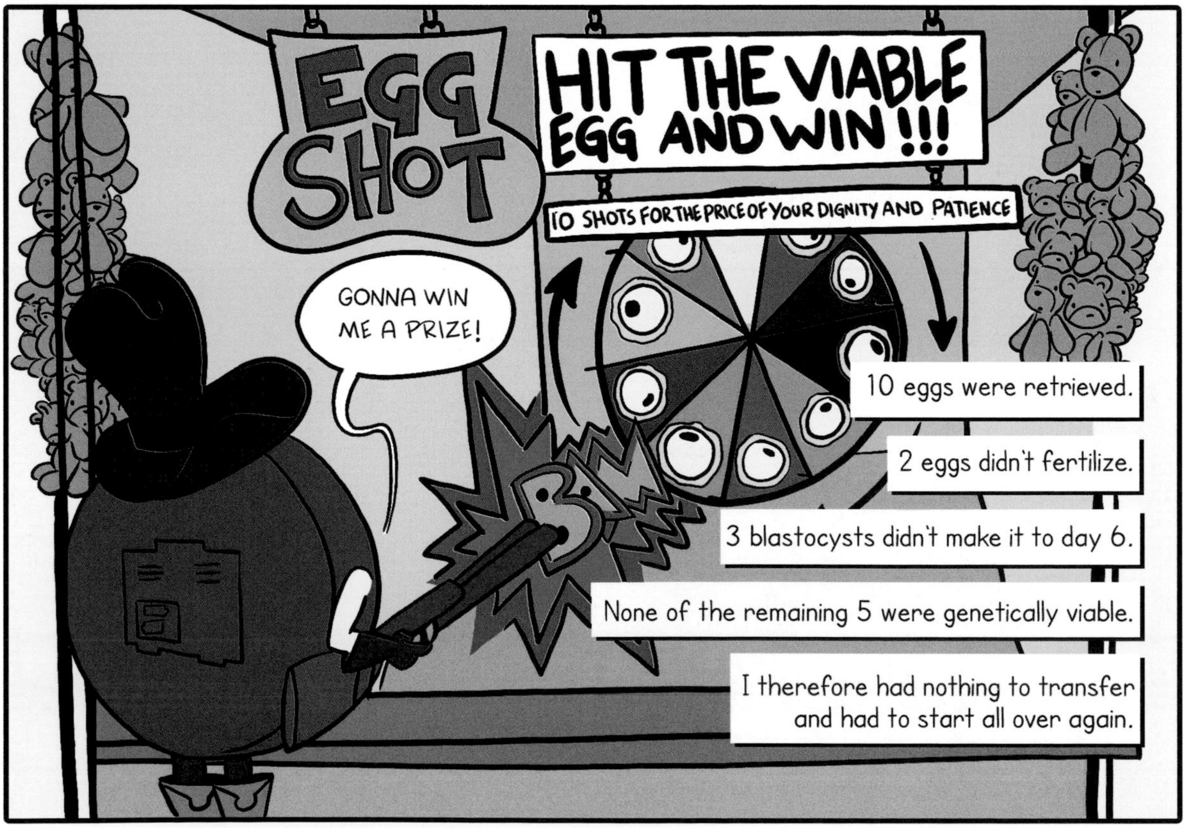
EGG SHOT
HIT THE VIABLE EGG AND WIN!!!
10 SHOTS FOR THE PRICE OF YOUR DIGNITY AND PATIENCE
GONNA WIN ME A PRIZE!
BAM
10 eggs were retrieved.
2 eggs didn't fertilize.
3 blastocysts didn't make it to day 6.
None of the remaining 5 were genetically viable.
I therefore had nothing to transfer and had to start all over again.

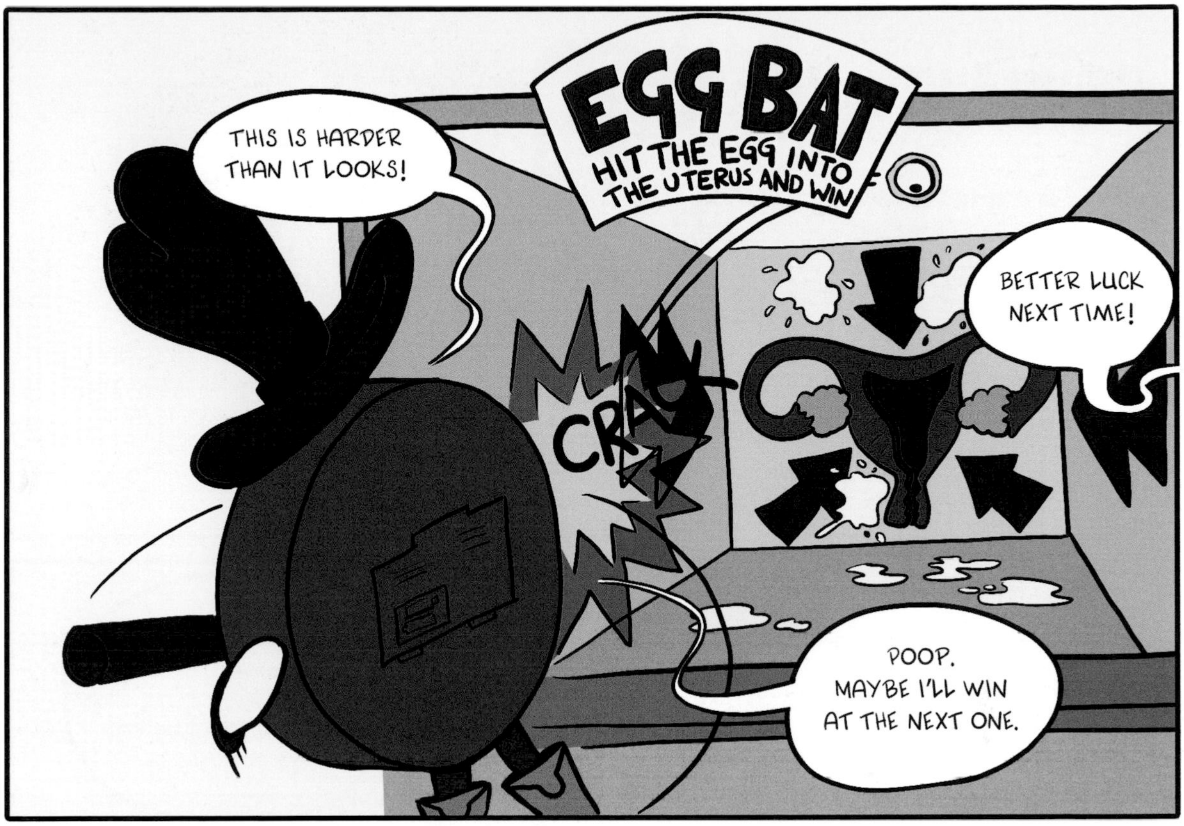
THIS IS HARDER THAN IT LOOKS!
EGG BAT
HIT THE EGG INTO THE UTERUS AND WIN
CRA
BETTER LUCK NEXT TIME!
POOP. MAYBE I'LL WIN AT THE NEXT ONE.

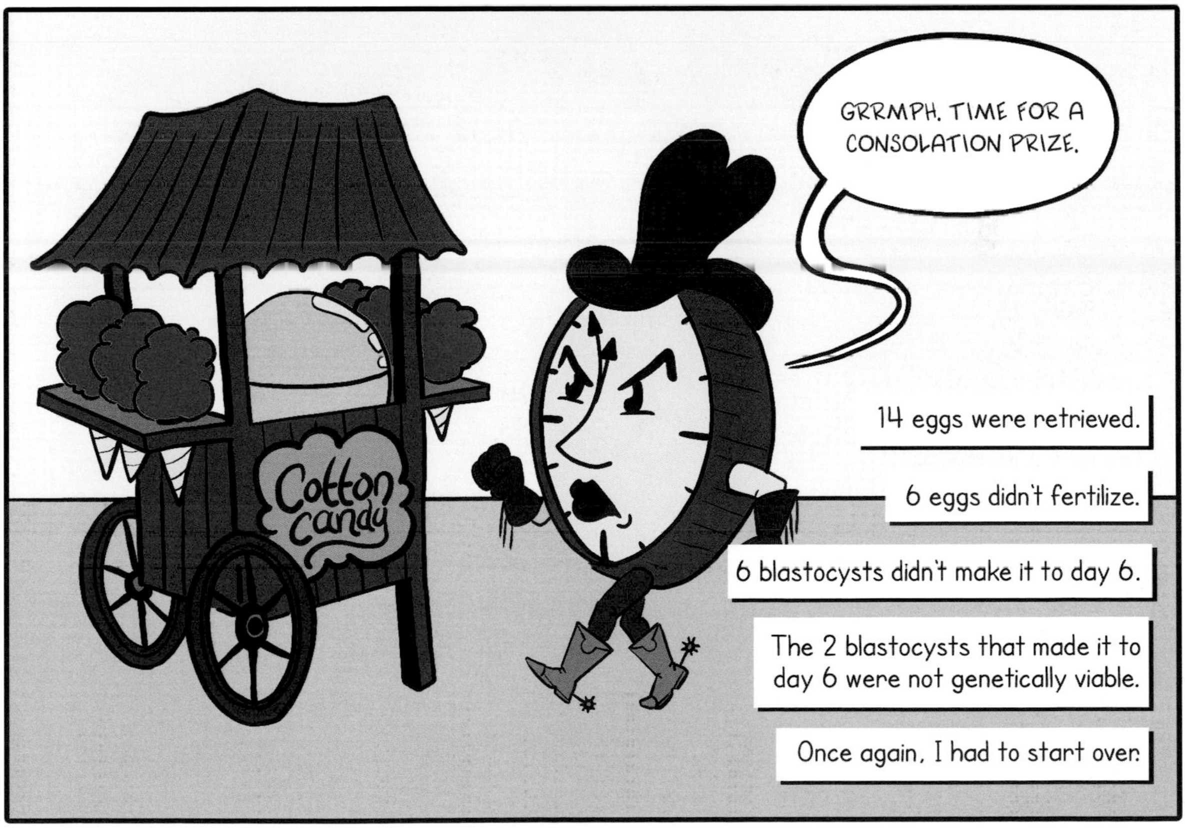
GRRMPH. TIME FOR A CONSOLATION PRIZE.
Cotton candy
14 eggs were retrieved.
6 eggs didn't fertilize.
6 blastocysts didn't make it to day 6.
The 2 blastocysts that made it to day 6 were not genetically viable.
Once again, I had to start over.

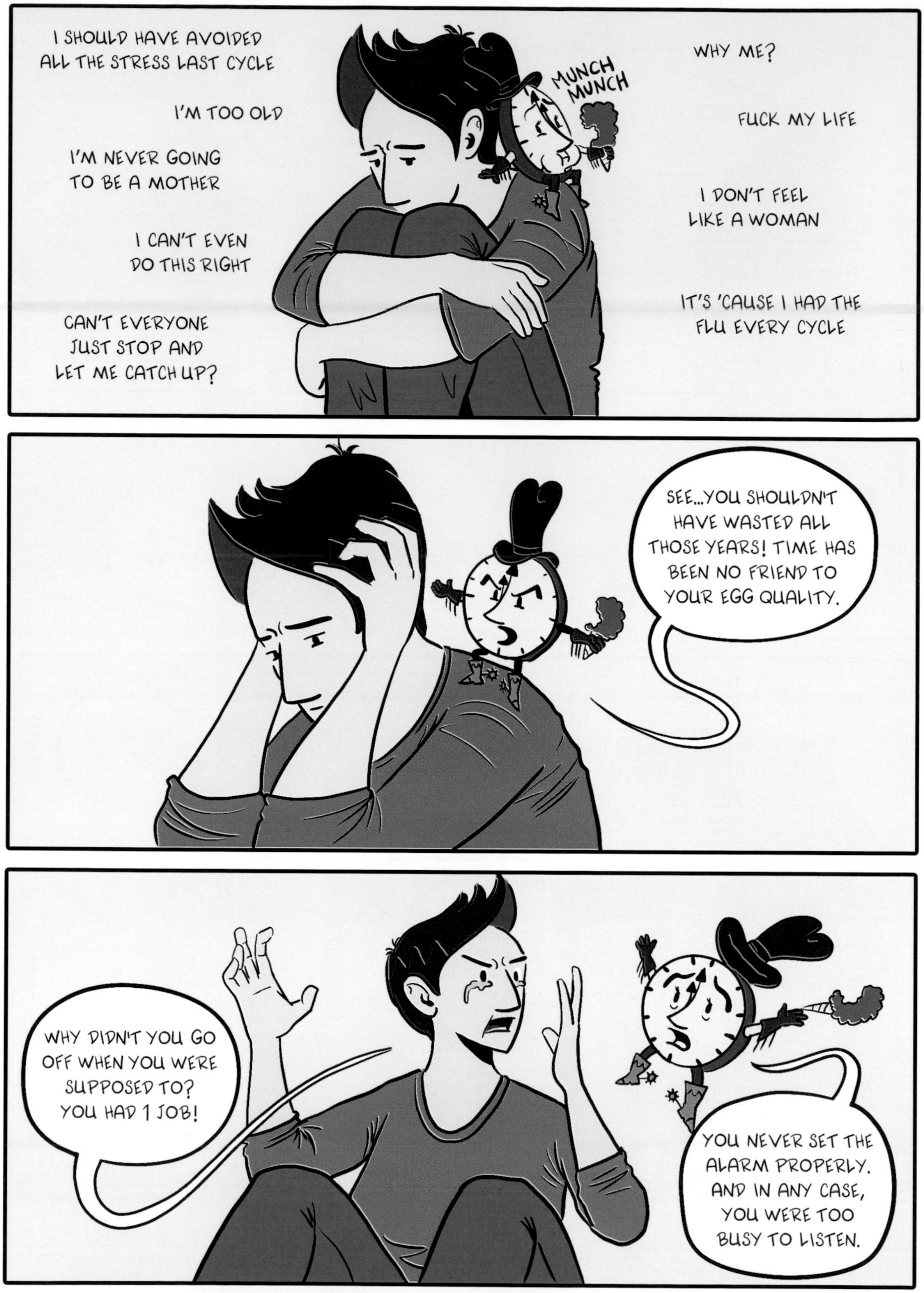
I SHOULD HAVE AVOIDED ALL THE STRESS LAST CYCLE
I'M TOO OLD
I'M NEVER GOING TO BE A MOTHER
I CAN'T EVEN DO THIS RIGHT
CAN'T EVERYONE JUST STOP AND LET ME CATCH UP?
MUNCH MUNCH
WHY ME?
FUCK MY LIFE
I DON'T FEEL LIKE A WOMAN
IT'S 'CAUSE I HAD THE FLU EVERY CYCLE
SEE...YOU SHOULDN'T HAVE WASTED ALL THOSE YEARS! TIME HAS BEEN NO FRIEND TO YOUR EGG QUALITY.
WHY DIDN'T YOU GO OFF WHEN YOU WERE SUPPOSED TO? YOU HAD 1 JOB!
YOU NEVER SET THE ALARM PROPERLY. AND IN ANY CASE, YOU WERE TOO BUSY TO LISTEN.

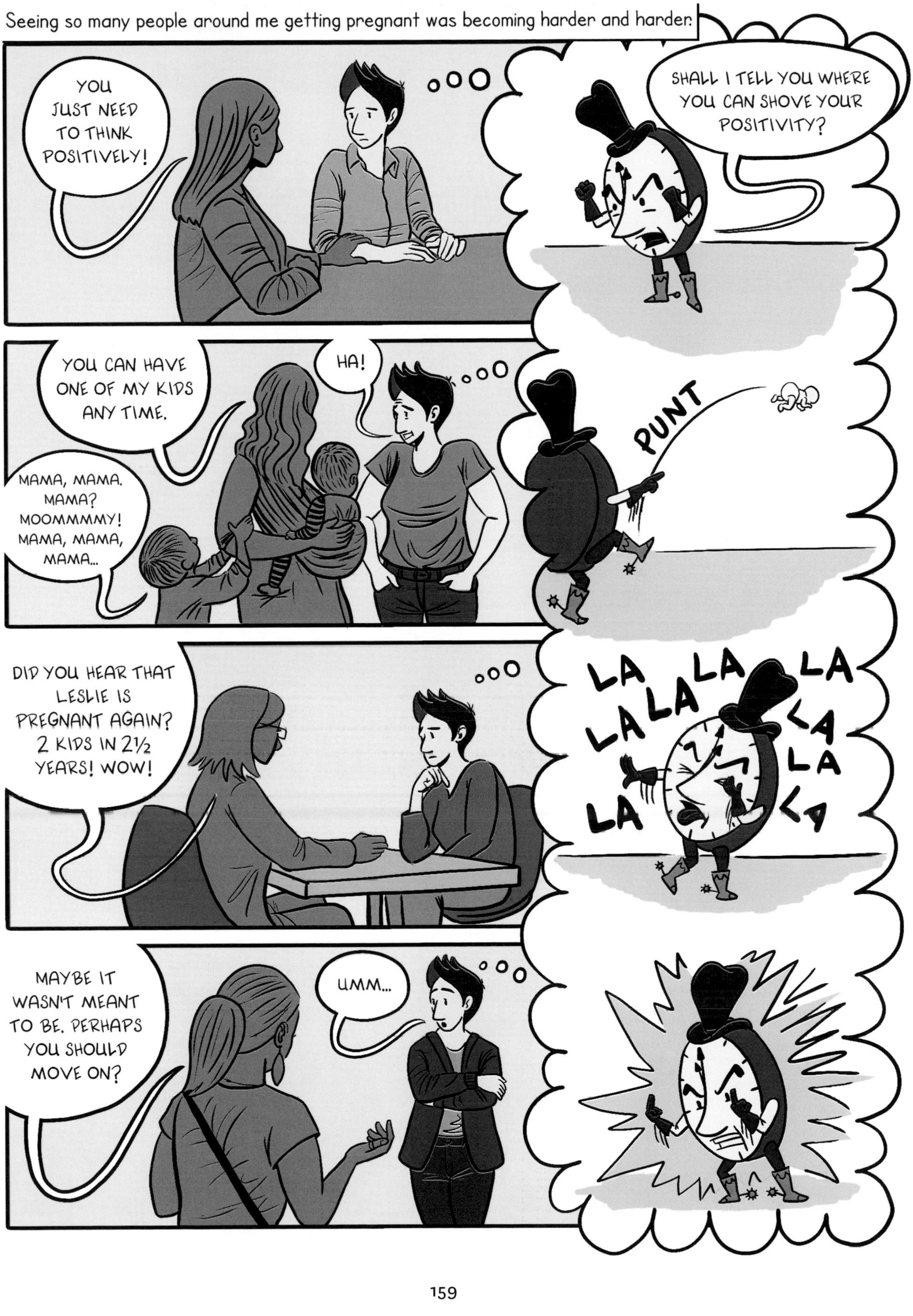
Seeing so many people around me getting pregnant was becoming harder and harder.
YOU JUST NEED TO THINK POSITIVELY!
SHALL I TELL YOU WHERE YOU CAN SHOVE YOUR POSITIVITY?
YOU CAN HAVE ONE OF MY KIDS ANY TIME.
HA!
MAMA, MAMA. MAMA? MOOMMMMY! MAMA, MAMA, MAMA...
PUNT
DID YOU HEAR THAT LESLIE IS PREGNANT AGAIN? 2 KIDS IN 2½ YEARS! WOW!
LA LA LA LA LA LA LA LA LA LA
MAYBE IT WASN'T MEANT TO BE. PERHAPS YOU SHOULD MOVE ON?
UMM...

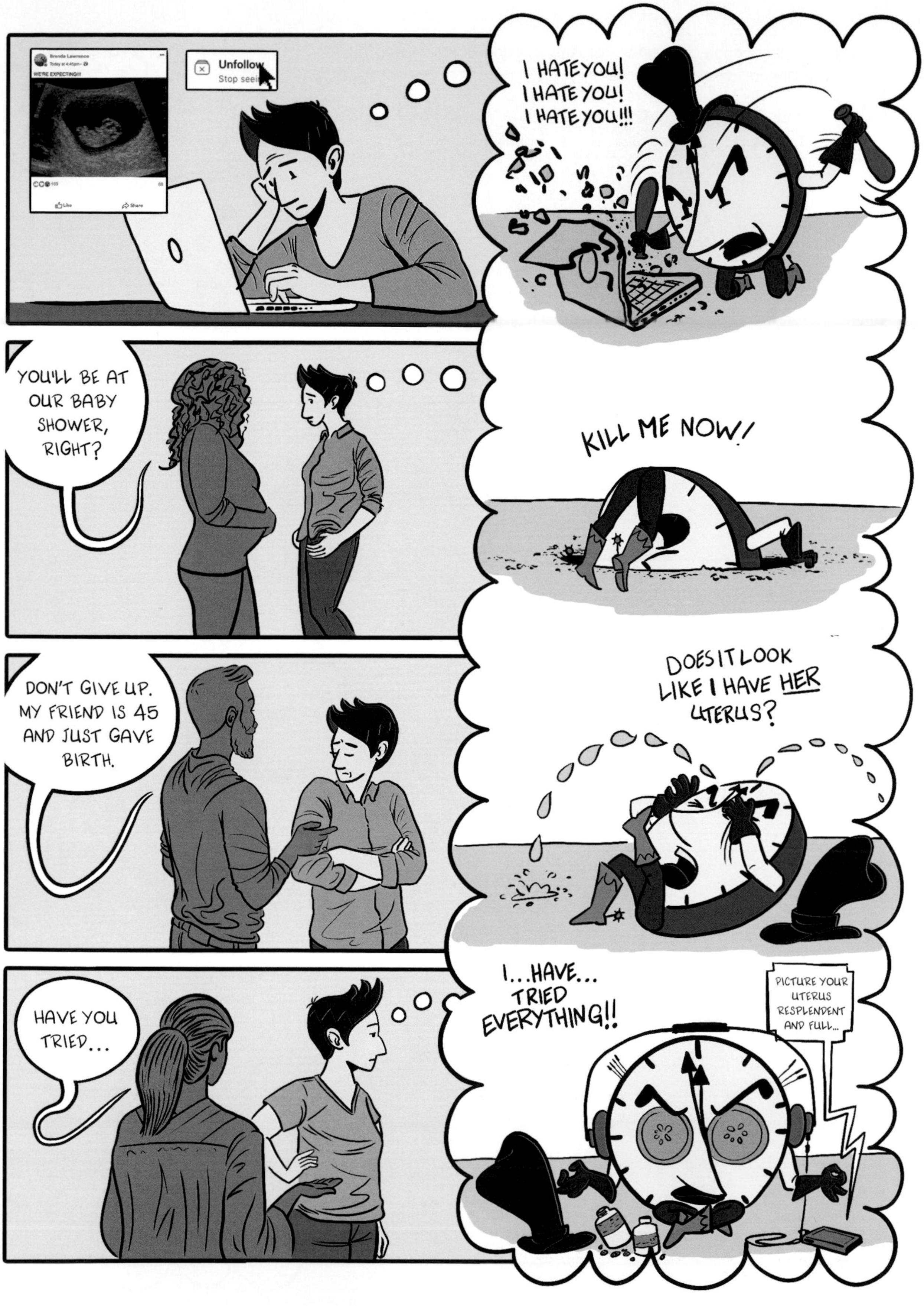
Brenda Lawrence
WE'RE EXPECTING!!!
Like
Share
Unfollow
I HATE YOU!
I HATE YOU!
I HATE YOU!!!
YOU'LL BE AT OUR BABY SHOWER, RIGHT?
KILL ME NOW!
DON'T GIVE UP. MY FRIEND IS 45 AND JUST GAVE BIRTH.
DOES IT LOOK LIKE I HAVE HER UTERUS?
HAVE YOU TRIED...
I...HAVE... TRIED EVERYTHING!!
PICTURE YOUR UTERUS RESPLENDENT AND FULL...

Some comments were easier to ignore—mostly because they didn't happen all that often for me. There was one comment, though, that recurred constantly and became my biggest trigger:

"HAVE YOU THOUGHT ABOUT ADOPTING?"

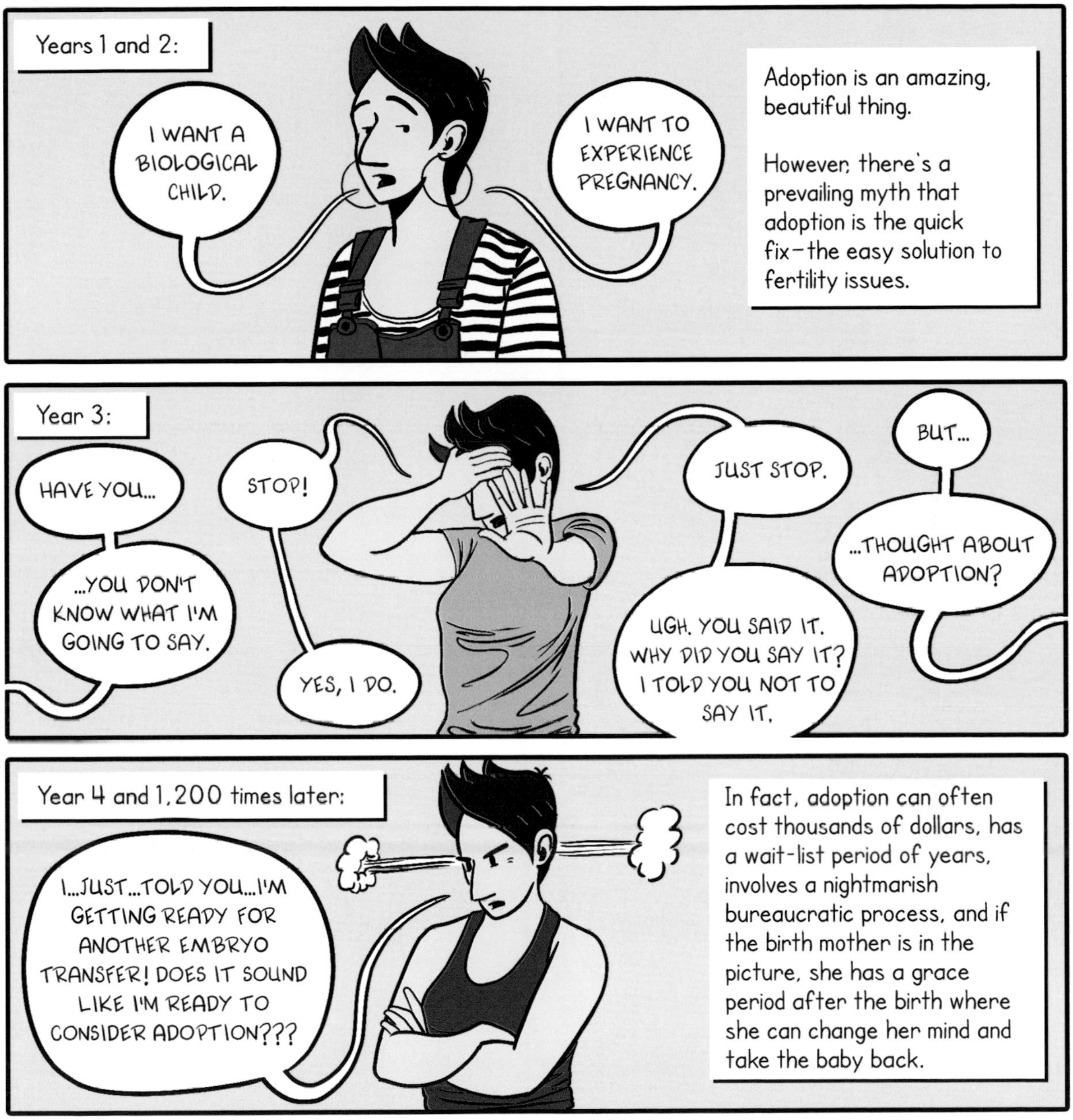

Years 1 and 2:
I WANT A BIOLOGICAL CHILD.
I WANT TO EXPERIENCE PREGNANCY.
Adoption is an amazing, beautiful thing.
However, there's a prevailing myth that adoption is the quick fix—the easy solution to fertility issues.
Year 3:
HAVE YOU...
...YOU DON'T KNOW WHAT I'M GOING TO SAY.
STOP!
YES, I DO.
JUST STOP.
BUT...
...THOUGHT ABOUT ADOPTION?
UGH. YOU SAID IT. WHY DID YOU SAY IT? I TOLD YOU NOT TO SAY IT.
Year 4 and 1,200 times later:
I...JUST...TOLD YOU...I'M GETTING READY FOR ANOTHER EMBRYO TRANSFER! DOES IT SOUND LIKE I'M READY TO CONSIDER ADOPTION???
In fact, adoption can often cost thousands of dollars, has a wait-list period of years, involves a nightmarish bureaucratic process, and if the birth mother is in the picture, she has a grace period after the birth where she can change her mind and take the baby back.

There is a stigma for women struggling with infertility, single women, or people in LGBTQ+ relationships around choosing pregnancy over adoption. Somehow it's thought that we are turning our backs on humanity. Couples who conceive easily are never asked about adoption. There are countless children who need a home. Regardless of your fertility level or relationship status, if you are considering bringing a child into your home, adoption should be an option put on the table as part of that initial discussion. Children up for adoption are not a consolation prize. They are to be cherished by people who truly want to adopt—not because they felt it was a distant-second alternative to conceiving.

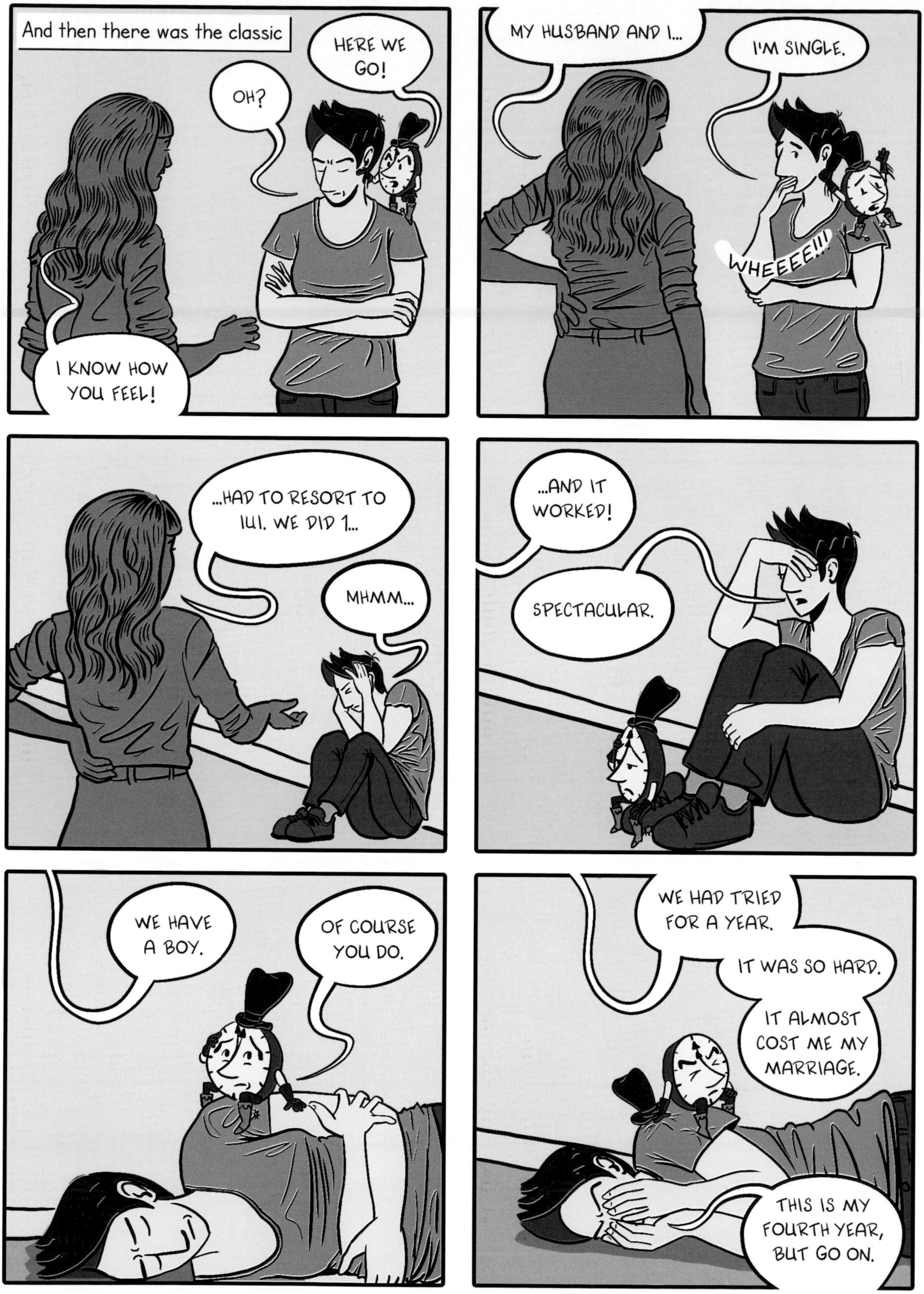
And then there was the classic
OH?
HERE WE GO!
I KNOW HOW YOU FEEL!
MY HUSBAND AND I...
I'M SINGLE.
WHEEEE!!!
...HAD TO RESORT TO IUI. WE DID 1...
MHMM...
...AND IT WORKED!
SPECTACULAR.
WE HAVE A BOY.
OF COURSE YOU DO.
WE HAD TRIED FOR A YEAR.
IT WAS SO HARD.
IT ALMOST COST ME MY MARRIAGE.
THIS IS MY FOURTH YEAR, BUT GO ON.

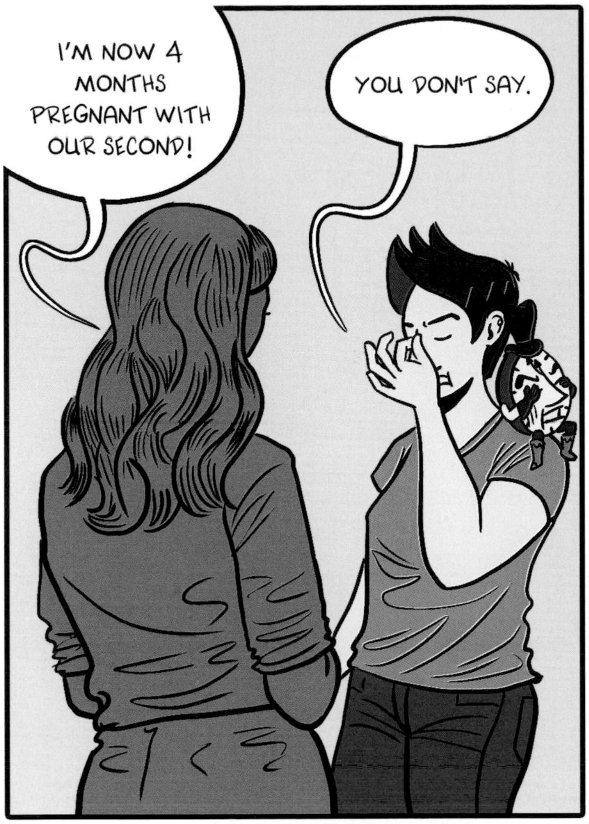
I'M NOW 4 MONTHS PREGNANT WITH OUR SECOND!
YOU DON'T SAY.

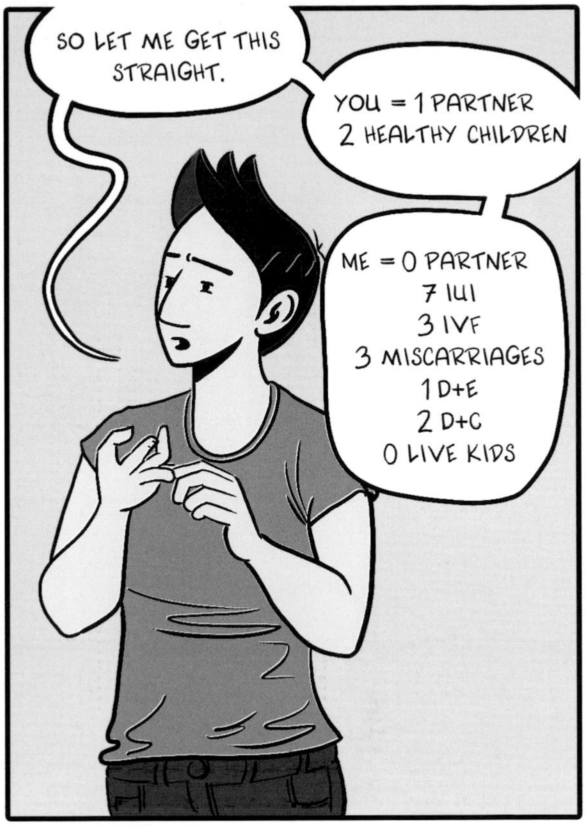
SO LET ME GET THIS STRAIGHT.
YOU = 1 PARTNER
2 HEALTHY CHILDREN
ME = 0 PARTNER
7 IUI
3 IVF
3 MISCARRIAGES
1 D+E
2 D+C
0 LIVE KIDS

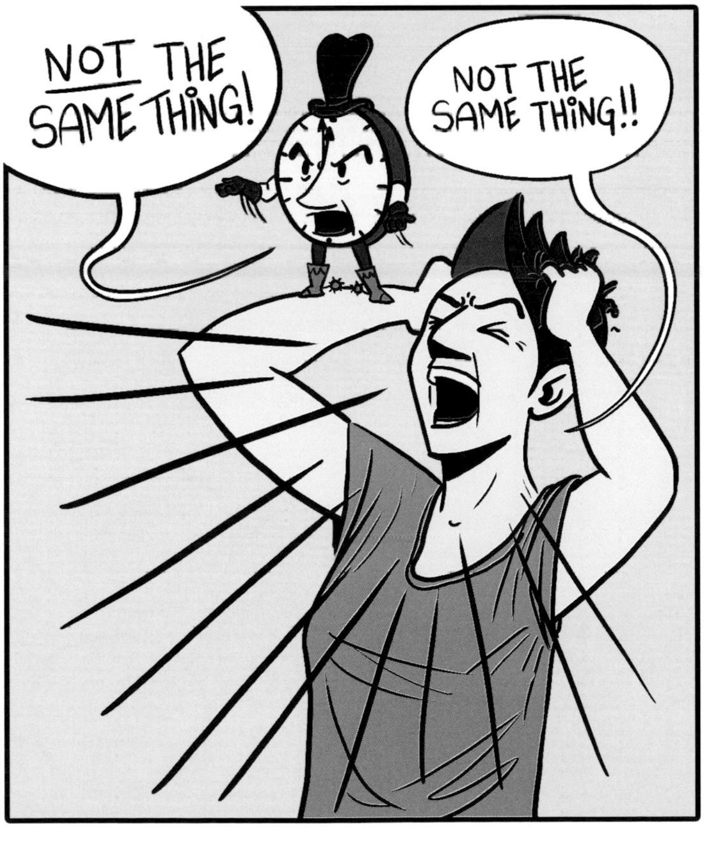
NOT THE SAME THING!
NOT THE SAME THING!!

The knee-jerk emotions that reared their head at every turn shocked me by their virulence and spitefulness. I didn't recognize myself. I wasn't a mean, jealous, vengeful, or bitter person. And yet here I was—exactly that (on the inside anyway). The almost-daily barrage of well-meaning comments and suggestions became acid-tipped daggers thrown at my heart and gut.

I felt a lot of shame and guilt around these vicious feelings. It was especially tricky to navigate the choppy waters of frustration and self-preservation while simultaneously trying to remember that loving, concerned friends, family, and acquaintances didn't want to see me in pain, and wanted to comfort and support me.

I decided to ask people in various (in)fertility groups on social media what comments triggered them.

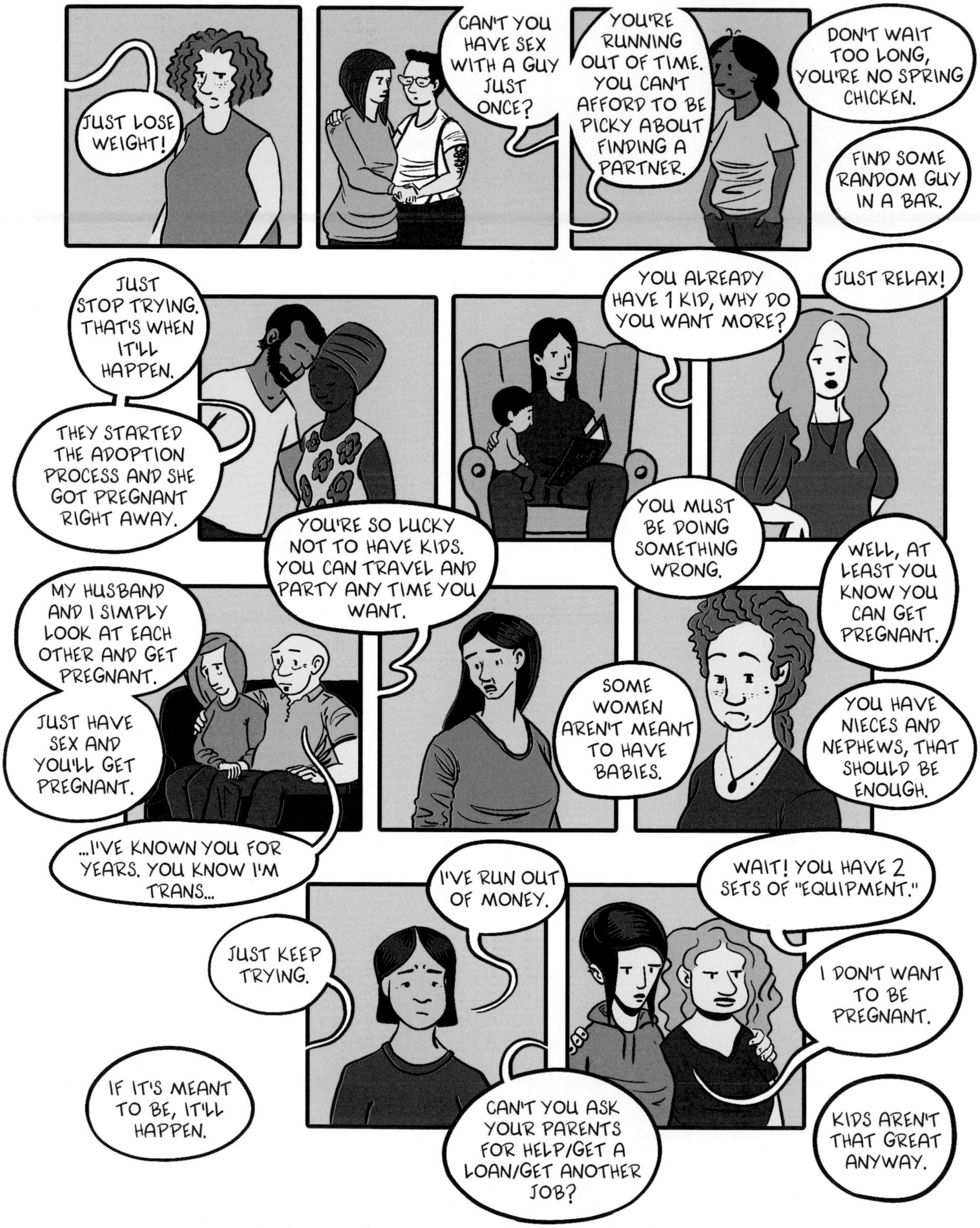
JUST LOSE WEIGHT!
CAN'T YOU HAVE SEX WITH A GUY JUST ONCE?
YOU'RE RUNNING OUT OF TIME. YOU CAN'T AFFORD TO BE PICKY ABOUT FINDING A PARTNER.
DON'T WAIT TOO LONG, YOU'RE NO SPRING CHICKEN.
FIND SOME RANDOM GUY IN A BAR.
JUST STOP TRYING. THAT'S WHEN IT'LL HAPPEN.
THEY STARTED THE ADOPTION PROCESS AND SHE GOT PREGNANT RIGHT AWAY.
YOU ALREADY HAVE 1 KID, WHY DO YOU WANT MORE?
JUST RELAX!
YOU'RE SO LUCKY NOT TO HAVE KIDS. YOU CAN TRAVEL AND PARTY ANY TIME YOU WANT.
YOU MUST BE DOING SOMETHING WRONG.
WELL, AT LEAST YOU KNOW YOU CAN GET PREGNANT.
MY HUSBAND AND I SIMPLY LOOK AT EACH OTHER AND GET PREGNANT.
JUST HAVE SEX AND YOU'LL GET PREGNANT.
...I'VE KNOWN YOU FOR YEARS. YOU KNOW I'M TRANS...
SOME WOMEN AREN'T MEANT TO HAVE BABIES.
YOU HAVE NIECES AND NEPHEWS, THAT SHOULD BE ENOUGH.
I'VE RUN OUT OF MONEY.
JUST KEEP TRYING.
IF IT'S MEANT TO BE, IT'LL HAPPEN.
CAN'T YOU ASK YOUR PARENTS FOR HELP/GET A LOAN/GET ANOTHER JOB?
WAIT! YOU HAVE 2 SETS OF "EQUIPMENT."
I DON'T WANT TO BE PREGNANT.
KIDS AREN'T THAT GREAT ANYWAY.

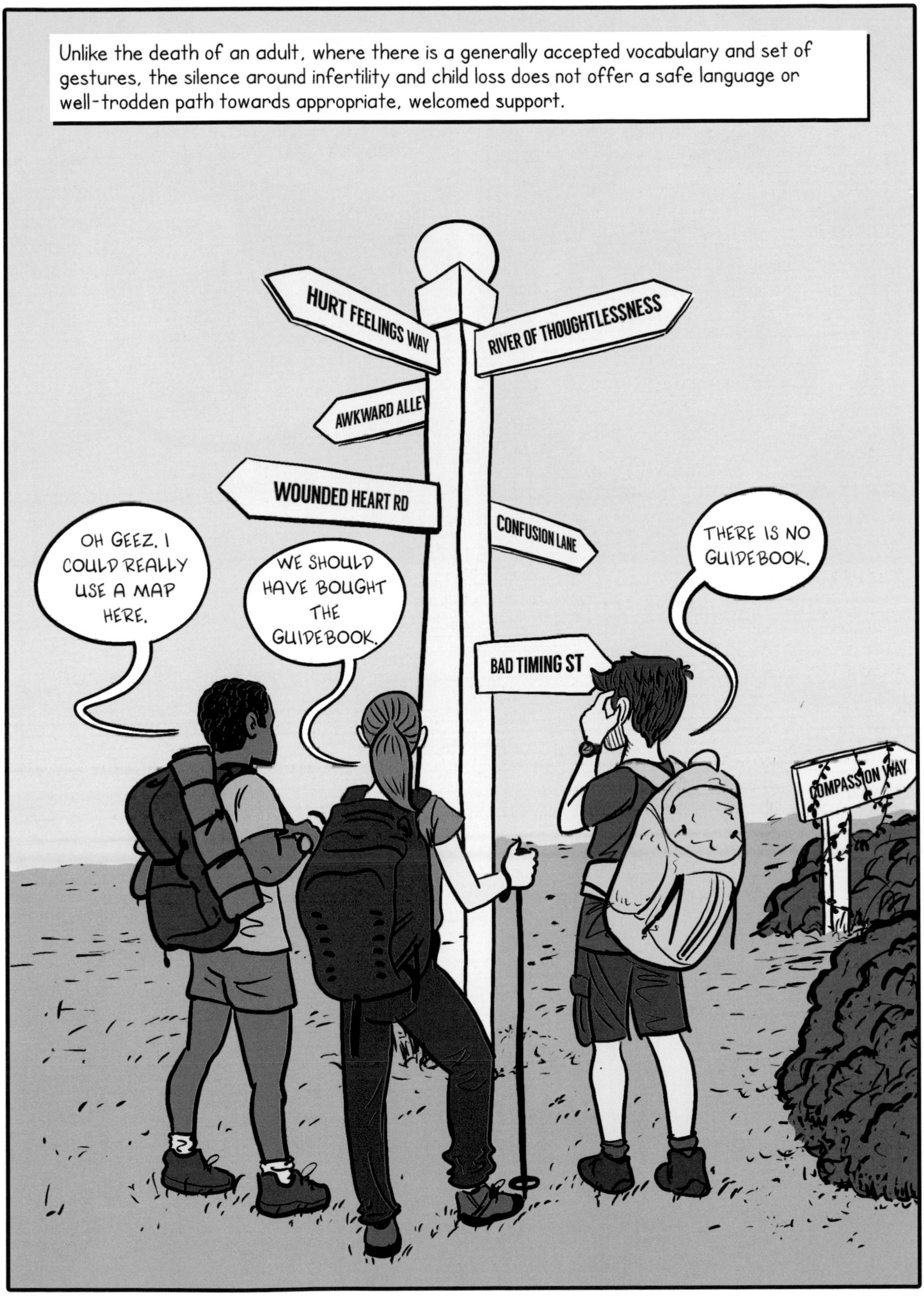
Unlike the death of an adult, where there is a generally accepted vocabulary and set of gestures, the silence around infertility and child loss does not offer a safe language or well-trodden path towards appropriate, welcomed support.
HURT FEELINGS WAY
RIVER OF THOUGHTLESSNESS
AWKWARD ALLEY
WOUNDED HEART RD
CONFUSION LANE
BAD TIMING ST
COMPASSION WAY
OH GEEZ. I COULD REALLY USE A MAP HERE.
WE SHOULD HAVE BOUGHT THE GUIDEBOOK.
THERE IS NO GUIDEBOOK.

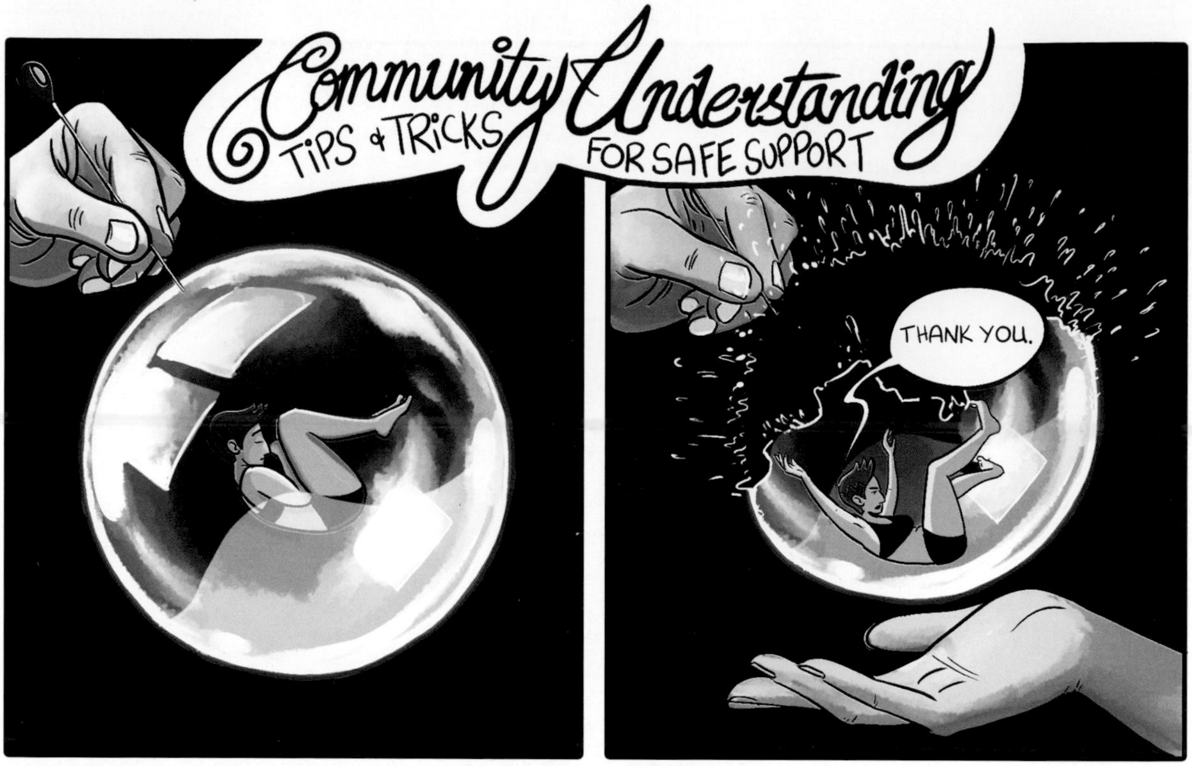
Community Understanding
TIPS & TRICKS FOR SAFE SUPPORT
THANK YOU.

It can be very difficult, if not impossible, to really understand what your friend/family member/colleague is going through. How do you support someone going through this journey?

Nothing you say or do will take away the pain. However, there are some very simple things you can do to ease it.

It all boils down to BE THERE, LISTEN, NOURISH, RESPECT.

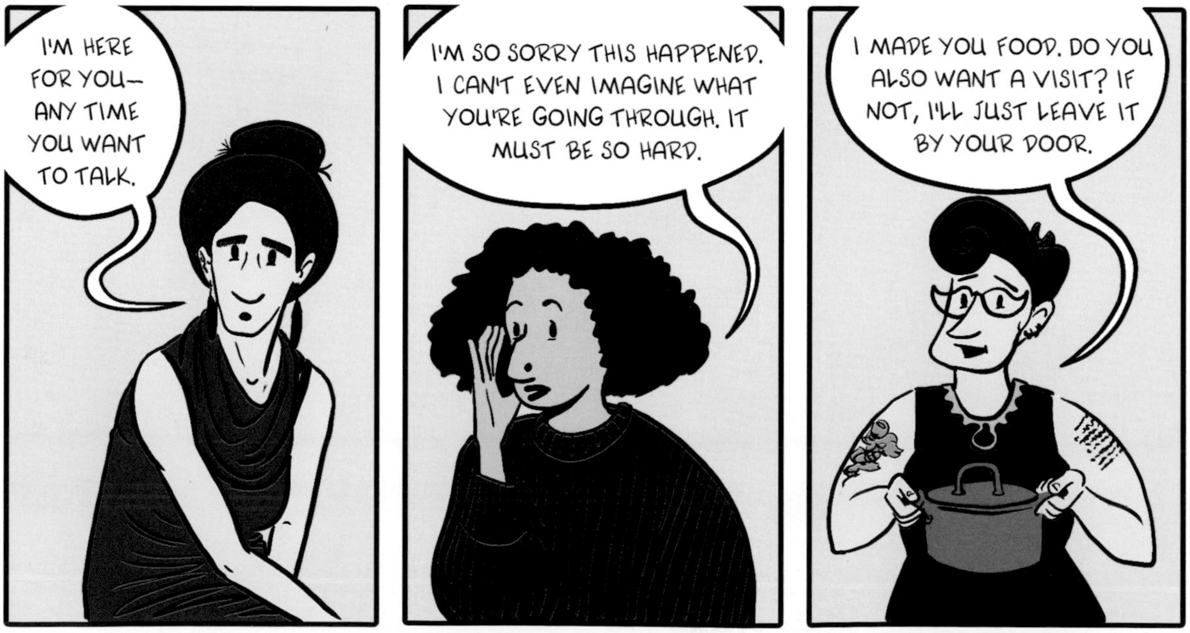
I'M HERE FOR YOU-- ANY TIME YOU WANT TO TALK.
I'M SO SORRY THIS HAPPENED. I CAN'T EVEN IMAGINE WHAT YOU'RE GOING THROUGH. IT MUST BE SO HARD.
I MADE YOU FOOD. DO YOU ALSO WANT A VISIT? IF NOT, I'LL JUST LEAVE IT BY YOUR DOOR.

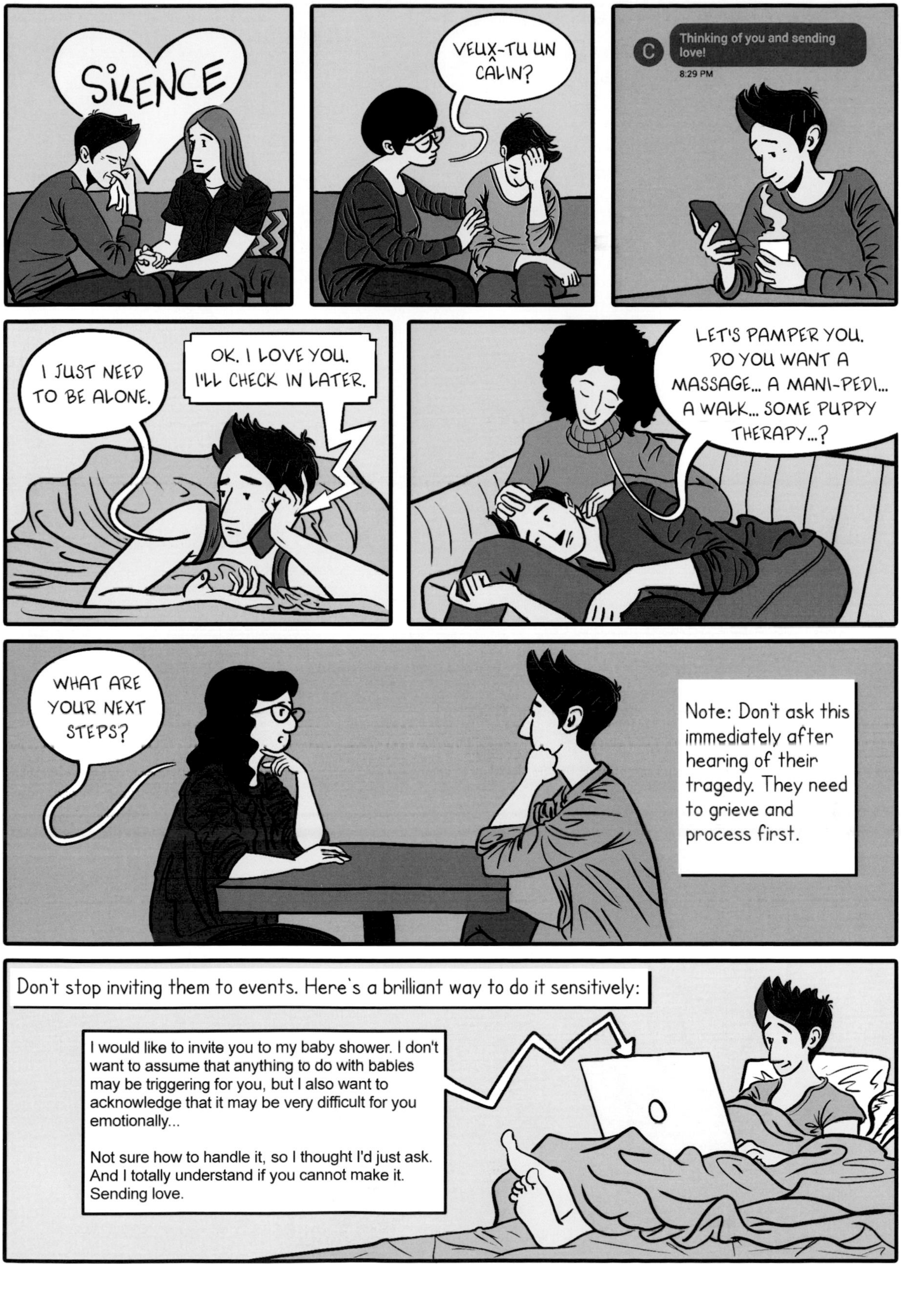
SILENCE
VEUX-TU UN CÂLIN?
Thinking of you and sending love!
8:29 PM
I JUST NEED TO BE ALONE.
OK. I LOVE YOU. I'LL CHECK IN LATER.
LET'S PAMPER YOU. DO YOU WANT A MASSAGE... A MANI-PEDI... A WALK... SOME PUPPY THERAPY...?
WHAT ARE YOUR NEXT STEPS?
Note: Don't ask this immediately after hearing of their tragedy. They need to grieve and process first.
Don't stop inviting them to events. Here's a brilliant way to do it sensitively:
I would like to invite you to my baby shower. I don't want to assume that anything to do with babies may be triggering for you, but I also want to acknowledge that it may be very difficult for you emotionally...
Not sure how to handle it, so I thought I'd just ask. And I totally understand if you cannot make it. Sending love.

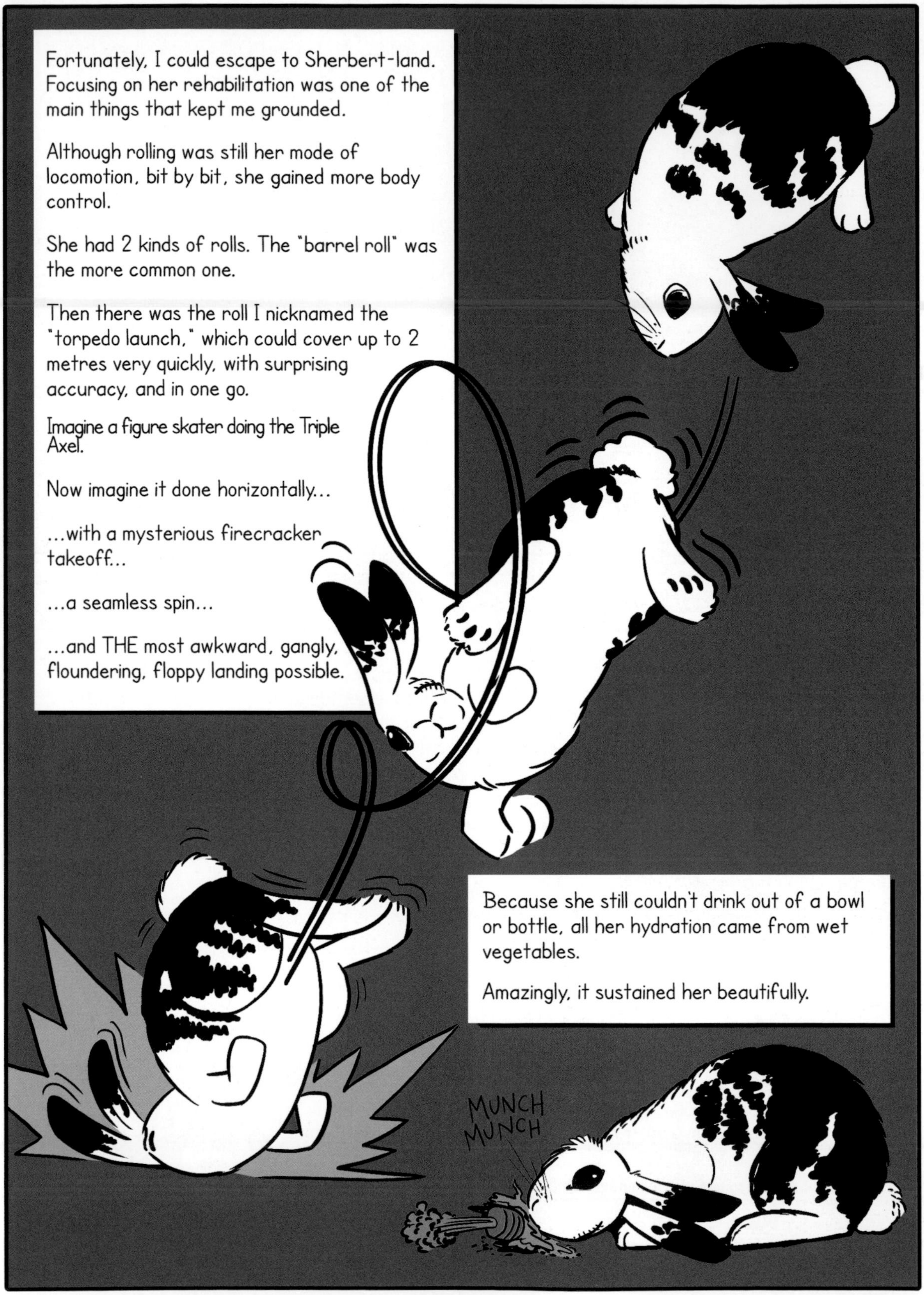
Fortunately, I could escape to Sherbert-land. Focusing on her rehabilitation was one of the main things that kept me grounded.
Although rolling was still her mode of locomotion, bit by bit, she gained more body control.
She had 2 kinds of rolls. The "barrel roll" was the more common one.
Then there was the roll I nicknamed the "torpedo launch," which could cover up to 2 metres very quickly, with surprising accuracy, and in one go.
Imagine a figure skater doing the Triple Axel.
Now imagine it done horizontally...
...with a mysterious firecracker takeoff...
...a seamless spin...
...and THE most awkward, gangly, floundering, floppy landing possible.
Because she still couldn't drink out of a bowl or bottle, all her hydration came from wet vegetables.
Amazingly, it sustained her beautifully.
MUNCH MUNCH

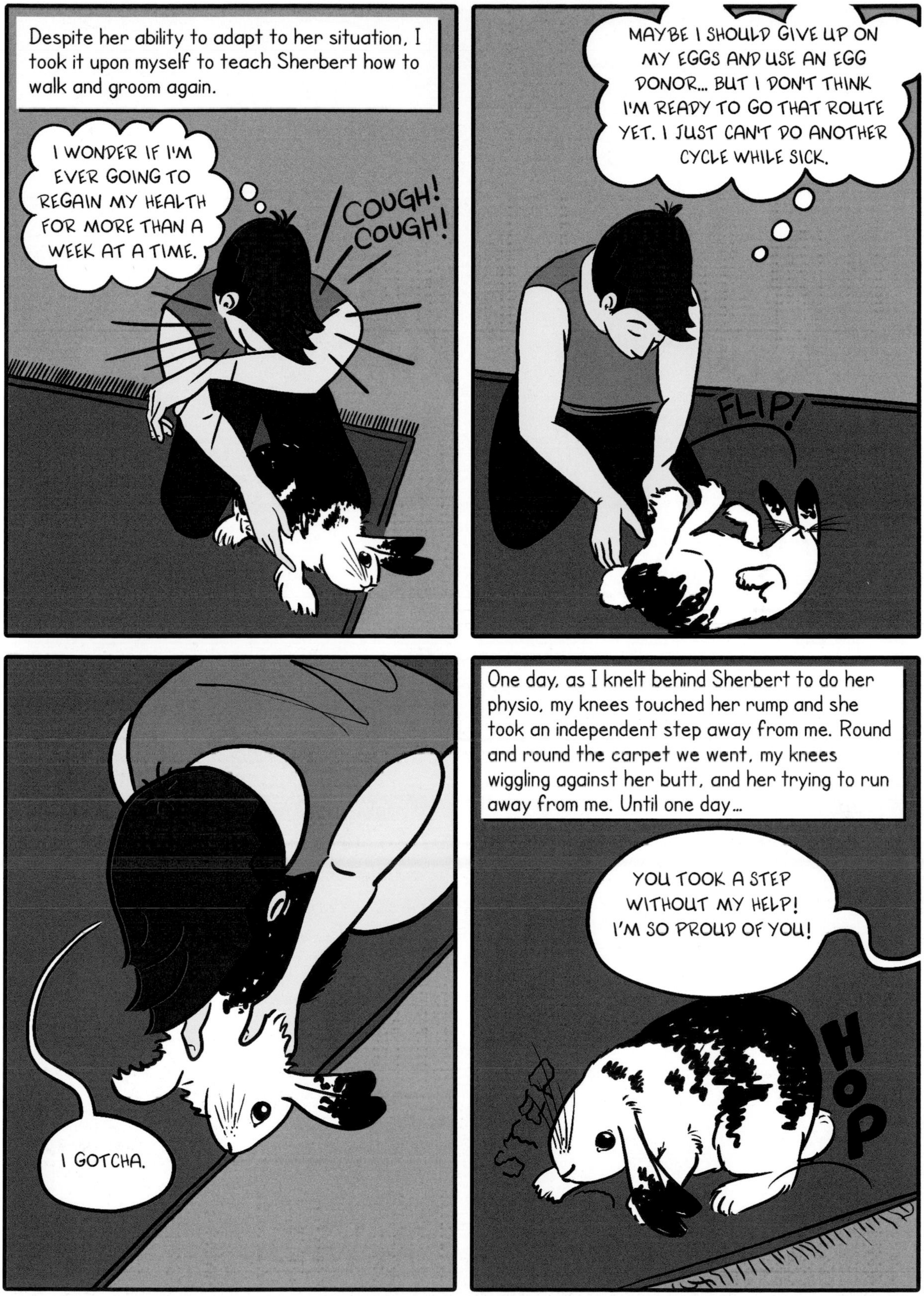
Despite her ability to adapt to her situation, I took it upon myself to teach Sherbert how to walk and groom again.
I WONDER IF I'M EVER GOING TO REGAIN MY HEALTH FOR MORE THAN A WEEK AT A TIME.
COUGH! COUGH!
MAYBE I SHOULD GIVE UP ON MY EGGS AND USE AN EGG DONOR... BUT I DON'T THINK I'M READY TO GO THAT ROUTE YET. I JUST CAN'T DO ANOTHER CYCLE WHILE SICK.
FLIP!
I GOTCHA.
One day, as I knelt behind Sherbert to do her physio, my knees touched her rump and she took an independent step away from me. Round and round the carpet we went, my knees wiggling against her butt, and her trying to run away from me. Until one day...
YOU TOOK A STEP WITHOUT MY HELP! I'M SO PROUD OF YOU!
HOP

She had other funny reflexes when I touched her.

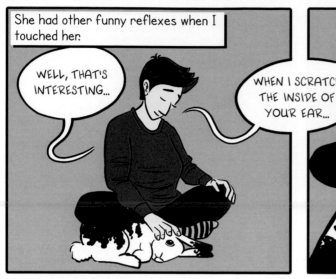

WELL, THAT'S INTERESTING...

WHEN I SCRATCH THE INSIDE OF YOUR EAR...

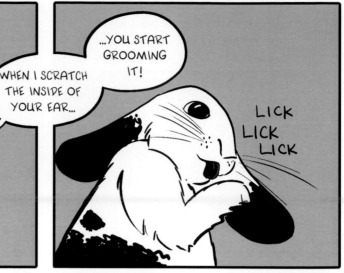

...YOU START GROOMING IT!

LICK LICK LICK

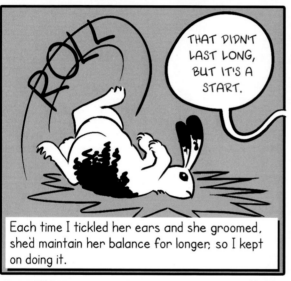

ROLL

THAT DIDN'T LAST LONG, BUT IT'S A START.

Each time I tickled her ears and she groomed, she'd maintain her balance for longer, so I kept on doing it.

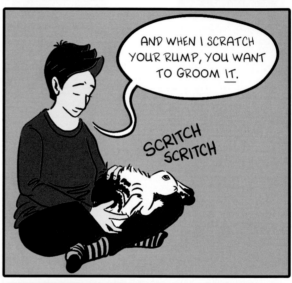

AND WHEN I SCRATCH YOUR RUMP, YOU WANT TO GROOM IT.

SCRITCH SCRITCH

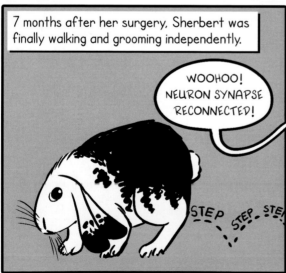

7 months after her surgery, Sherbert was finally walking and grooming independently.

WOOHOO! NEURON SYNAPSE RECONNECTED!

STEP STEP STE

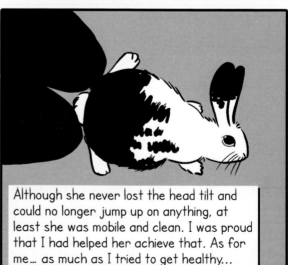

Although she never lost the head tilt and could no longer jump up on anything, at least she was mobile and clean. I was proud that I had helped her achieve that. As for me... as much as I tried to get healthy...

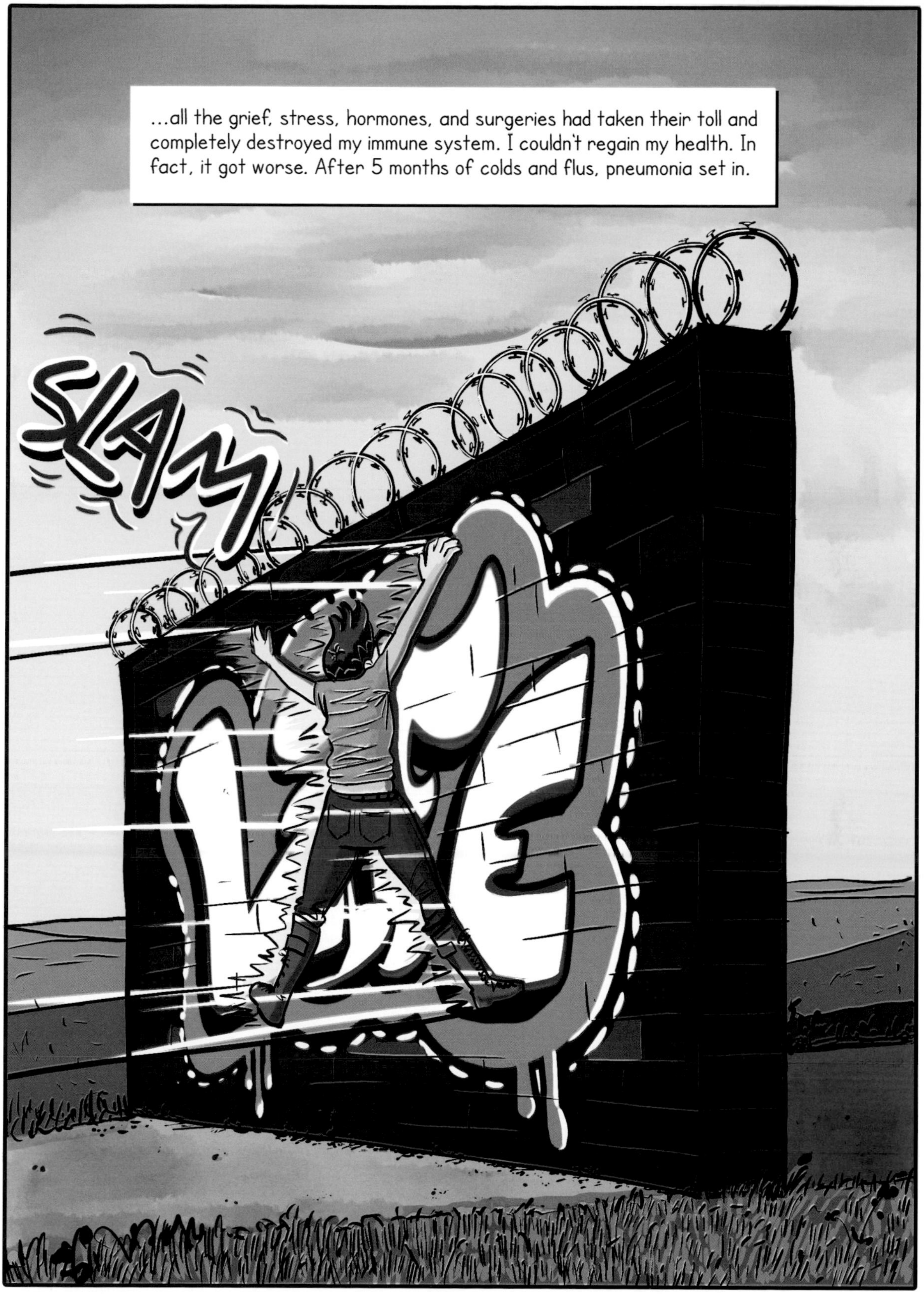
...all the grief, stress, hormones, and surgeries had taken their toll and completely destroyed my immune system. I couldn't regain my health. In fact, it got worse. After 5 months of colds and flus, pneumonia set in.
SLAM

Chapter 5

Leila

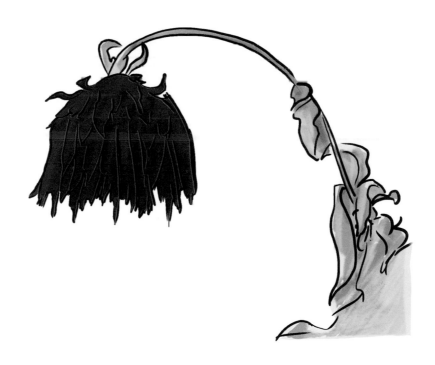

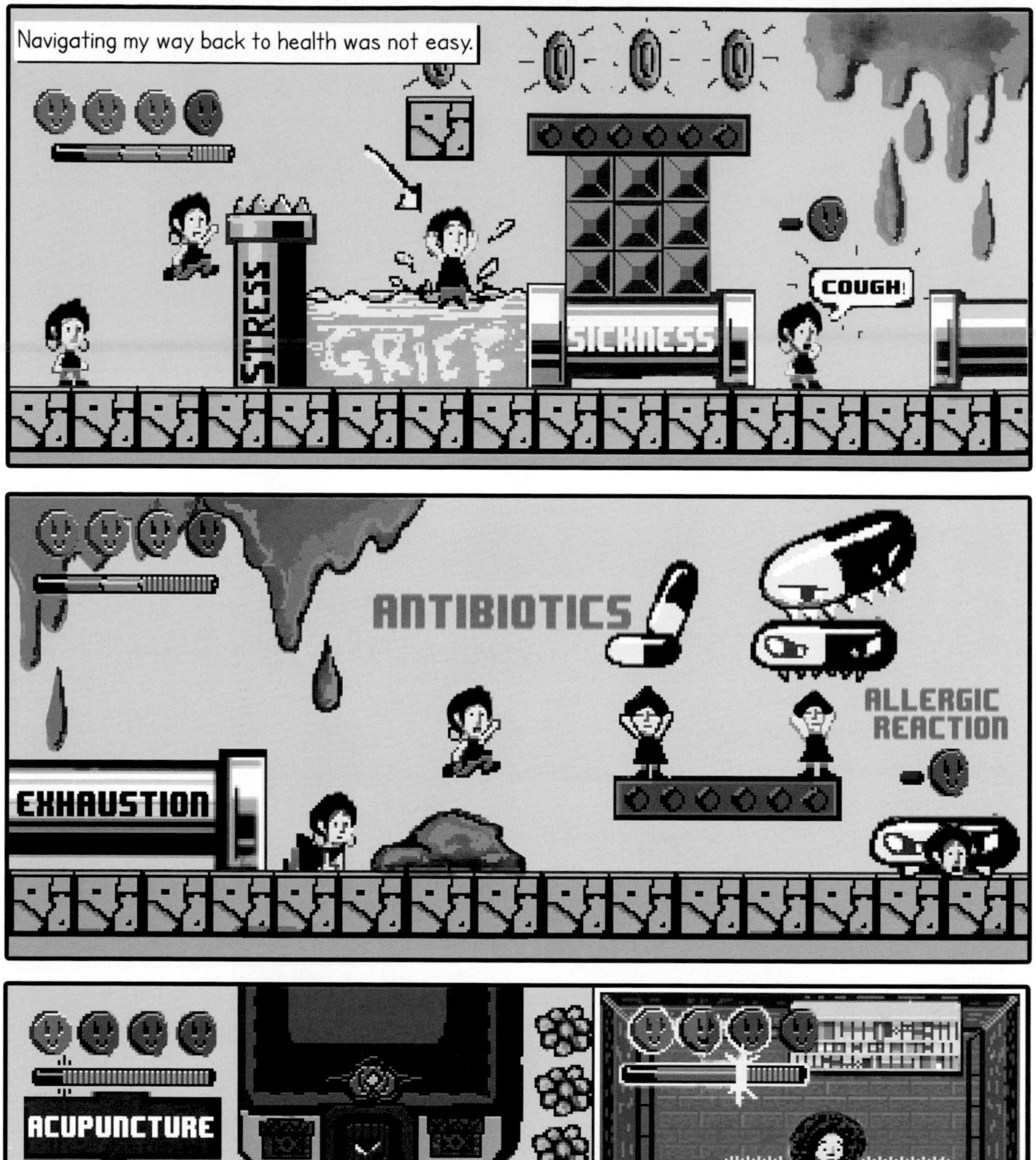
Navigating my way back to health was not easy.
STRESS
GRIEF
SICKNESS
COUGH!
ANTIBIOTICS
ALLERGIC REACTION
EXHAUSTION
ACUPUNCTURE
AHHHHHH

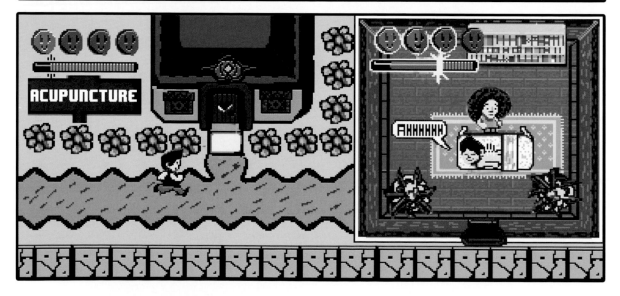

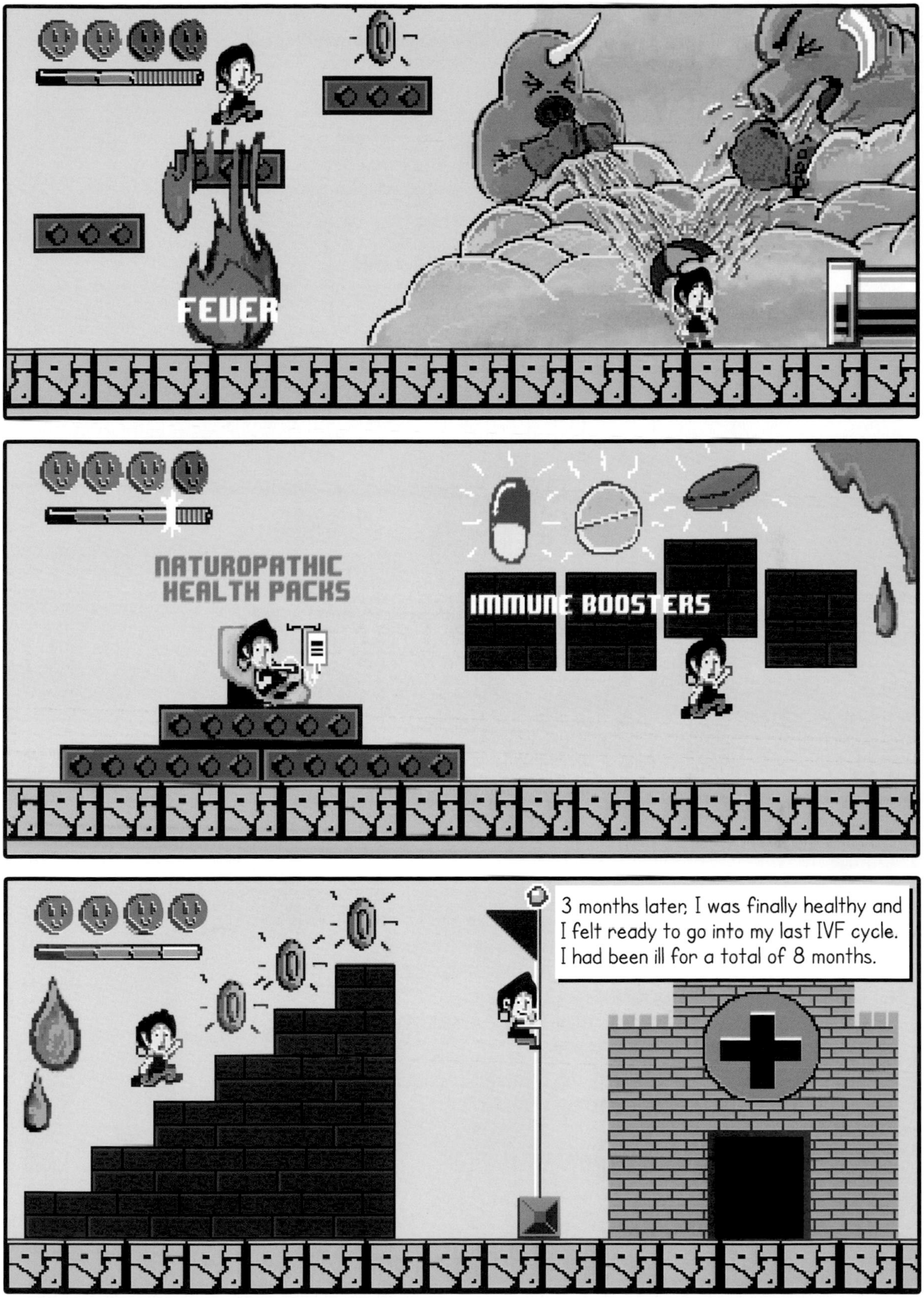
FEVER
NATUROPATHIC HEALTH PACKS
IMMUNE BOOSTERS
3 months later, I was finally healthy and I felt ready to go into my last IVF cycle. I had been ill for a total of 8 months.

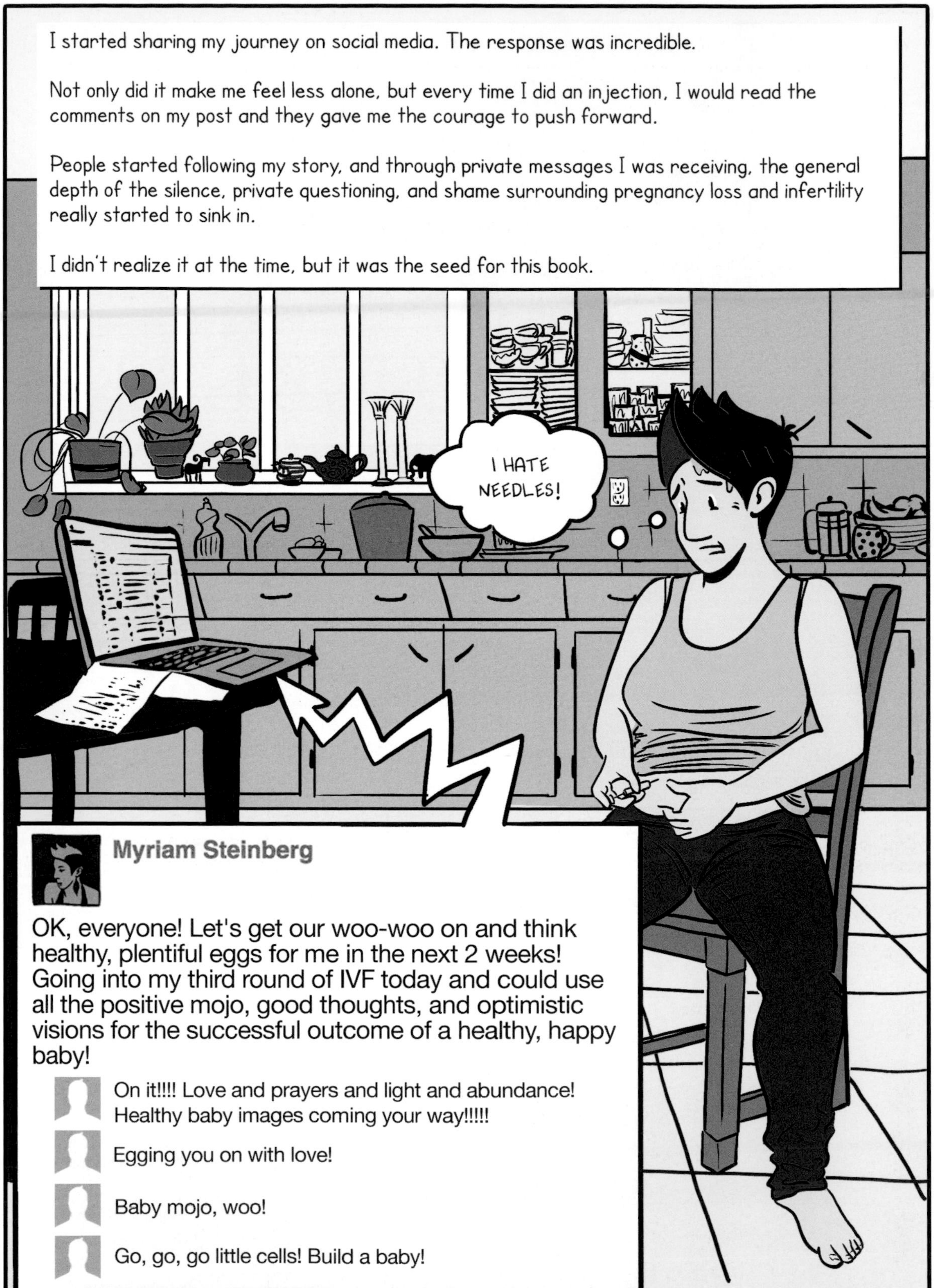
I started sharing my journey on social media. The response was incredible.
Not only did it make me feel less alone, but every time I did an injection, I would read the comments on my post and they gave me the courage to push forward.
People started following my story, and through private messages I was receiving, the general depth of the silence, private questioning, and shame surrounding pregnancy loss and infertility really started to sink in.
I didn't realize it at the time, but it was the seed for this book.
I HATE NEEDLES!
Myriam Steinberg
OK, everyone! Let's get our woo-woo on and think healthy, plentiful eggs for me in the next 2 weeks! Going into my third round of IVF today and could use all the positive mojo, good thoughts, and optimistic visions for the successful outcome of a healthy, happy baby!
On it!!!! Love and prayers and light and abundance! Healthy baby images coming your way!!!!!
Egging you on with love!
Baby mojo, woo!
Go, go, go little cells! Build a baby!

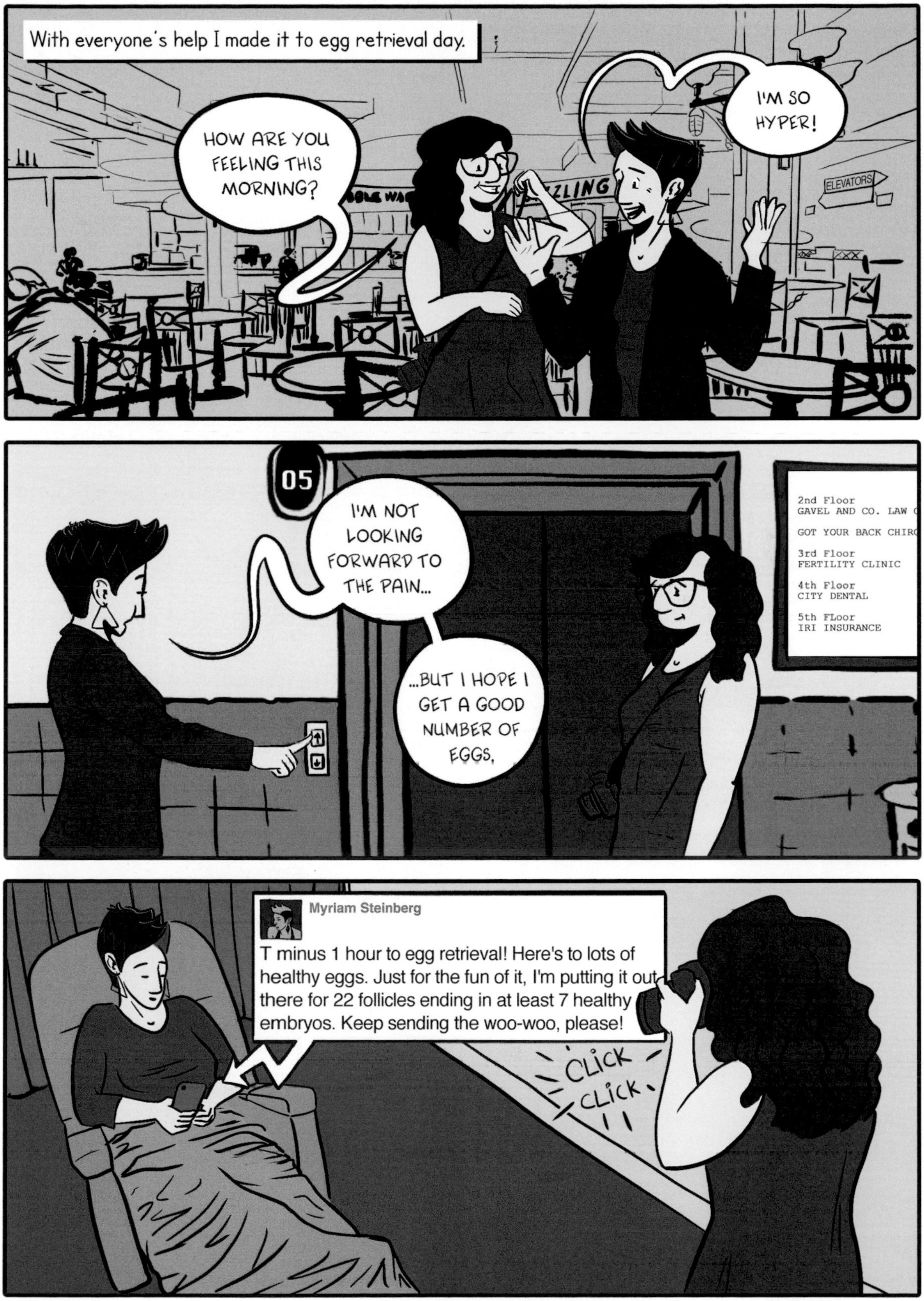
With everyone's help I made it to egg retrieval day.
HOW ARE YOU FEELING THIS MORNING?
I'M SO HYPER!
ELEVATORS
05
I'M NOT LOOKING FORWARD TO THE PAIN...
...BUT I HOPE I GET A GOOD NUMBER OF EGGS.
2nd Floor
GAVEL AND CO. LAW
GOT YOUR BACK CHIR
3rd Floor
FERTILITY CLINIC
4th Floor
CITY DENTAL
5th FLoor
IRI INSURANCE
Myriam Steinberg
T minus 1 hour to egg retrieval! Here's to lots of healthy eggs. Just for the fun of it, I'm putting it out there for 22 follicles ending in at least 7 healthy embryos. Keep sending the woo-woo, please!
CLICK
CLICK

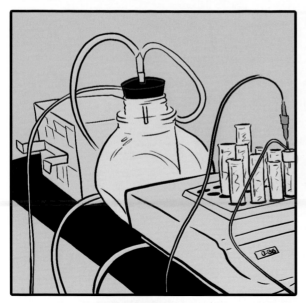

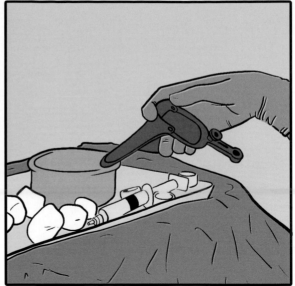

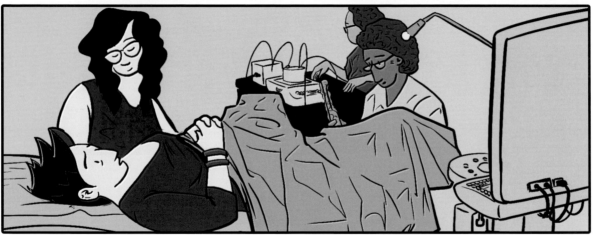

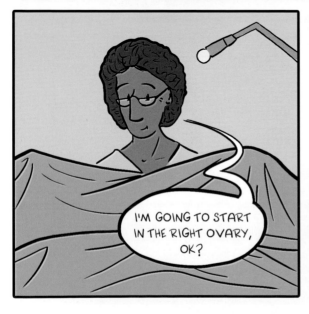

I'M GOING TO START IN THE RIGHT OVARY, OK?

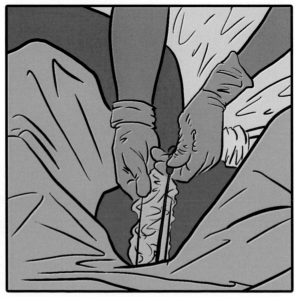

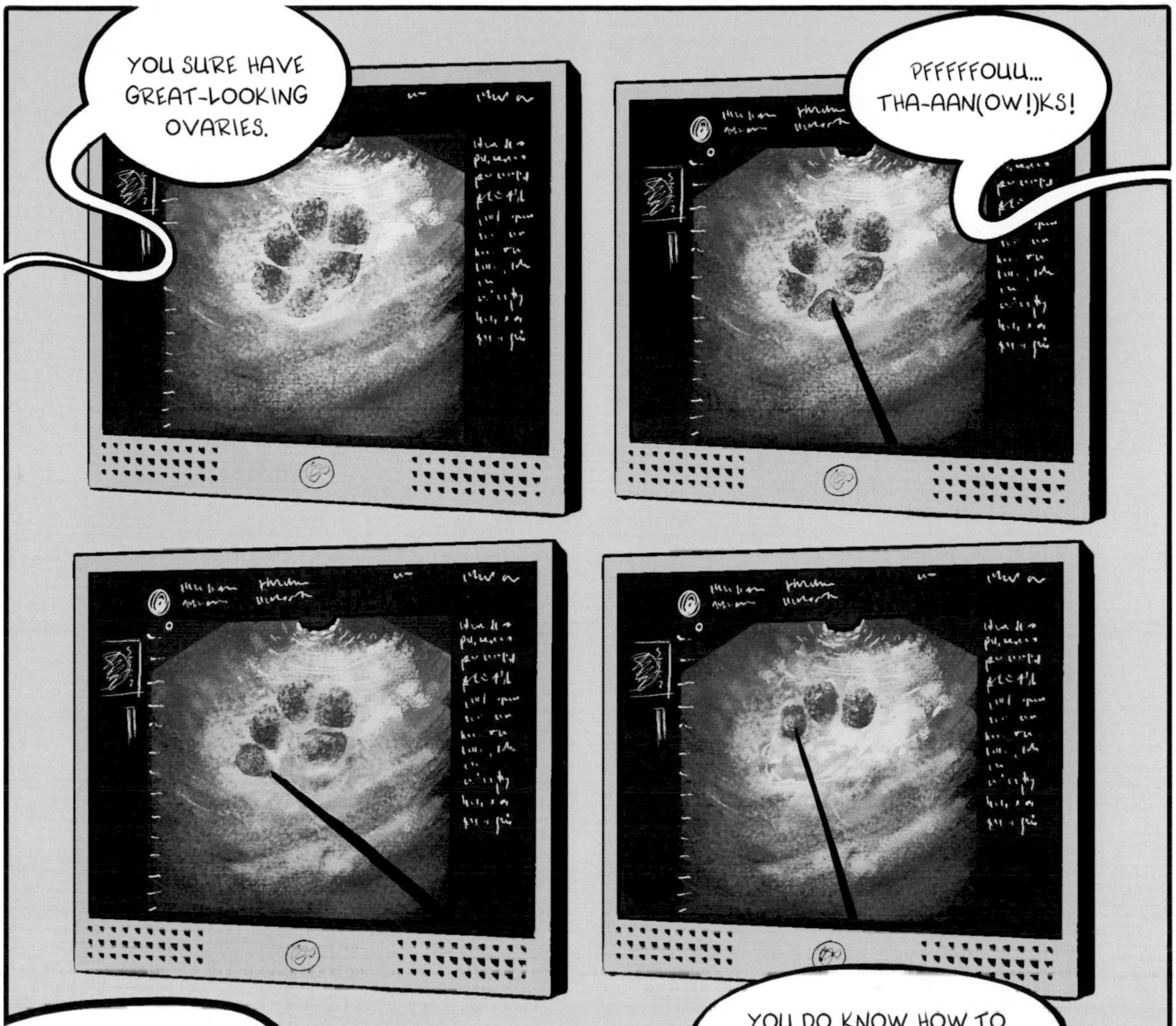
YOU SURE HAVE GREAT-LOOKING OVARIES.
PFFFFFOUU... THA-AAN(OW!)KS!

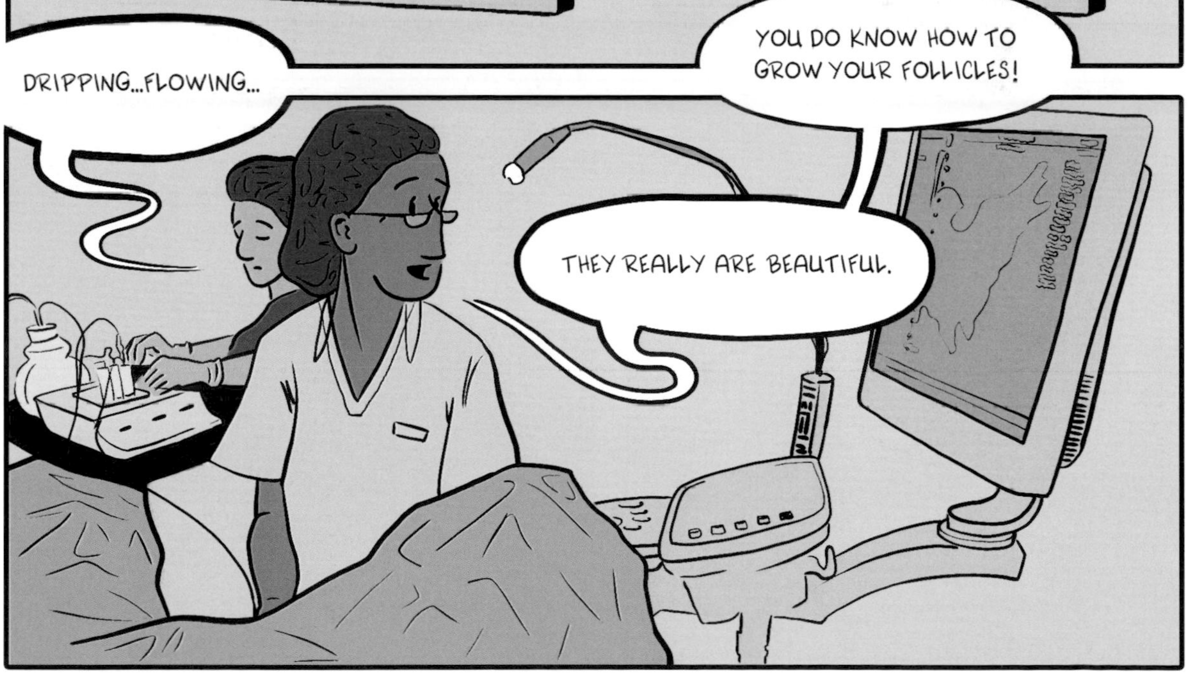
DRIPPING...FLOWING...
YOU DO KNOW HOW TO GROW YOUR FOLLICLES!
THEY REALLY ARE BEAUTIFUL.

I'M GOING TO GO TO THE LEFT SIDE NOW.
CAN WE TAKE A LITTLE BREAK?
OF COURSE!
HERE'S SOME UNICORN FART SPARKLES TO MAKE YOU FEEL BETTER!
MMMM! SMELLS LIKE CANDY!
HOW MANY EGGS ARE THERE SO FAR?
I DON'T KNOW. I JUST DRAIN EVERYTHING I CAN SEE.
THE EGG IS MICROSCOPIC RIGHT NOW, SO YOU ONLY SEE THE FLUID.

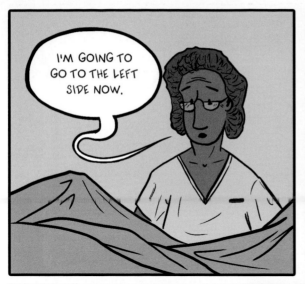

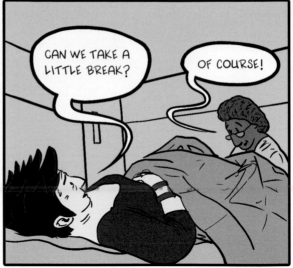

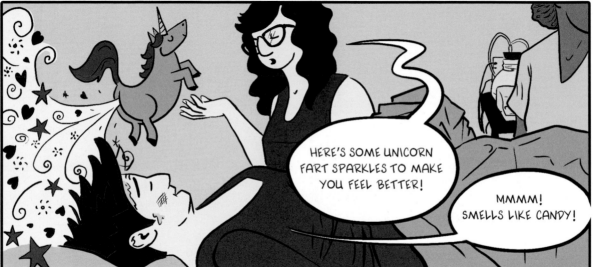

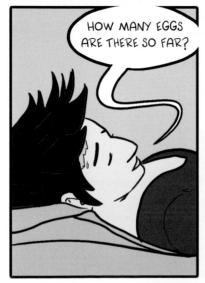

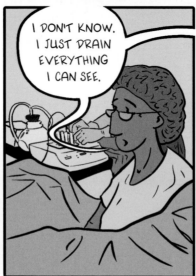

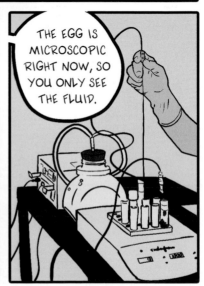

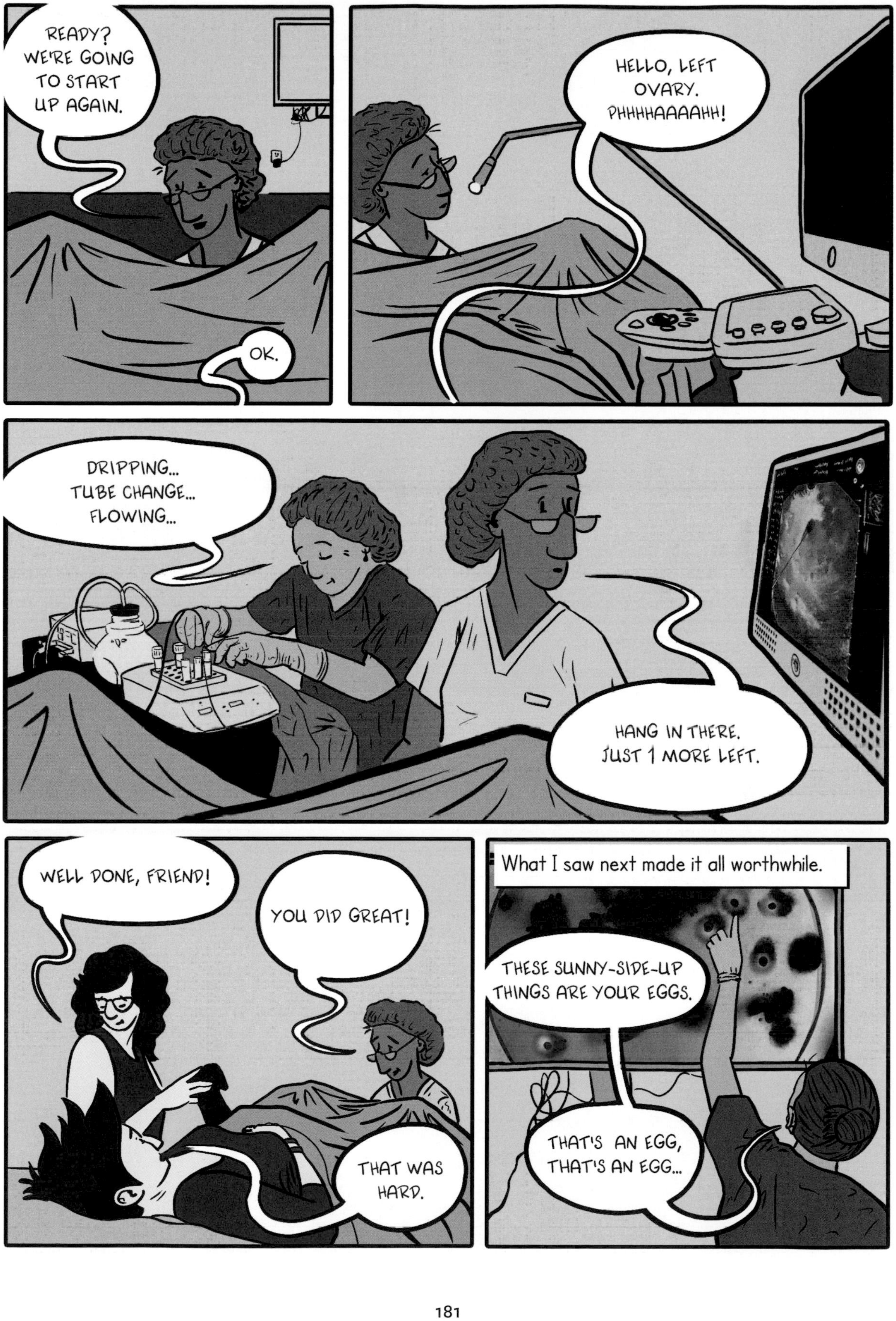
READY? WE'RE GOING TO START UP AGAIN.
OK.
HELLO, LEFT OVARY. PHHHHAAAAHH!
DRIPPING... TUBE CHANGE... FLOWING...
HANG IN THERE. JUST 1 MORE LEFT.
WELL DONE, FRIEND!
YOU DID GREAT!
THAT WAS HARD.
What I saw next made it all worthwhile.
THESE SUNNY-SIDE-UP THINGS ARE YOUR EGGS.
THAT'S AN EGG, THAT'S AN EGG...

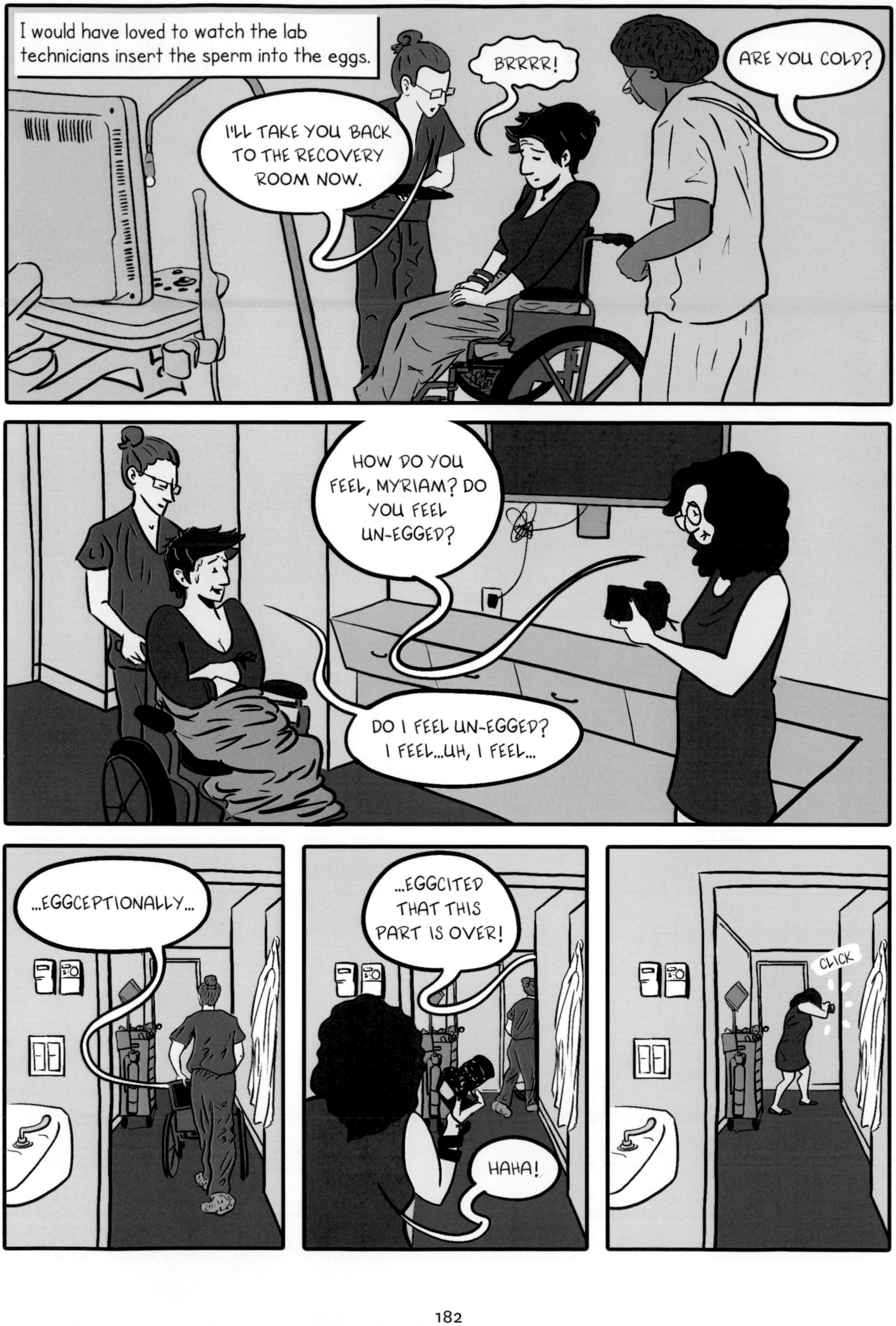
I would have loved to watch the lab technicians insert the sperm into the eggs.
I'LL TAKE YOU BACK TO THE RECOVERY ROOM NOW.
BRRRR!
ARE YOU COLD?
HOW DO YOU FEEL, MYRIAM? DO YOU FEEL UN-EGGED?
DO I FEEL UN-EGGED? I FEEL...UH, I FEEL...
...EGGCEPTIONALLY...
...EGGCITED THAT THIS PART IS OVER!
HAHA!
CLICK

REC
SO, MYRIAM. YOU'RE ON DRUGS...
REC
I'M SO ON DRUGS RIGHT NOW... I SURE AM!
I'M SO TIRED!
REC
WELL, THEY DID JUST SUCK OUT ALL YOUR EGGS.
YEAH... LOOKS LIKE THERE WERE AT LEAST 20 EGGS.
18, ACTUALLY. JUST GOT THE NUMBER FROM THE LAB.
OH, THAT'S GREAT! THANKS!
18 LITTLE EGGIES!
AND NOW THEY GET FERTILIZED.
AND IN 5 OR 6 DAYS WE SEE HOW MANY SURVIVE AND GROW INTO BLASTOCYSTS AND...
...ARE BIG ENOUGH TO GET BIOPSIED AND TESTED.
HOPEFULLY I'LL END UP WITH THOSE 7 HEALTHY EMBRYOS TO CHOOSE FROM!

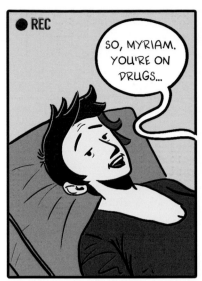

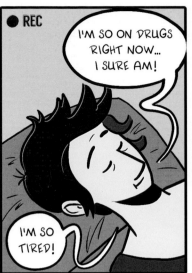

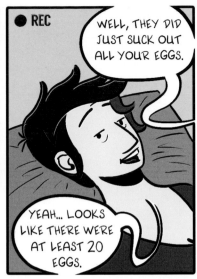

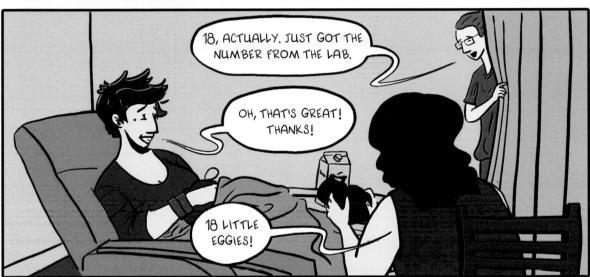

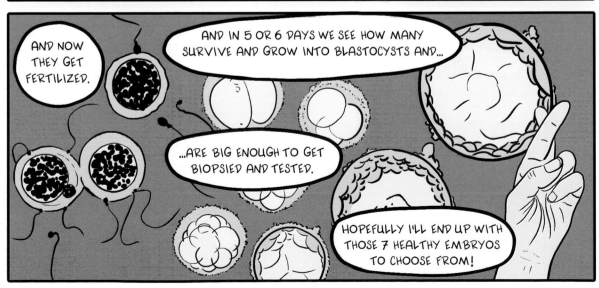

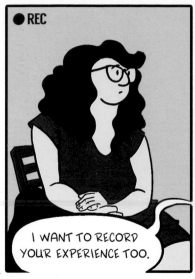

● REC

I WANT TO RECORD YOUR EXPERIENCE TOO.

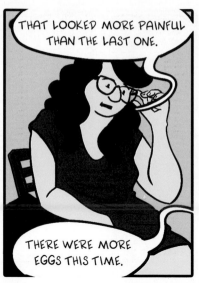

THAT LOOKED MORE PAINFUL THAN THE LAST ONE.

THERE WERE MORE EGGS THIS TIME.

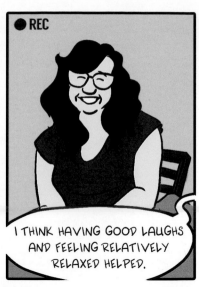

● REC

I THINK HAVING GOOD LAUGHS AND FEELING RELATIVELY RELAXED HELPED.

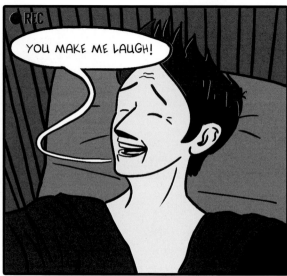

● REC

YOU MAKE ME LAUGH!

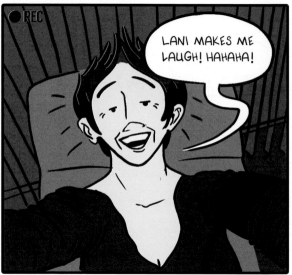

● REC

LANI MAKES ME LAUGH! HAHAHA!

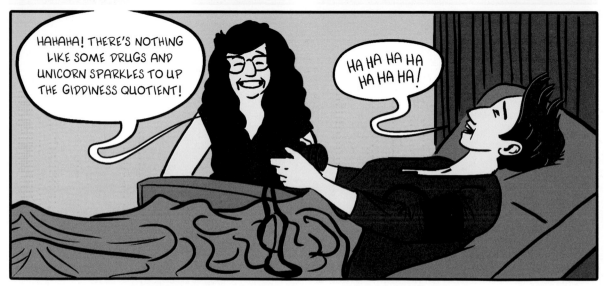

HAHAHA! THERE'S NOTHING LIKE SOME DRUGS AND UNICORN SPARKLES TO UP THE GIDDINESS QUOTIENT!

HA HA HA HA HA HA HA!

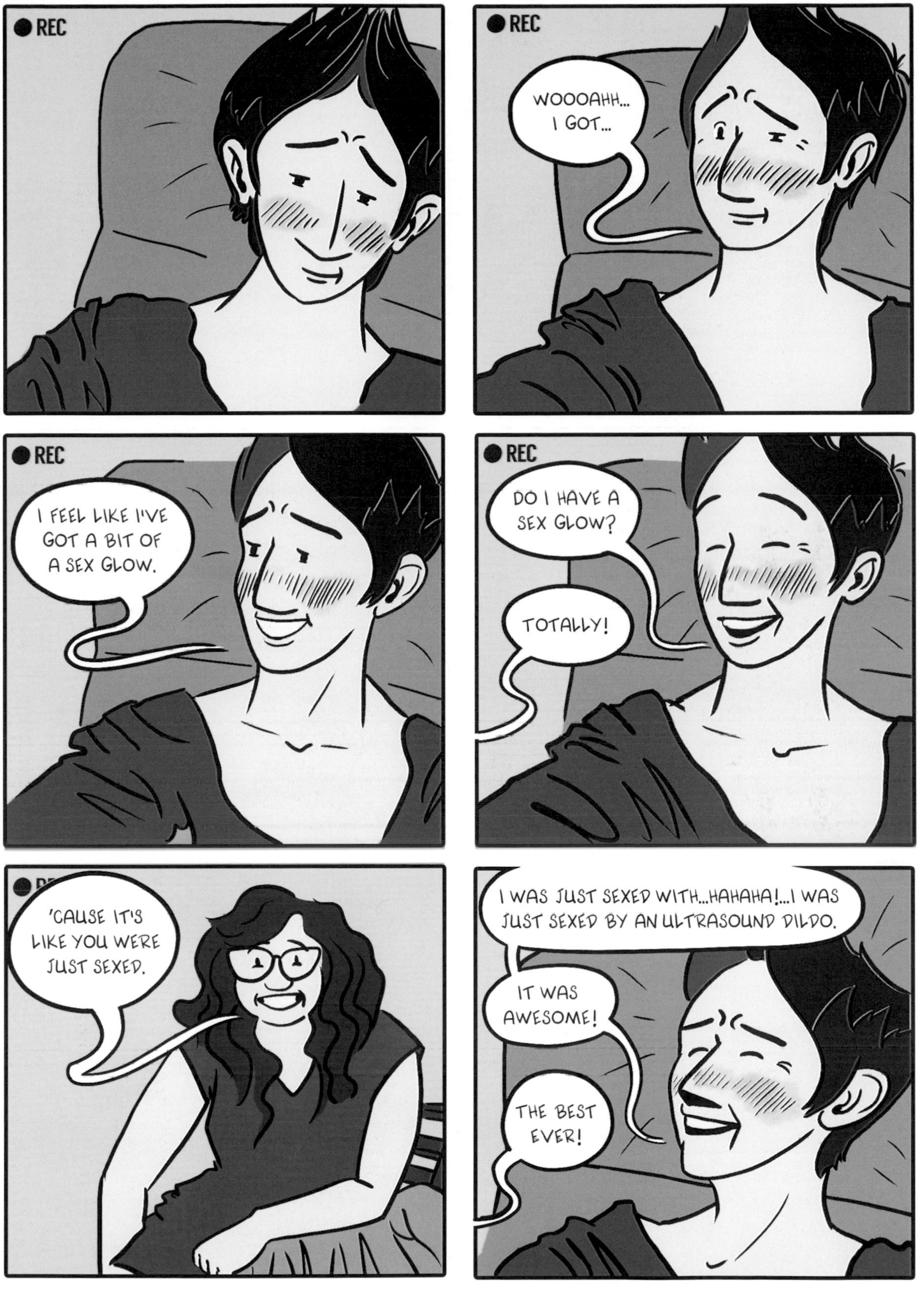
REC
REC
WOOOAHH... I GOT...
REC
I FEEL LIKE I'VE GOT A BIT OF A SEX GLOW.
REC
DO I HAVE A SEX GLOW?
TOTALLY!
'CAUSE IT'S LIKE YOU WERE JUST SEXED.
I WAS JUST SEXED WITH...HAHAHA!...I WAS JUST SEXED BY AN ULTRASOUND DILDO.
IT WAS AWESOME!
THE BEST EVER!

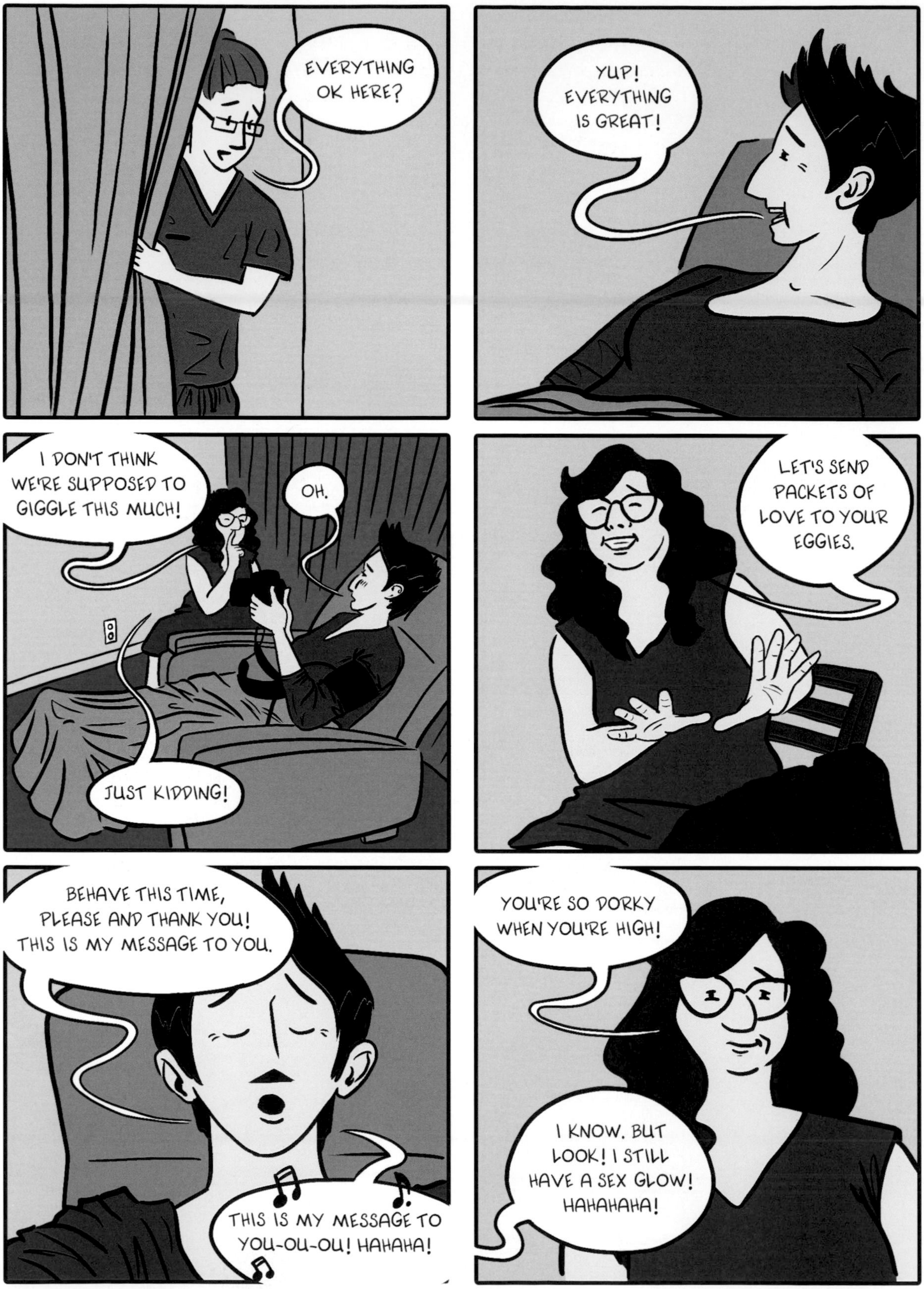
EVERYTHING OK HERE?
YUP! EVERYTHING IS GREAT!
I DON'T THINK WE'RE SUPPOSED TO GIGGLE THIS MUCH!
OH.
JUST KIDDING!
LET'S SEND PACKETS OF LOVE TO YOUR EGGIES.
BEHAVE THIS TIME, PLEASE AND THANK YOU! THIS IS MY MESSAGE TO YOU.
THIS IS MY MESSAGE TO YOU-OU-OU! HAHAHA!
YOU'RE SO DORKY WHEN YOU'RE HIGH!
I KNOW. BUT LOOK! I STILL HAVE A SEX GLOW! HAHAHAHA!

As I waited for the genetic test results, there were a few drugs I had to take to prepare my body in case there was an embryo transfer. Amongst them were progesterone and estrogen suppositories.

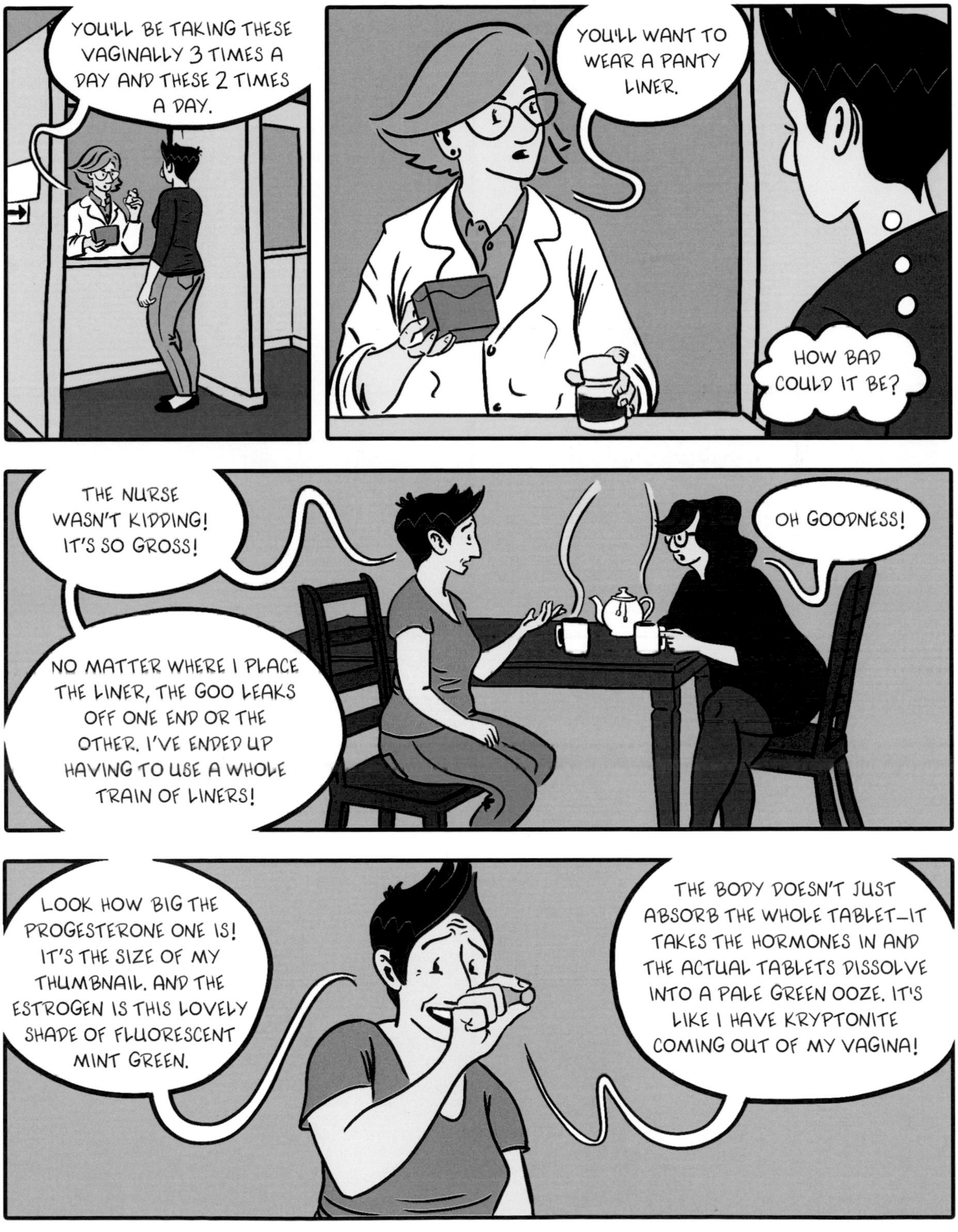
YOU'LL BE TAKING THESE VAGINALLY 3 TIMES A DAY AND THESE 2 TIMES A DAY.
YOU'LL WANT TO WEAR A PANTY LINER.
HOW BAD COULD IT BE?
THE NURSE WASN'T KIDDING! IT'S SO GROSS!
NO MATTER WHERE I PLACE THE LINER, THE GOO LEAKS OFF ONE END OR THE OTHER. I'VE ENDED UP HAVING TO USE A WHOLE TRAIN OF LINERS!
OH GOODNESS!
LOOK HOW BIG THE PROGESTERONE ONE IS! IT'S THE SIZE OF MY THUMBNAIL. AND THE ESTROGEN IS THIS LOVELY SHADE OF FLUORESCENT MINT GREEN.
THE BODY DOESN'T JUST ABSORB THE WHOLE TABLET—IT TAKES THE HORMONES IN AND THE ACTUAL TABLETS DISSOLVE INTO A PALE GREEN OOZE. IT'S LIKE I HAVE KRYPTONITE COMING OUT OF MY VAGINA!

And then there were the progesterone shots in the butt, which, if there was a pregnancy, had to continue for the first 12 weeks of gestation. This was the one thing I couldn't bring myself to do on my own. Thank goodness for community! Each person had their own style.

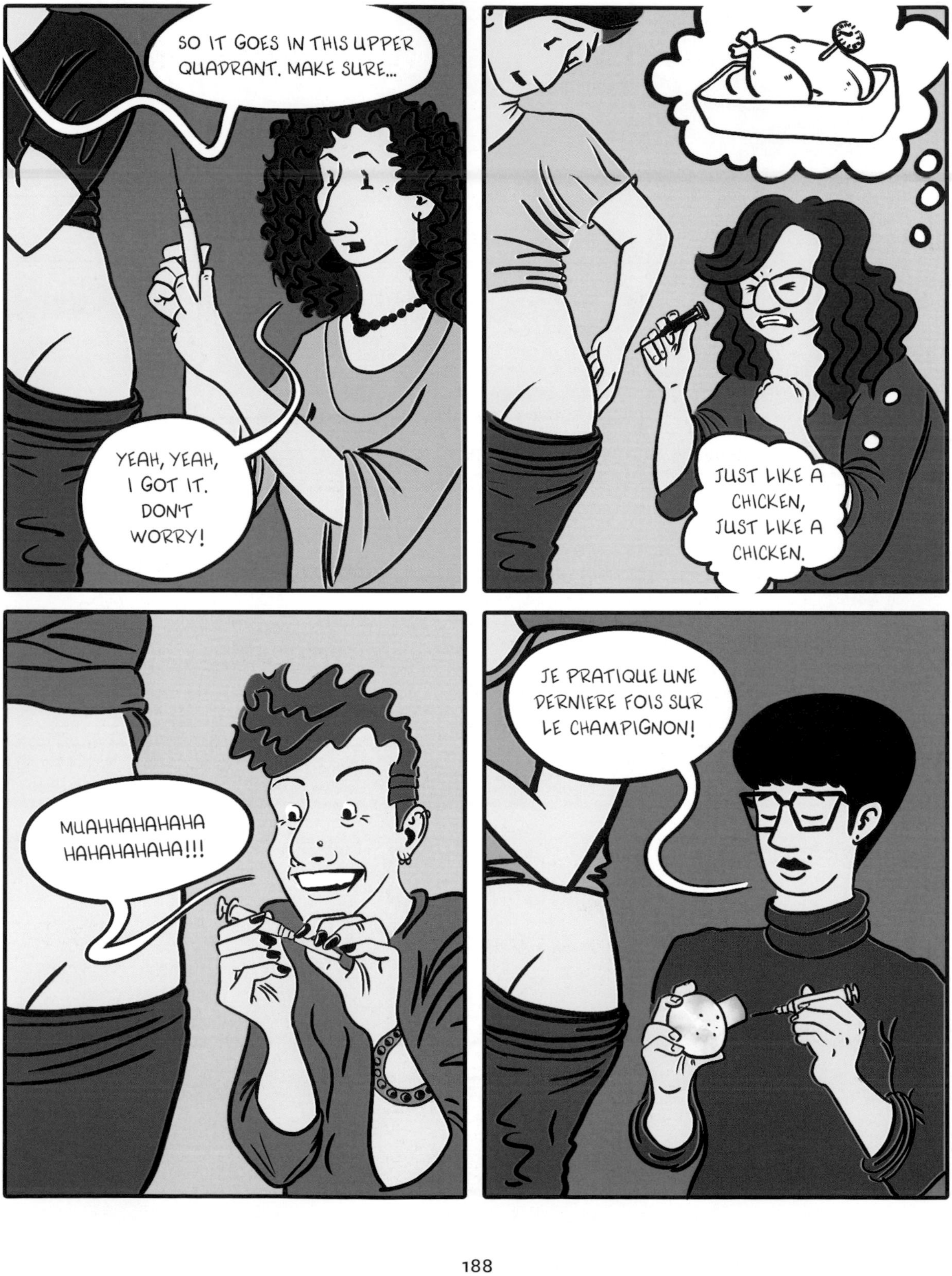

SO IT GOES IN THIS UPPER QUADRANT. MAKE SURE...
YEAH, YEAH, I GOT IT. DON'T WORRY!
JUST LIKE A CHICKEN, JUST LIKE A CHICKEN.
MUAHHHAHAHAHA HAHAHAHAHA!!!
JE PRATIQUE UNE DERNIERE FOIS SUR LE CHAMPIGNON!

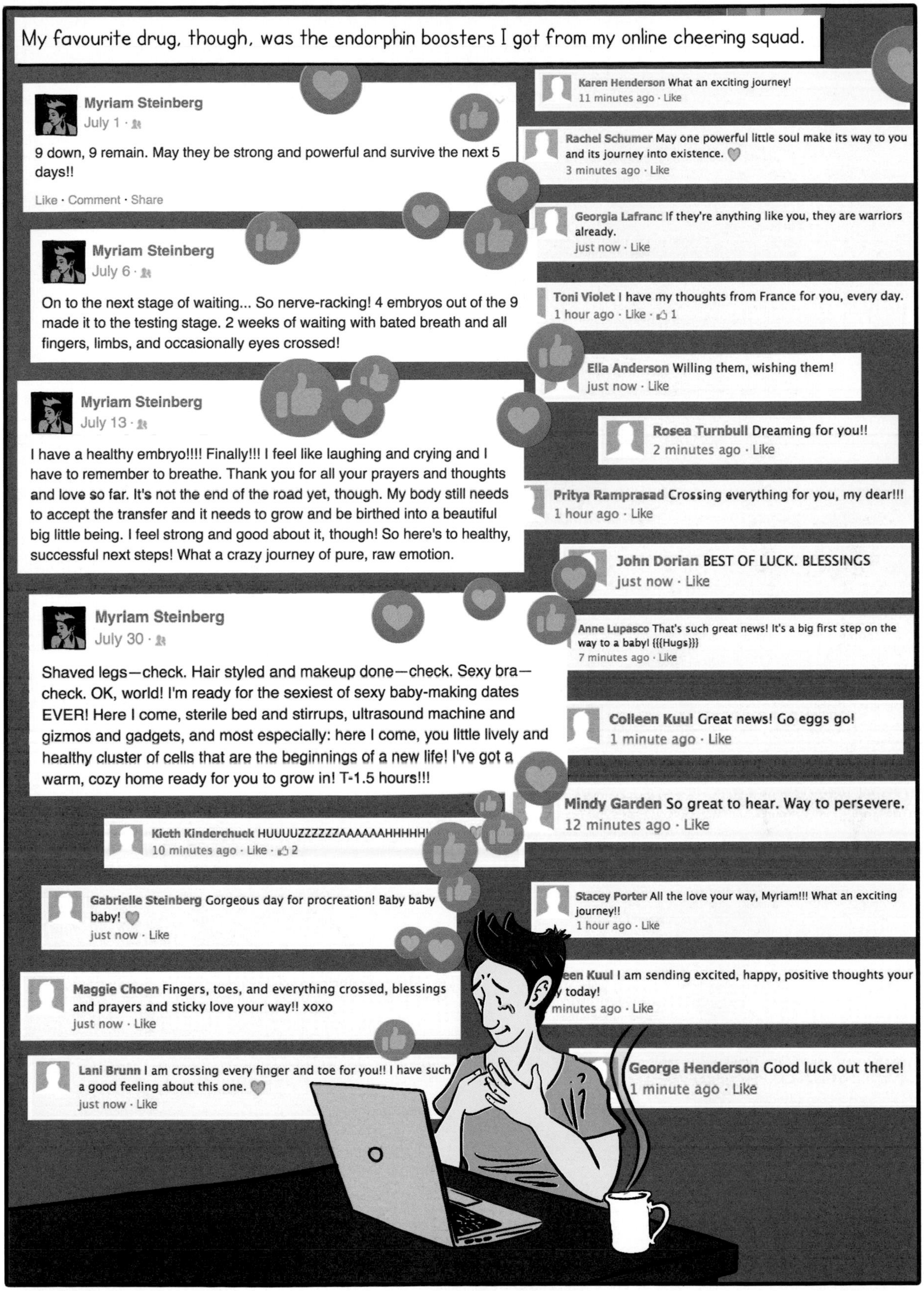

My favourite drug, though, was the endorphin boosters I got from my online cheering squad.
Myriam Steinberg
July 1 ·
9 down, 9 remain. May they be strong and powerful and survive the next 5 days!!
Like · Comment · Share
Myriam Steinberg
July 6 ·
On to the next stage of waiting... So nerve-racking! 4 embryos out of the 9 made it to the testing stage. 2 weeks of waiting with bated breath and all fingers, limbs, and occasionally eyes crossed!
Myriam Steinberg
July 13 ·
I have a healthy embryo!!!! Finally!!! I feel like laughing and crying and I have to remember to breathe. Thank you for all your prayers and thoughts and love so far. It's not the end of the road yet, though. My body still needs to accept the transfer and it needs to grow and be birthed into a beautiful big little being. I feel strong and good about it, though! So here's to healthy, successful next steps! What a crazy journey of pure, raw emotion.
Myriam Steinberg
July 30 ·
Shaved legs—check. Hair styled and makeup done—check. Sexy bra—check. OK, world! I'm ready for the sexiest of sexy baby-making dates EVER! Here I come, sterile bed and stirrups, ultrasound machine and gizmos and gadgets, and most especially: here I come, you little lively and healthy cluster of cells that are the beginnings of a new life! I've got a warm, cozy home ready for you to grow in! T-1.5 hours!!!
Kieth Kinderchuck HUUUUZZZZZZAAAAAAHHHHH
10 minutes ago · Like · 2
Gabrielle Steinberg Gorgeous day for procreation! Baby baby baby!
just now · Like
Maggie Choen Fingers, toes, and everything crossed, blessings and prayers and sticky love your way!! xoxo
just now · Like
Lani Brunn I am crossing every finger and toe for you!! I have such a good feeling about this one.
just now · Like
Karen Henderson What an exciting journey!
11 minutes ago · Like
Rachel Schumer May one powerful little soul make its way to you and its journey into existence.
3 minutes ago · Like
Georgia Lafranc If they're anything like you, they are warriors already.
just now · Like
Toni Violet I have my thoughts from France for you, every day.
1 hour ago · Like · 1
Ella Anderson Willing them, wishing them!
just now · Like
Rosea Turnbull Dreaming for you!!
2 minutes ago · Like
Pritya Ramprasad Crossing everything for you, my dear!!!
1 hour ago · Like
John Dorian BEST OF LUCK. BLESSINGS
just now · Like
Anne Lupasco That's such great news! It's a big first step on the way to a baby! {{{Hugs}}}
7 minutes ago · Like
Colleen Kuul Great news! Go eggs go!
1 minute ago · Like
Mindy Garden So great to hear. Way to persevere.
12 minutes ago · Like
Stacey Porter All the love your way, Myriam!!! What an exciting journey!!
1 hour ago · Like
een Kuul I am sending excited, happy, positive thoughts your
y today!
minutes ago · Like
George Henderson Good luck out there!
1 minute ago · Like

Finally, it was transfer day. The procedure was simple and fast.

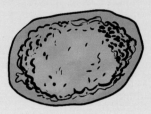

The most amazing thing was seeing the embryo onscreen as the embryologist was prepping it...

...and sucking it into the catheter that would bring the embryo into the procedure room.

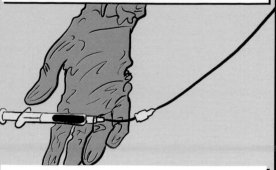

That cluster of cells, circles within circles, truly circles of life, was a human in the making.

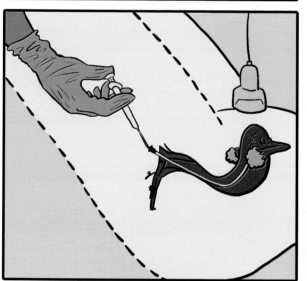

YOU SEE THAT WHITE BUBBLE THERE? THE EMBRYO SHOULD BE IN THAT NEIGHBOURHOOD.

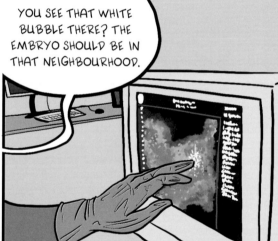

GOOD LUCK!

I HAVE AN EMBRYO INSIDE ME! AN ACTUAL BABY-TO-BE.

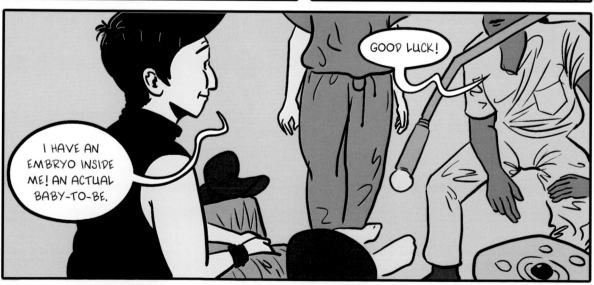

AND NOW WE WAIT.
CROSSING FINGERS FOR YOU. LARRY AND I ARE GOING TO START TRYING FOR NUMBER 2 IN NOVEMBER OR DECEMBER.
HE WANTS A SUMMER BABY. I'M NOT SURE WHY. SOMETHING ABOUT HOROSCOPES. HE'S REALLY INTO THEM. NOT SO MUCH MY THING, BUT WHATEVER FLOATS HIS BOAT I GUESS.
I'VE TRIED TELLING HIM THAT THERE'S NO GUARANTEES THAT WE'LL GET PREGNANT RIGHT AWAY EVEN THOUGH THAT'S WHAT HAPPENED WITH OUR FIRST KID, BUT HE WANTS TO TRY ANYWAYS. I DON'T KNOW IF I'M QUITE READY YET. I MEAN, I JUST GOT MY BODY BACK FROM THE FIRST PREGNANCY AND I JUST STOPPED BREASTFEEDING.
!
ZAP!!
I THINK IT TOOK.
IT WOULD BE NICE
TO WAIT A BIT
AND...
I HEAR THAT KIDS WITH
BIG AGE GAPS BETWEEN
...IT'S A GIRL!
IT'S NICE TO BE
OUTSIDE AND GET

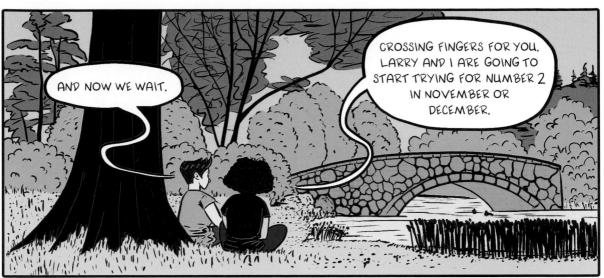

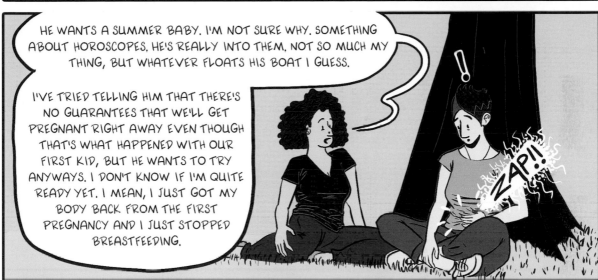

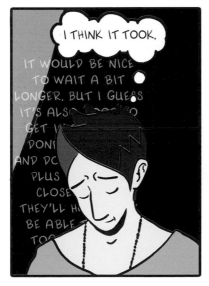

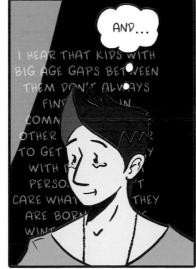

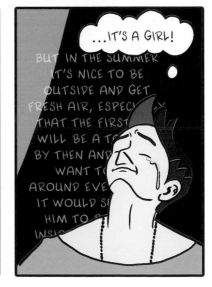

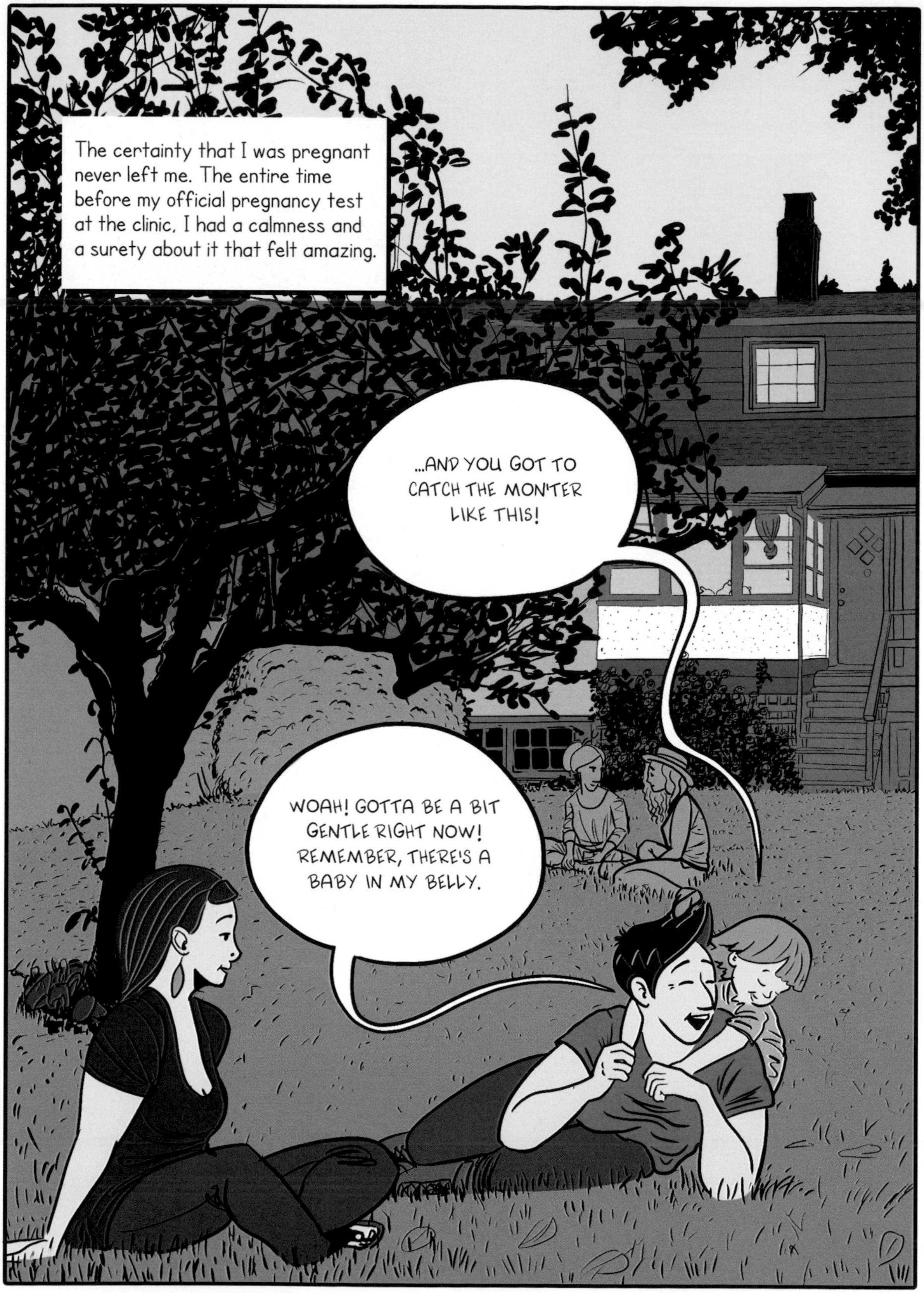
The certainty that I was pregnant never left me. The entire time before my official pregnancy test at the clinic, I had a calmness and a surety about it that felt amazing.
...AND YOU GOT TO CATCH THE MON'TER LIKE THIS!
WOAH! GOTTA BE A BIT GENTLE RIGHT NOW! REMEMBER, THERE'S A BABY IN MY BELLY.

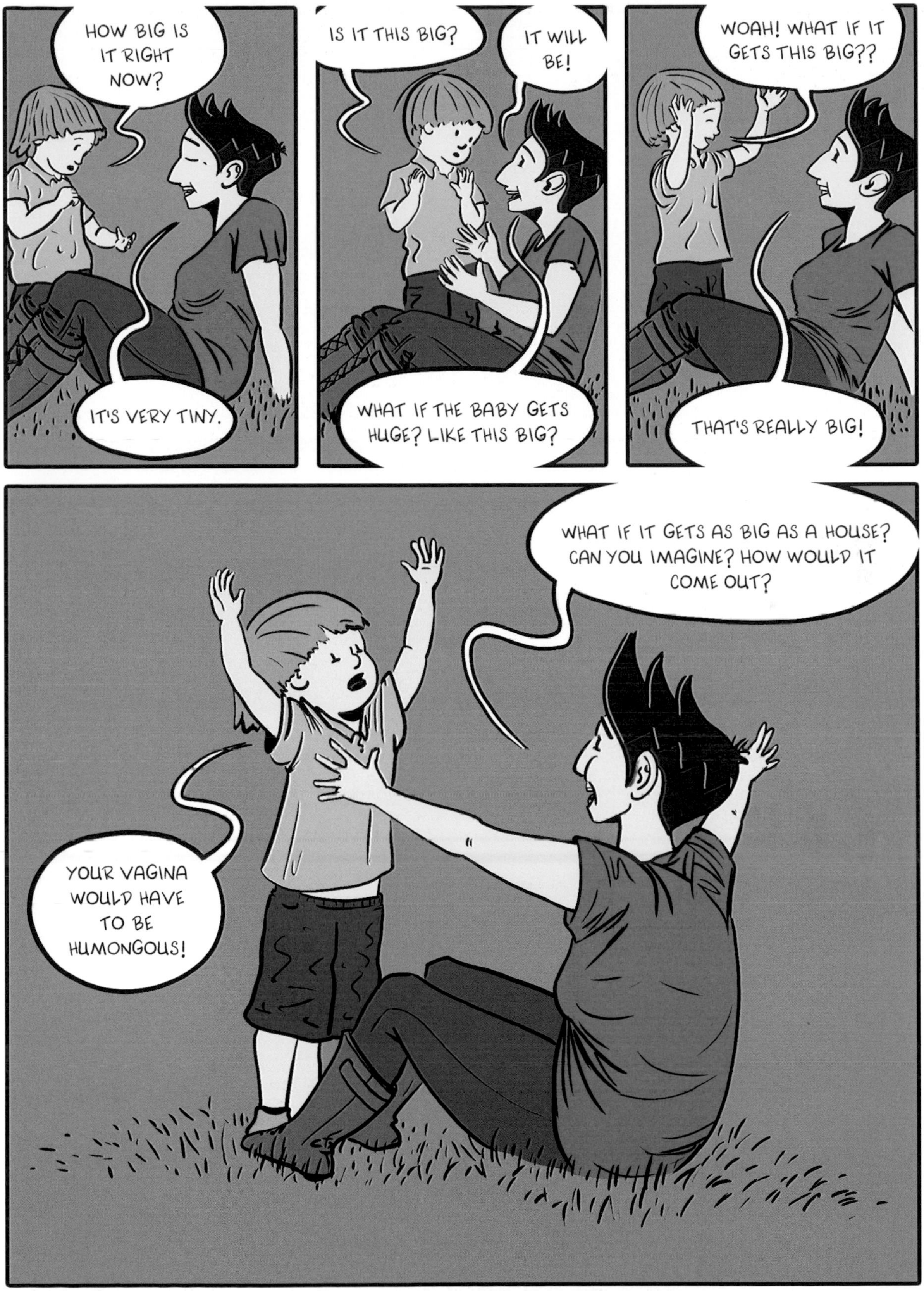
HOW BIG IS IT RIGHT NOW?
IT'S VERY TINY.
IS IT THIS BIG?
IT WILL BE!
WHAT IF THE BABY GETS HUGE? LIKE THIS BIG?
WOAH! WHAT IF IT GETS THIS BIG??
THAT'S REALLY BIG!
WHAT IF IT GETS AS BIG AS A HOUSE? CAN YOU IMAGINE? HOW WOULD IT COME OUT?
YOUR VAGINA WOULD HAVE TO BE HUMONGOUS!

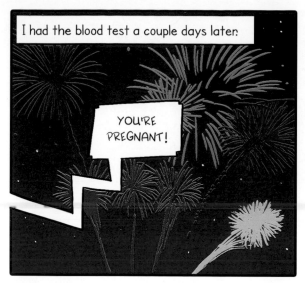

I had the blood test a couple days later.

YOU'RE PREGNANT!

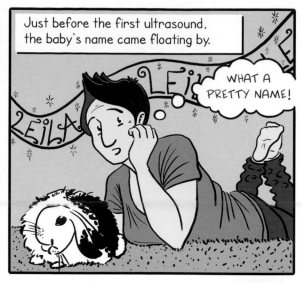

Just before the first ultrasound, the baby's name came floating by.

WHAT A PRETTY NAME!

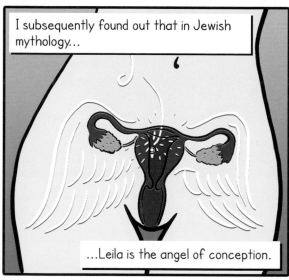

I subsequently found out that in Jewish mythology...

...Leila is the angel of conception.

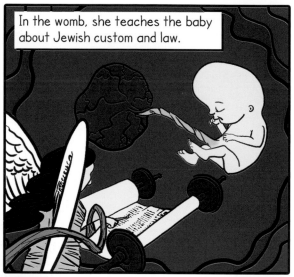

In the womb, she teaches the baby about Jewish custom and law.

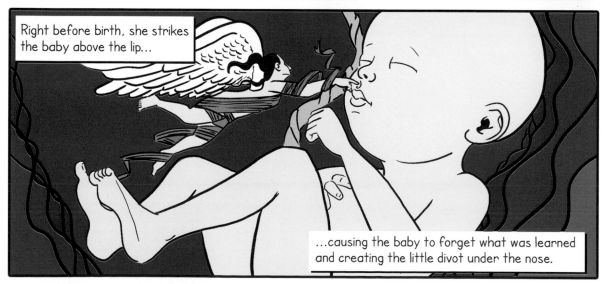

Right before birth, she strikes the baby above the lip...

...causing the baby to forget what was learned and creating the little divot under the nose.

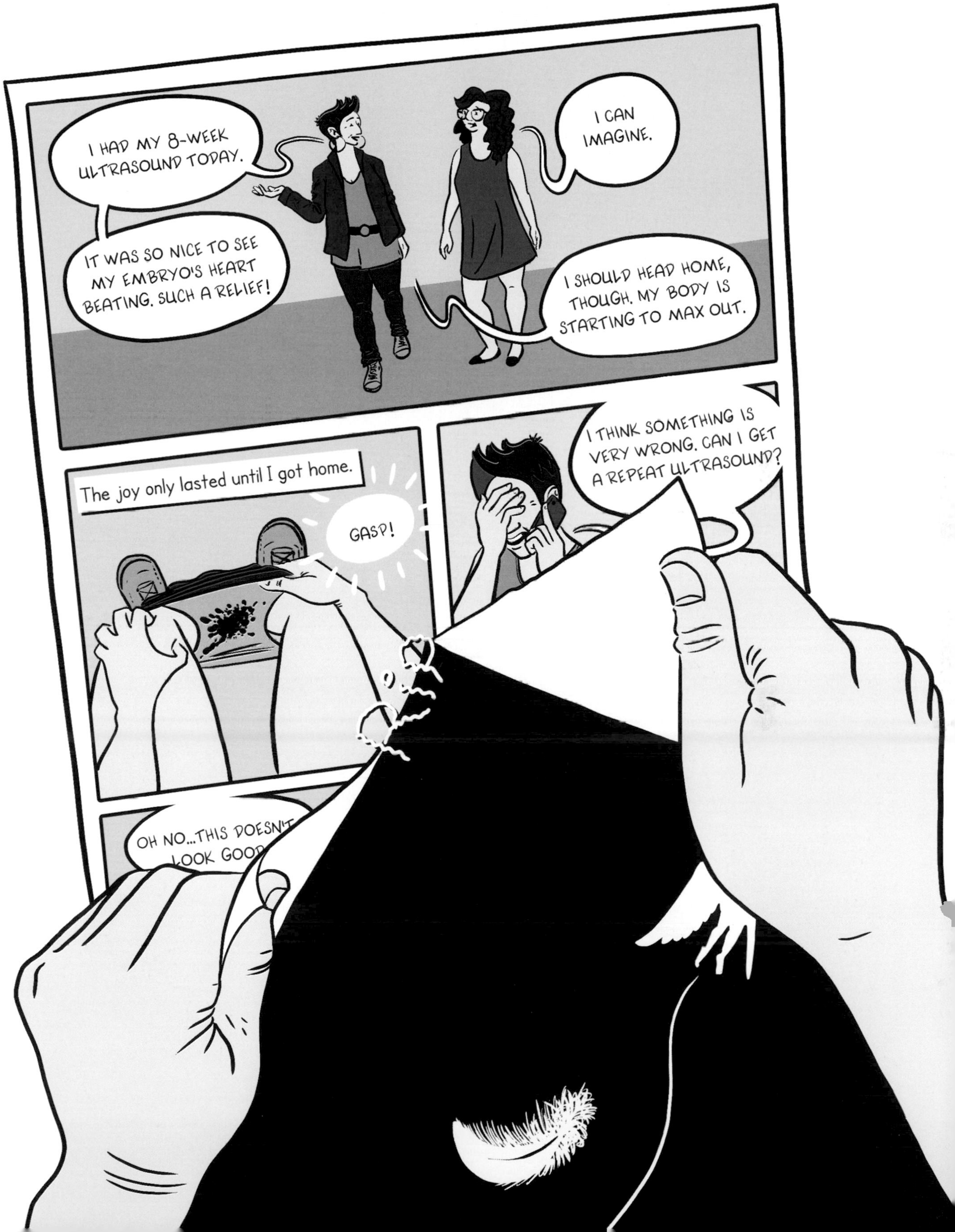
I HAD MY 8-WEEK ULTRASOUND TODAY.
IT WAS SO NICE TO SEE MY EMBRYO'S HEART BEATING. SUCH A RELIEF!
I CAN IMAGINE.
I SHOULD HEAD HOME, THOUGH. MY BODY IS STARTING TO MAX OUT.
The joy only lasted until I got home.
GASP!
I THINK SOMETHING IS VERY WRONG. CAN I GET A REPEAT ULTRASOUND?
OH NO...THIS DOESN'T LOOK GOOD

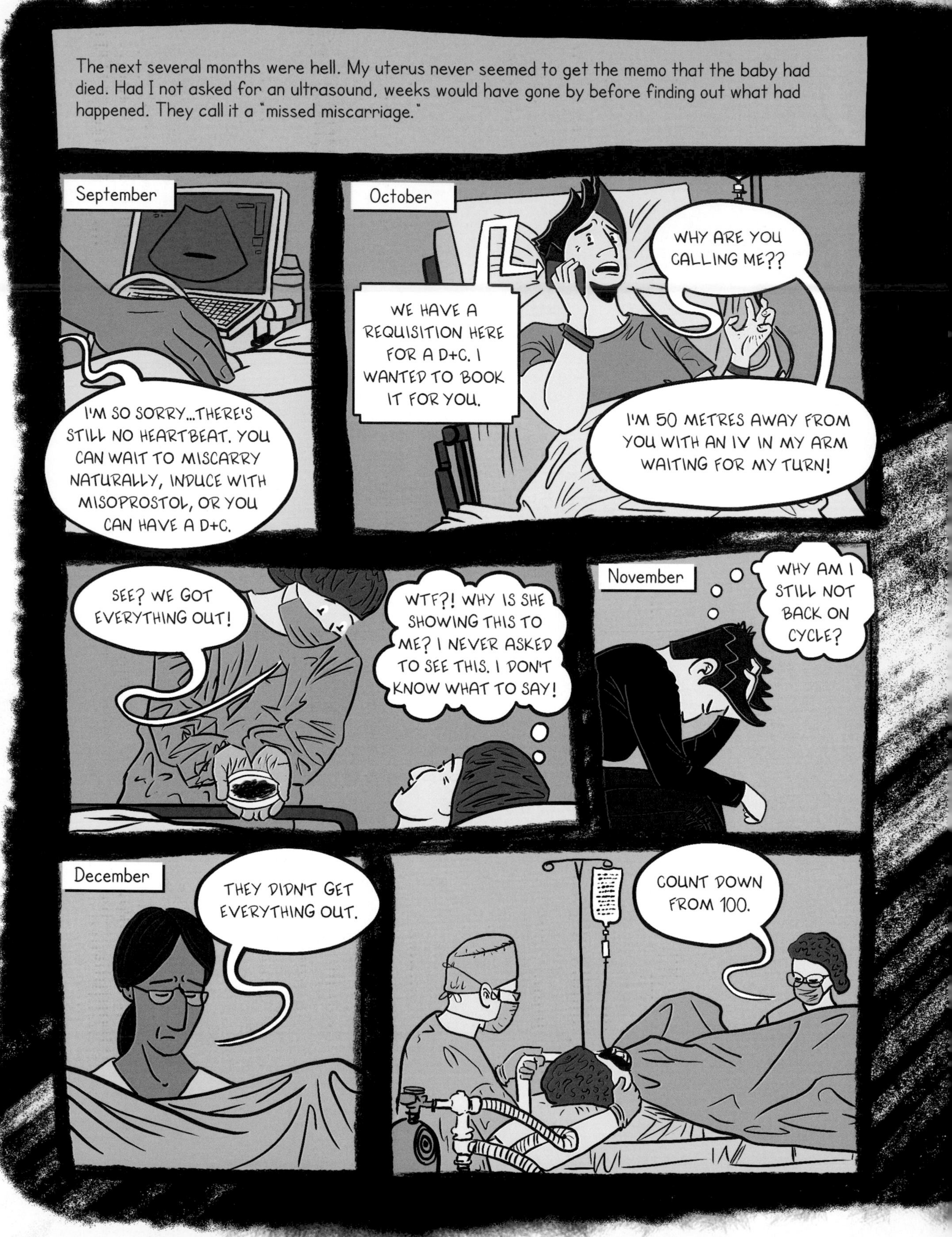

The next several months were hell. My uterus never seemed to get the memo that the baby had died. Had I not asked for an ultrasound, weeks would have gone by before finding out what had happened. They call it a "missed miscarriage."
September
I'M SO SORRY...THERE'S STILL NO HEARTBEAT. YOU CAN WAIT TO MISCARRY NATURALLY, INDUCE WITH MISOPROSTOL, OR YOU CAN HAVE A D+C.
October
WE HAVE A REQUISITION HERE FOR A D+C. I WANTED TO BOOK IT FOR YOU.
WHY ARE YOU CALLING ME??
I'M 50 METRES AWAY FROM YOU WITH AN IV IN MY ARM WAITING FOR MY TURN!
SEE? WE GOT EVERYTHING OUT!
WTF?! WHY IS SHE SHOWING THIS TO ME? I NEVER ASKED TO SEE THIS. I DON'T KNOW WHAT TO SAY!
November
WHY AM I STILL NOT BACK ON CYCLE?
December
THEY DIDN'T GET EVERYTHING OUT.
COUNT DOWN FROM 100.

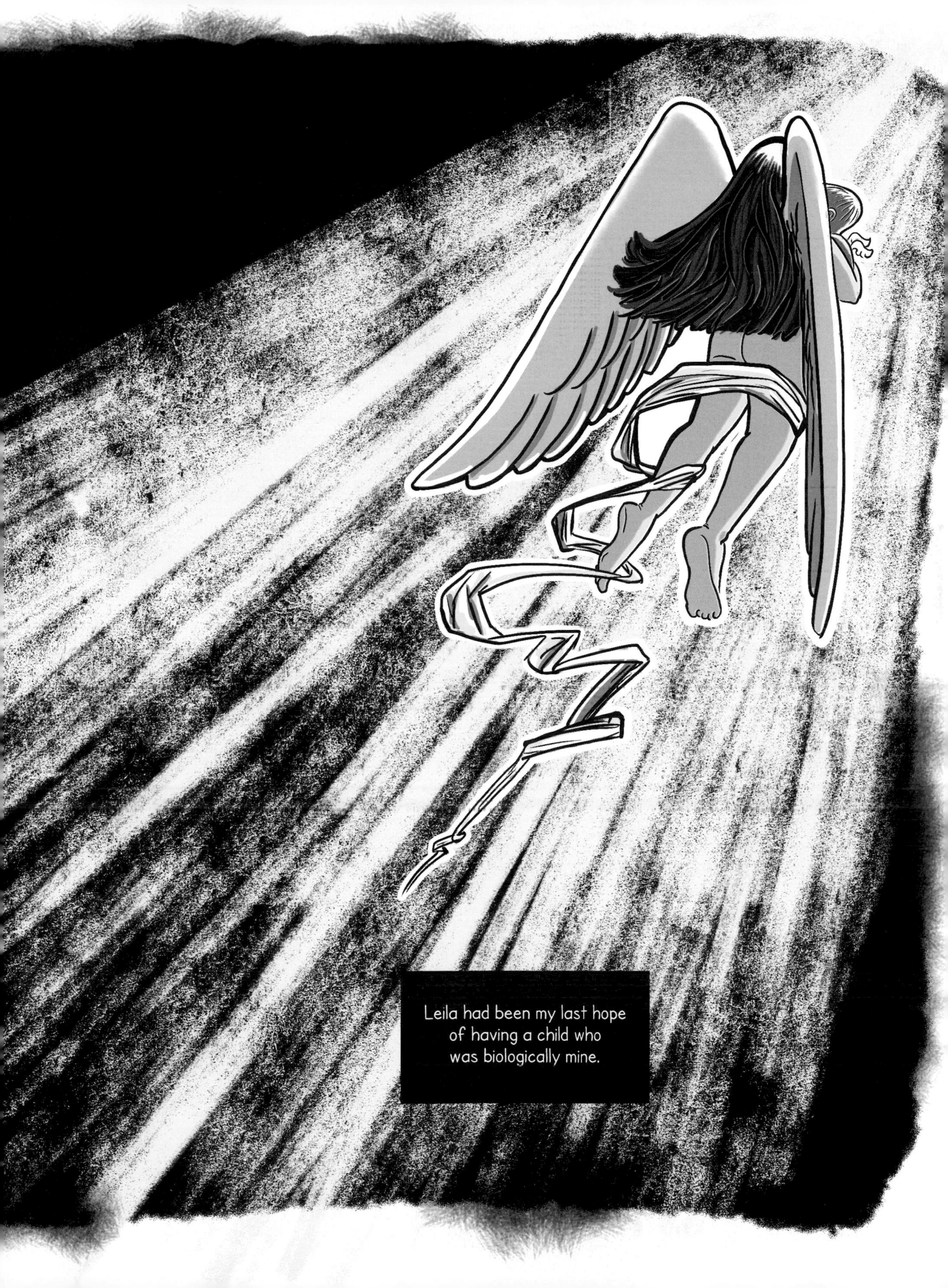
Leila had been my last hope of having a child who was biologically mine.

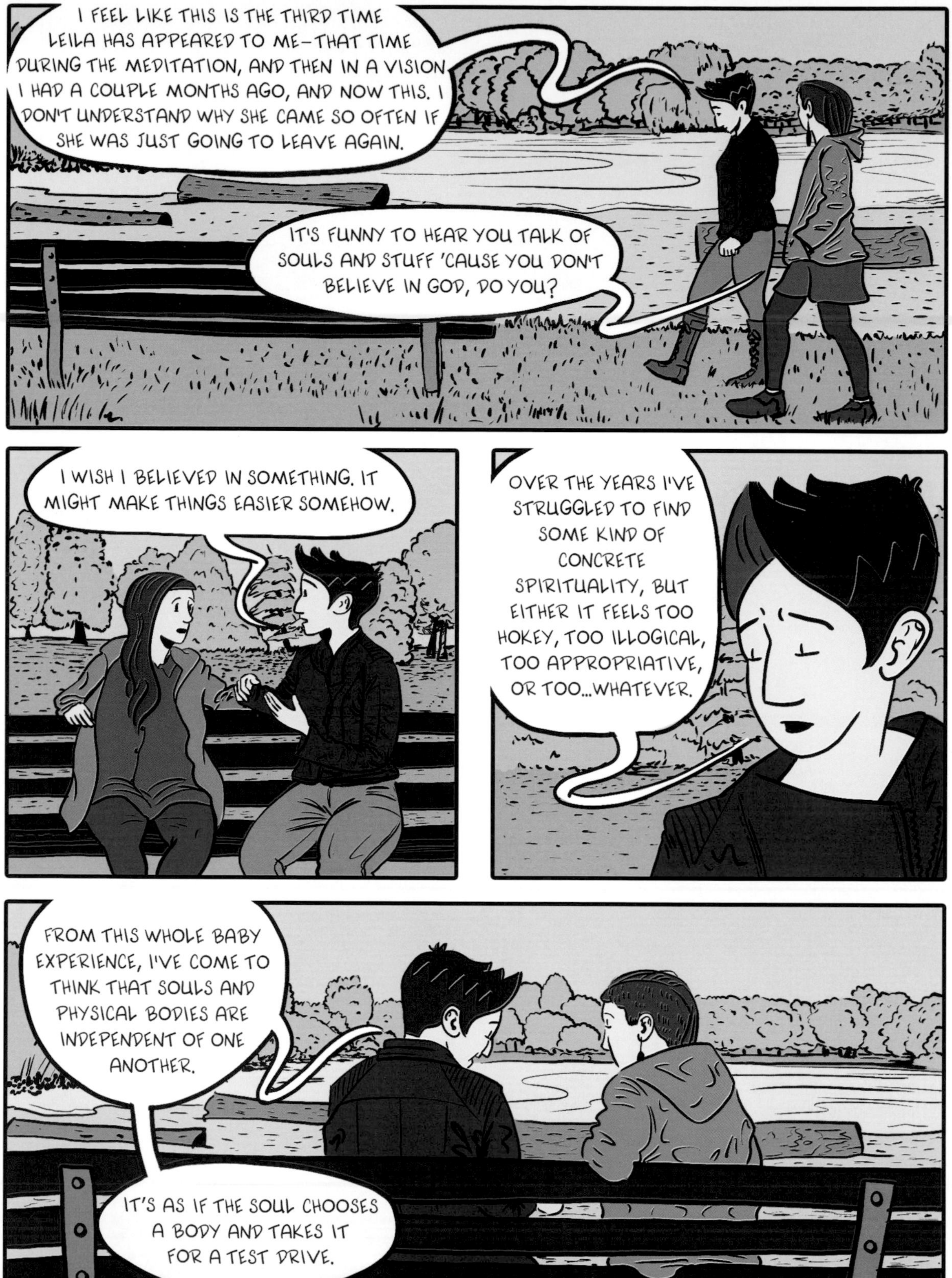
I FEEL LIKE THIS IS THE THIRD TIME LEILA HAS APPEARED TO ME—THAT TIME DURING THE MEDITATION, AND THEN IN A VISION I HAD A COUPLE MONTHS AGO, AND NOW THIS. I DON'T UNDERSTAND WHY SHE CAME SO OFTEN IF SHE WAS JUST GOING TO LEAVE AGAIN.
IT'S FUNNY TO HEAR YOU TALK OF SOULS AND STUFF 'CAUSE YOU DON'T BELIEVE IN GOD, DO YOU?
I WISH I BELIEVED IN SOMETHING. IT MIGHT MAKE THINGS EASIER SOMEHOW.
OVER THE YEARS I'VE STRUGGLED TO FIND SOME KIND OF CONCRETE SPIRITUALITY, BUT EITHER IT FEELS TOO HOKEY, TOO ILLOGICAL, TOO APPROPRIATIVE, OR TOO...WHATEVER.
FROM THIS WHOLE BABY EXPERIENCE, I'VE COME TO THINK THAT SOULS AND PHYSICAL BODIES ARE INDEPENDENT OF ONE ANOTHER.
IT'S AS IF THE SOUL CHOOSES A BODY AND TAKES IT FOR A TEST DRIVE.

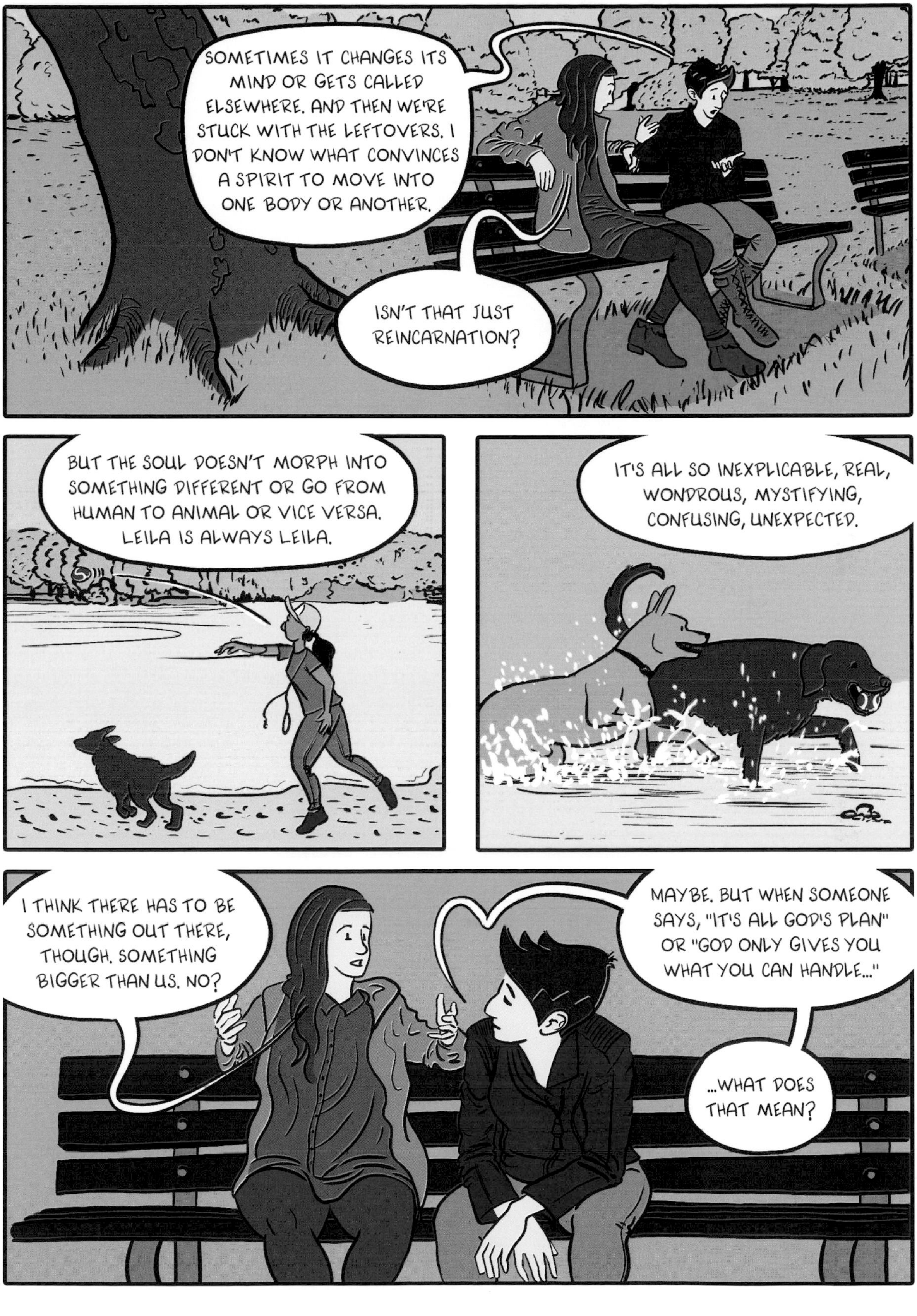
SOMETIMES IT CHANGES ITS MIND OR GETS CALLED ELSEWHERE. AND THEN WE'RE STUCK WITH THE LEFTOVERS. I DON'T KNOW WHAT CONVINCES A SPIRIT TO MOVE INTO ONE BODY OR ANOTHER.
ISN'T THAT JUST REINCARNATION?
BUT THE SOUL DOESN'T MORPH INTO SOMETHING DIFFERENT OR GO FROM HUMAN TO ANIMAL OR VICE VERSA. LEILA IS ALWAYS LEILA.
IT'S ALL SO INEXPLICABLE, REAL, WONDROUS, MYSTIFYING, CONFUSING, UNEXPECTED.
I THINK THERE HAS TO BE SOMETHING OUT THERE, THOUGH. SOMETHING BIGGER THAN US. NO?
MAYBE. BUT WHEN SOMEONE SAYS, "IT'S ALL GOD'S PLAN" OR "GOD ONLY GIVES YOU WHAT YOU CAN HANDLE..."
...WHAT DOES THAT MEAN?

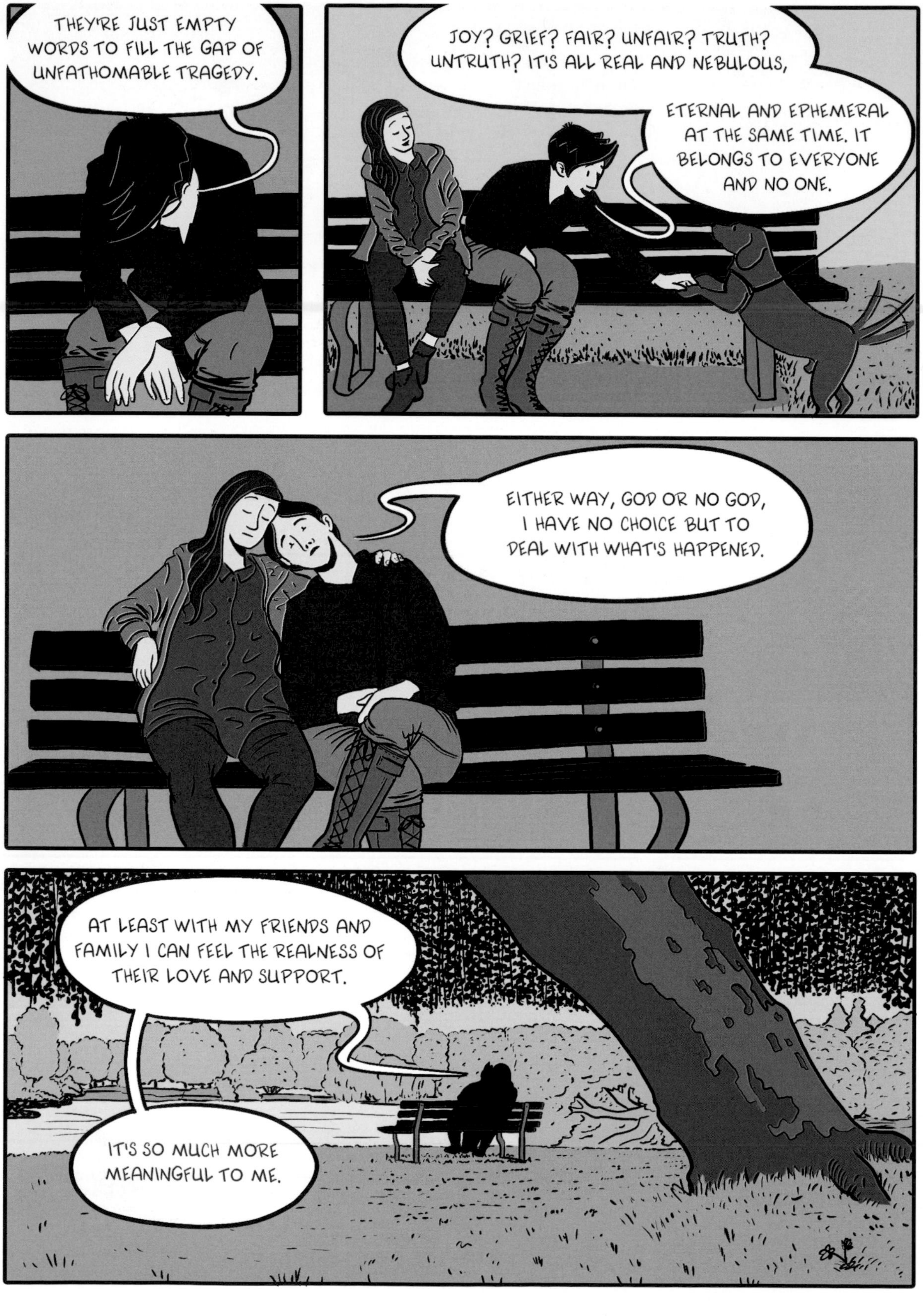
THEY'RE JUST EMPTY WORDS TO FILL THE GAP OF UNFATHOMABLE TRAGEDY.
JOY? GRIEF? FAIR? UNFAIR? TRUTH? UNTRUTH? IT'S ALL REAL AND NEBULOUS,
ETERNAL AND EPHEMERAL AT THE SAME TIME. IT BELONGS TO EVERYONE AND NO ONE.
EITHER WAY, GOD OR NO GOD, I HAVE NO CHOICE BUT TO DEAL WITH WHAT'S HAPPENED.
AT LEAST WITH MY FRIENDS AND FAMILY I CAN FEEL THE REALNESS OF THEIR LOVE AND SUPPORT.
IT'S SO MUCH MORE MEANINGFUL TO ME.

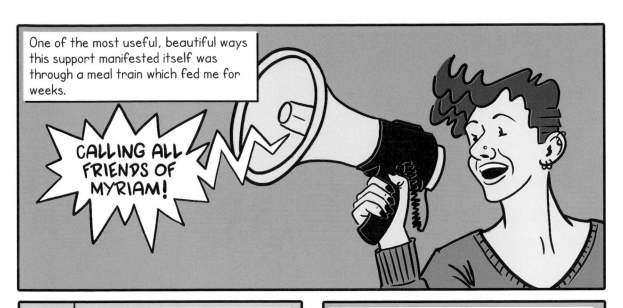

One of the most useful, beautiful ways this support manifested itself was through a meal train which fed me for weeks.

CALLING ALL FRIENDS OF MYRIAM!

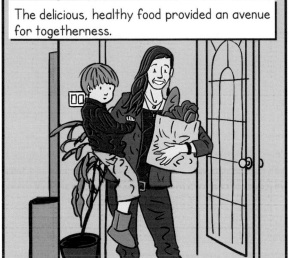

The delicious, healthy food provided an avenue for togetherness.

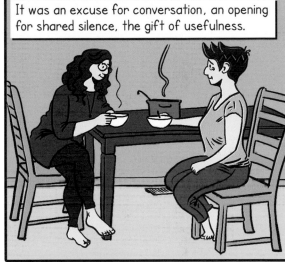

It was an excuse for conversation, an opening for shared silence, the gift of usefulness.

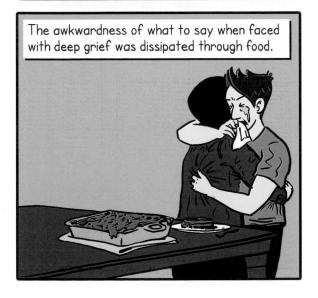

The awkwardness of what to say when faced with deep grief was dissipated through food.

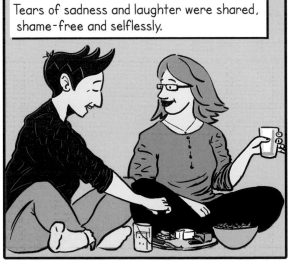

Tears of sadness and laughter were shared, shame-free and selflessly.

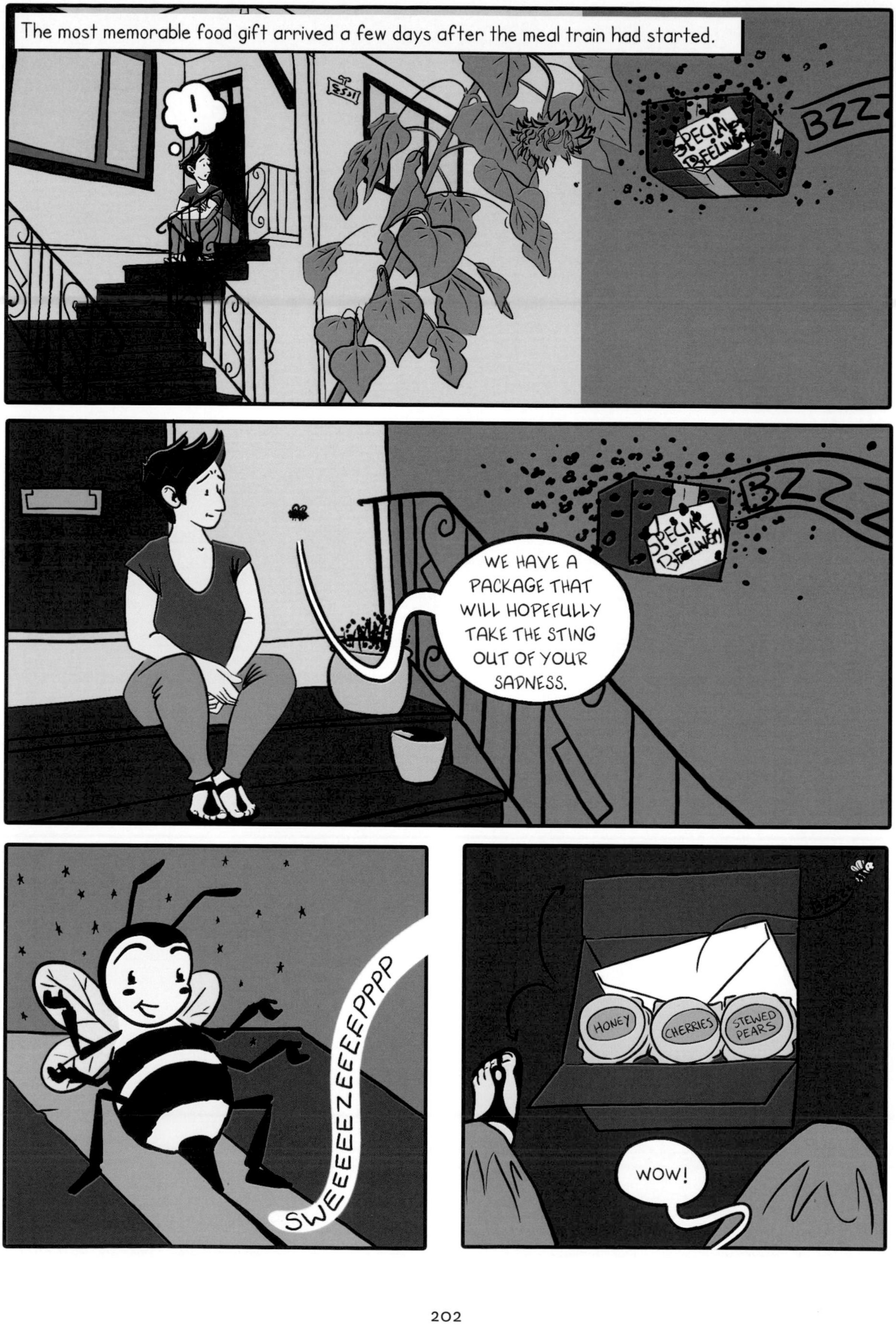
The most memorable food gift arrived a few days after the meal train had started.
!
BZZZ
BZZZ
WE HAVE A PACKAGE THAT WILL HOPEFULLY TAKE THE STING OUT OF YOUR SADNESS.
SWEEEEEZEEEEPPPP
HONEY
CHERRIES
STEWED PEARS
WOW!

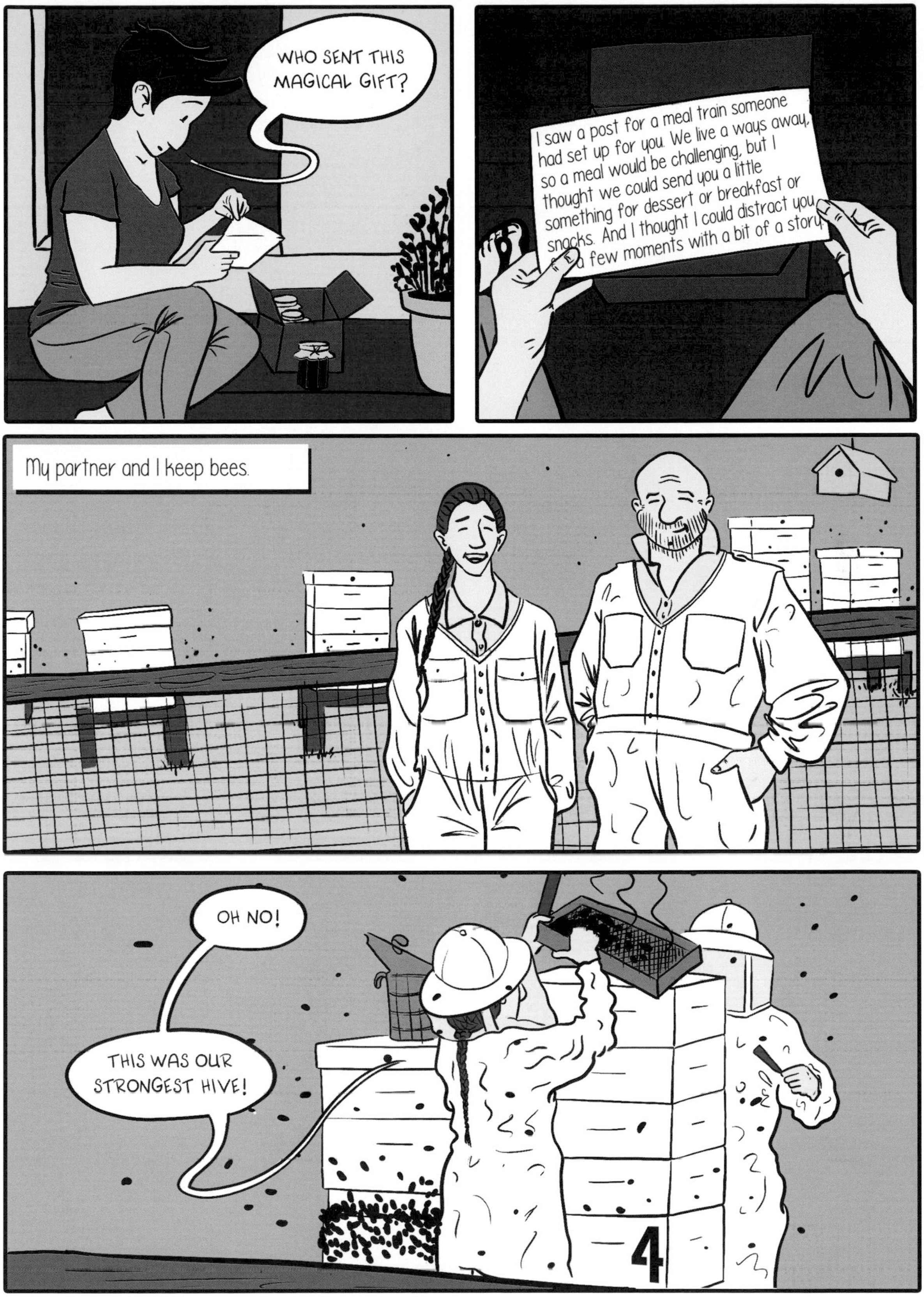
WHO SENT THIS MAGICAL GIFT?
I saw a post for a meal train someone had set up for you. We live a ways away, so a meal would be challenging, but I thought we could send you a little something for dessert or breakfast or snacks. And I thought I could distract you a few moments with a bit of a story
My partner and I keep bees.
OH NO!
THIS WAS OUR STRONGEST HIVE!
4

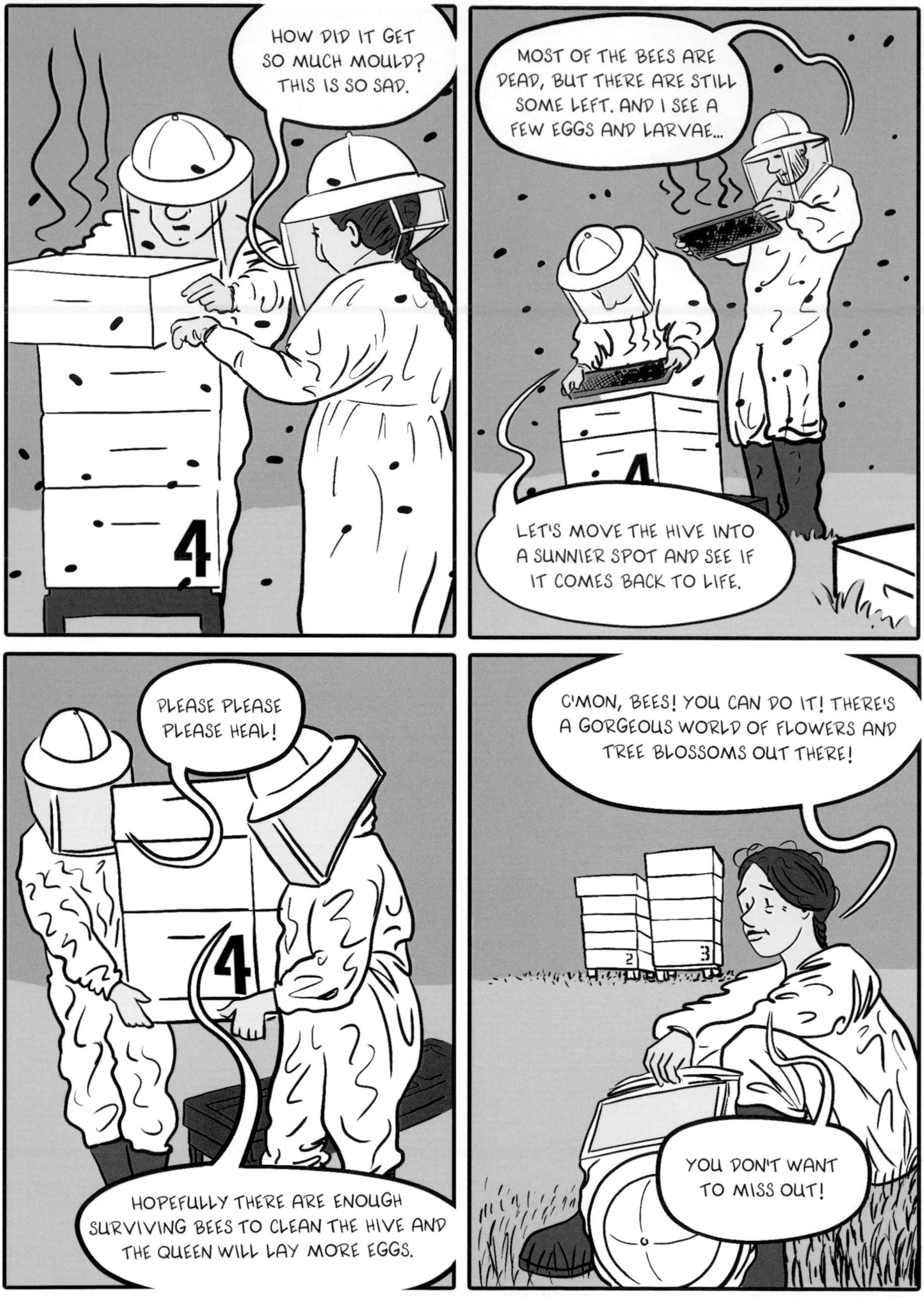
HOW DID IT GET SO MUCH MOULD? THIS IS SO SAD.
MOST OF THE BEES ARE DEAD, BUT THERE ARE STILL SOME LEFT. AND I SEE A FEW EGGS AND LARVAE...
LET'S MOVE THE HIVE INTO A SUNNIER SPOT AND SEE IF IT COMES BACK TO LIFE.
PLEASE PLEASE PLEASE HEAL!
HOPEFULLY THERE ARE ENOUGH SURVIVING BEES TO CLEAN THE HIVE AND THE QUEEN WILL LAY MORE EGGS.
C'MON, BEES! YOU CAN DO IT! THERE'S A GORGEOUS WORLD OF FLOWERS AND TREE BLOSSOMS OUT THERE!
YOU DON'T WANT TO MISS OUT!

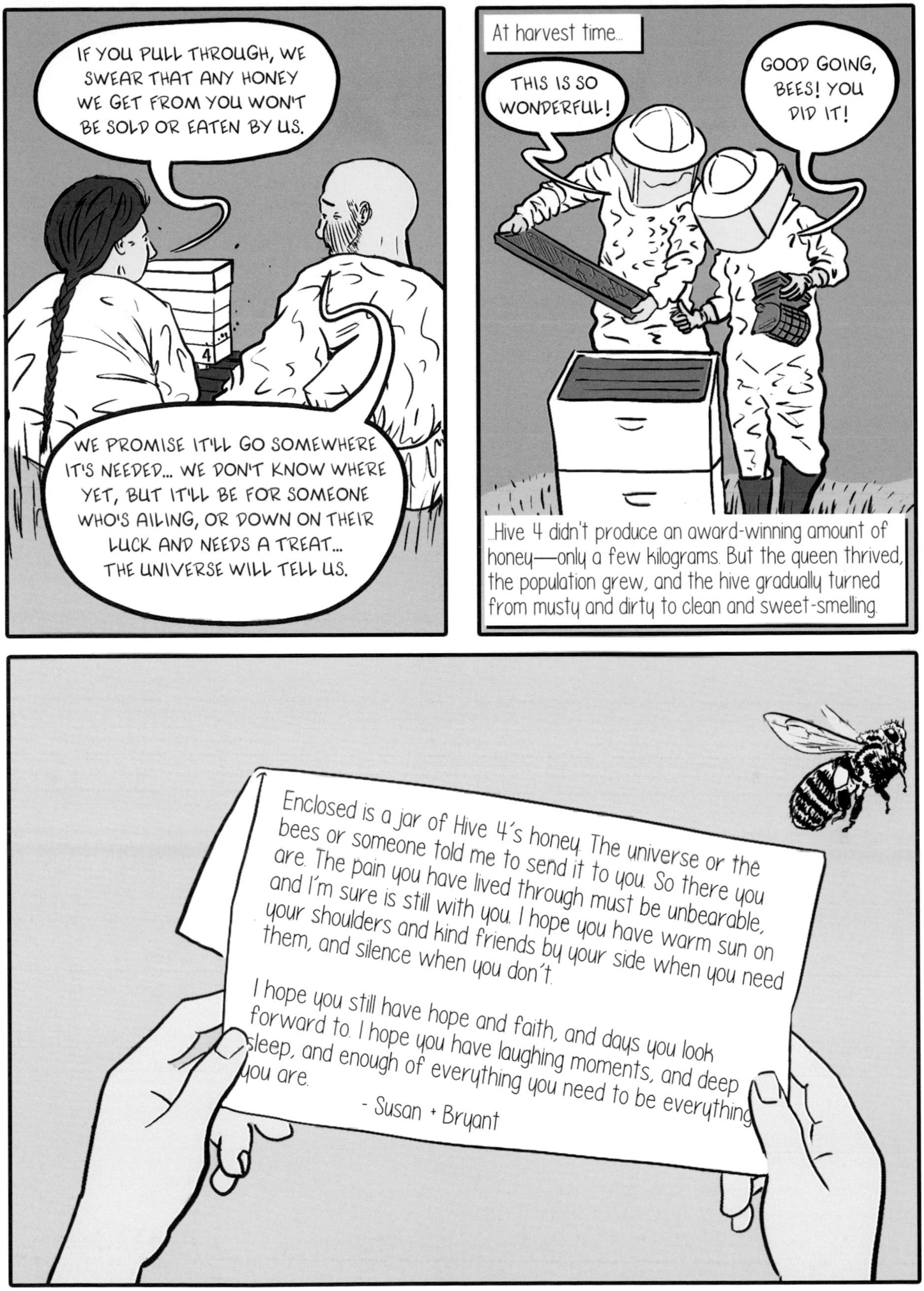
IF YOU PULL THROUGH, WE SWEAR THAT ANY HONEY WE GET FROM YOU WON'T BE SOLD OR EATEN BY US.
WE PROMISE IT'LL GO SOMEWHERE IT'S NEEDED... WE DON'T KNOW WHERE YET, BUT IT'LL BE FOR SOMEONE WHO'S AILING, OR DOWN ON THEIR LUCK AND NEEDS A TREAT... THE UNIVERSE WILL TELL US.
At harvest time...
THIS IS SO WONDERFUL!
GOOD GOING, BEES! YOU DID IT!
...Hive 4 didn't produce an award-winning amount of honey—only a few kilograms. But the queen thrived, the population grew, and the hive gradually turned from musty and dirty to clean and sweet-smelling.
Enclosed is a jar of Hive 4's honey. The universe or the bees or someone told me to send it to you. So there you are. The pain you have lived through must be unbearable, and I'm sure is still with you. I hope you have warm sun on your shoulders and kind friends by your side when you need them, and silence when you don't.
I hope you still have hope and faith, and days you look forward to. I hope you have laughing moments, and deep sleep, and enough of everything you need to be everything you are.
- Susan + Bryant

YEAR FOUR

DECEMBER 2017–APRIL 2018

Donor Eggs

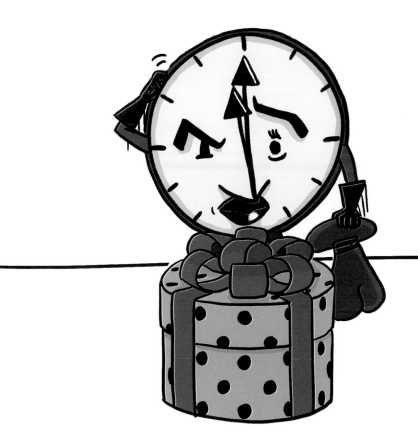

Chapter 6

Snoogy Wookums

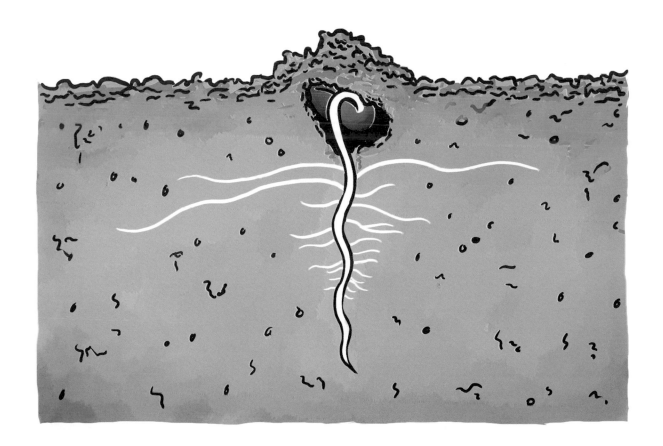

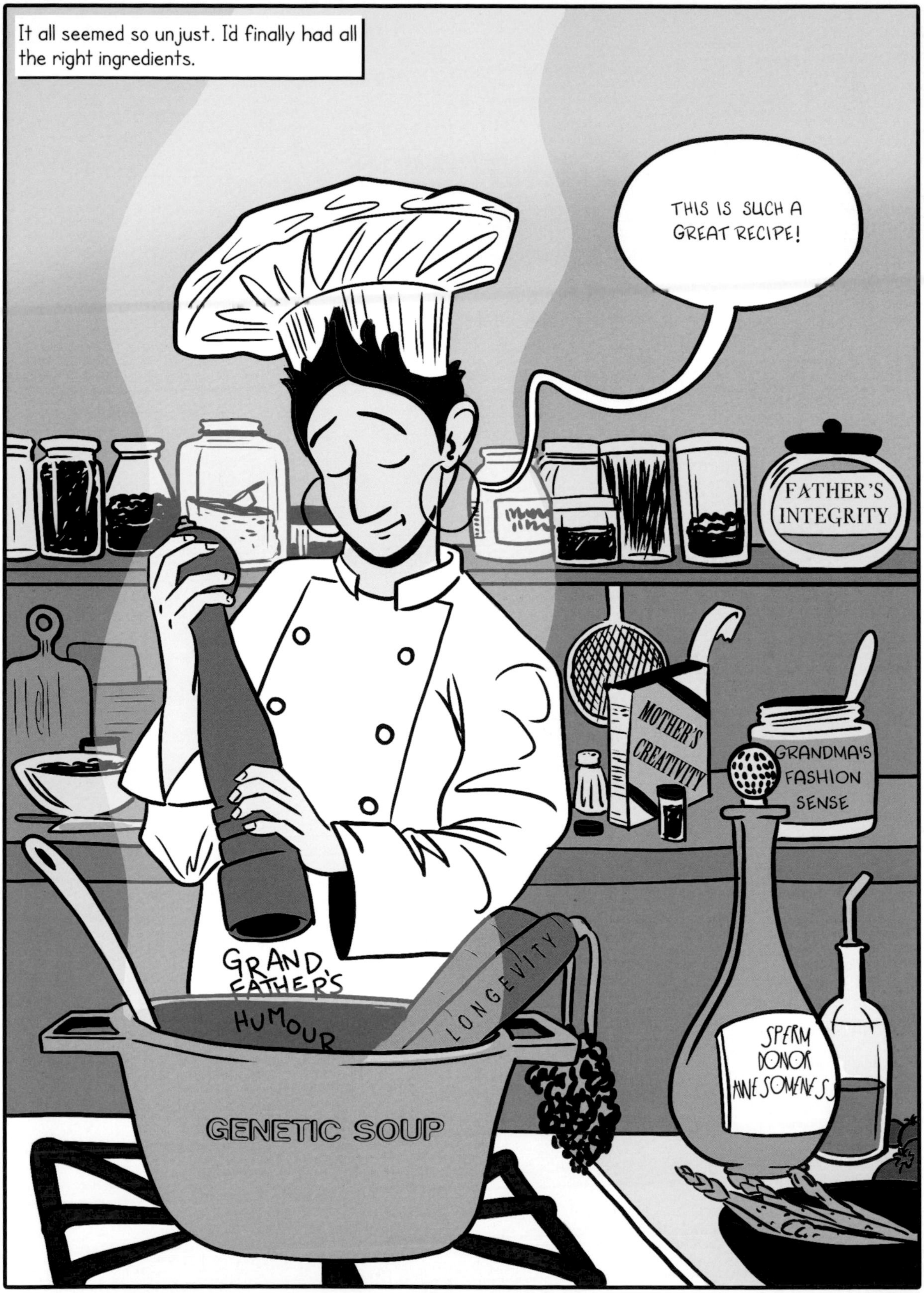
It all seemed so unjust. I'd finally had all the right ingredients.
THIS IS SUCH A GREAT RECIPE!
FATHER'S INTEGRITY
MOTHER'S CREATIVITY
GRANDMA'S FASHION SENSE
GRAND FATHER'S HUMOUR
LONGEVITY
SPERM DONOR AWESOMENESS
GENETIC SOUP

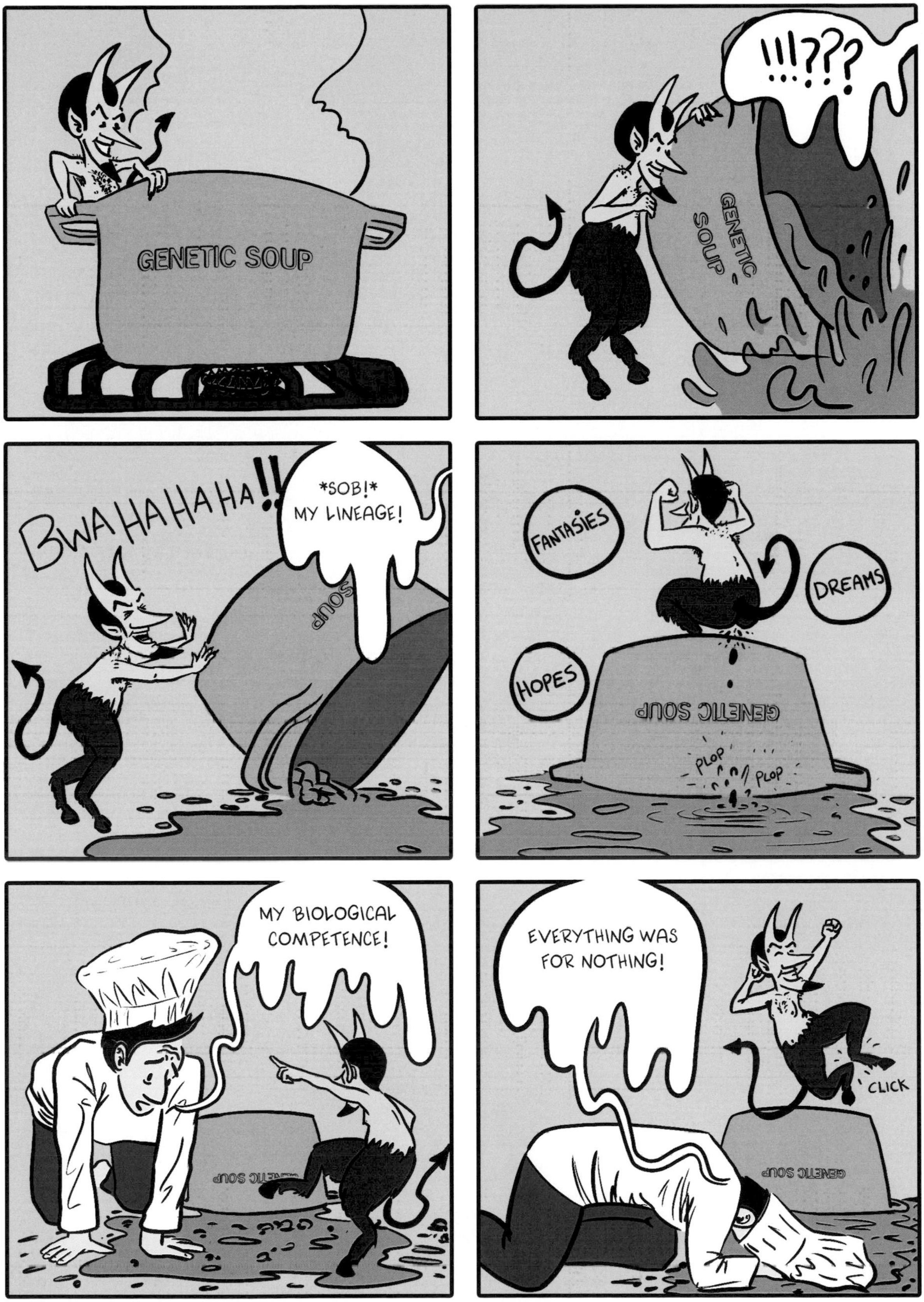
GENETIC SOUP
!!!???
GENETIC SOUP
BWAHAHAHAHA!!
SOB! MY LINEAGE!
SOUP
FANTASIES
DREAMS
HOPES
GENETIC SOUP
PLOP
PLOP
MY BIOLOGICAL COMPETENCE!
GENETIC SOUP
EVERYTHING WAS FOR NOTHING!
CLICK
GENETIC SOUP

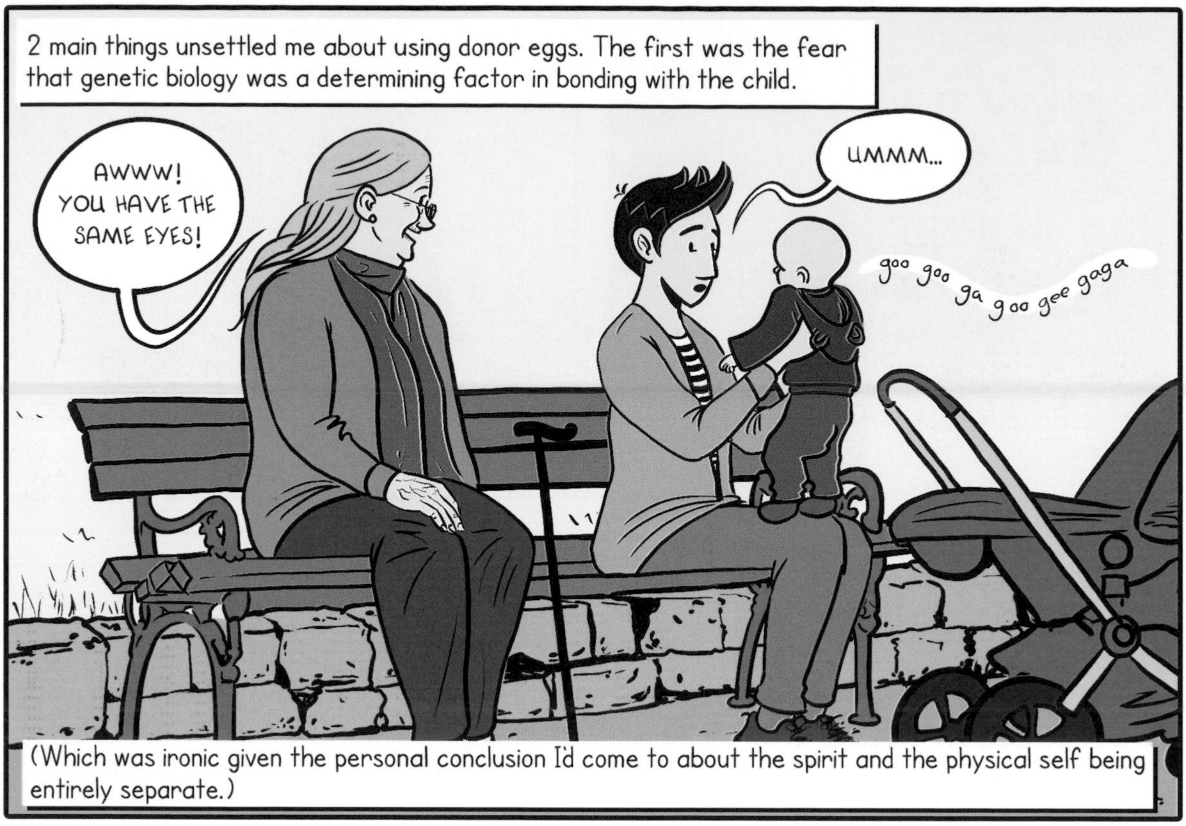
2 main things unsettled me about using donor eggs. The first was the fear that genetic biology was a determining factor in bonding with the child.
AWWW! YOU HAVE THE SAME EYES!
UMMM...
goo goo ga goo gee gaga
(Which was ironic given the personal conclusion I'd come to about the spirit and the physical self being entirely separate.)

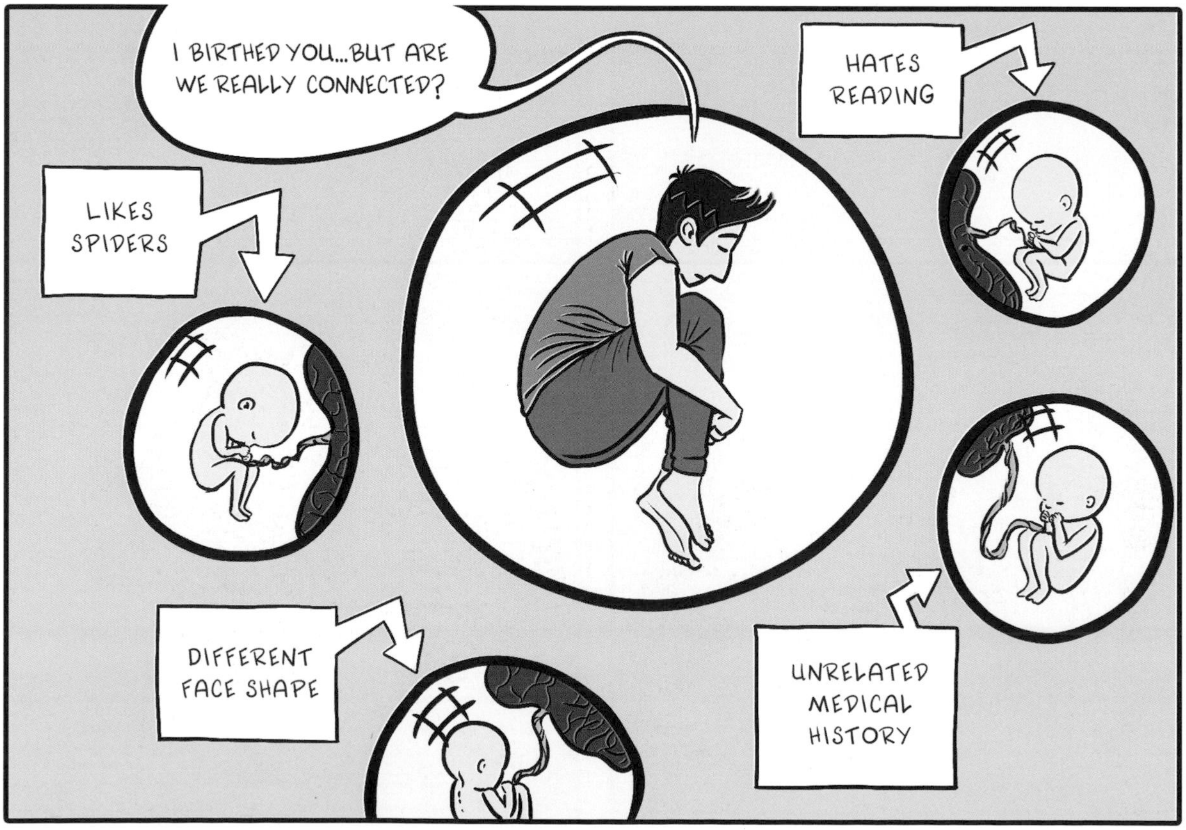
I BIRTHED YOU...BUT ARE WE REALLY CONNECTED?
HATES READING
LIKES SPIDERS
DIFFERENT FACE SHAPE
UNRELATED MEDICAL HISTORY

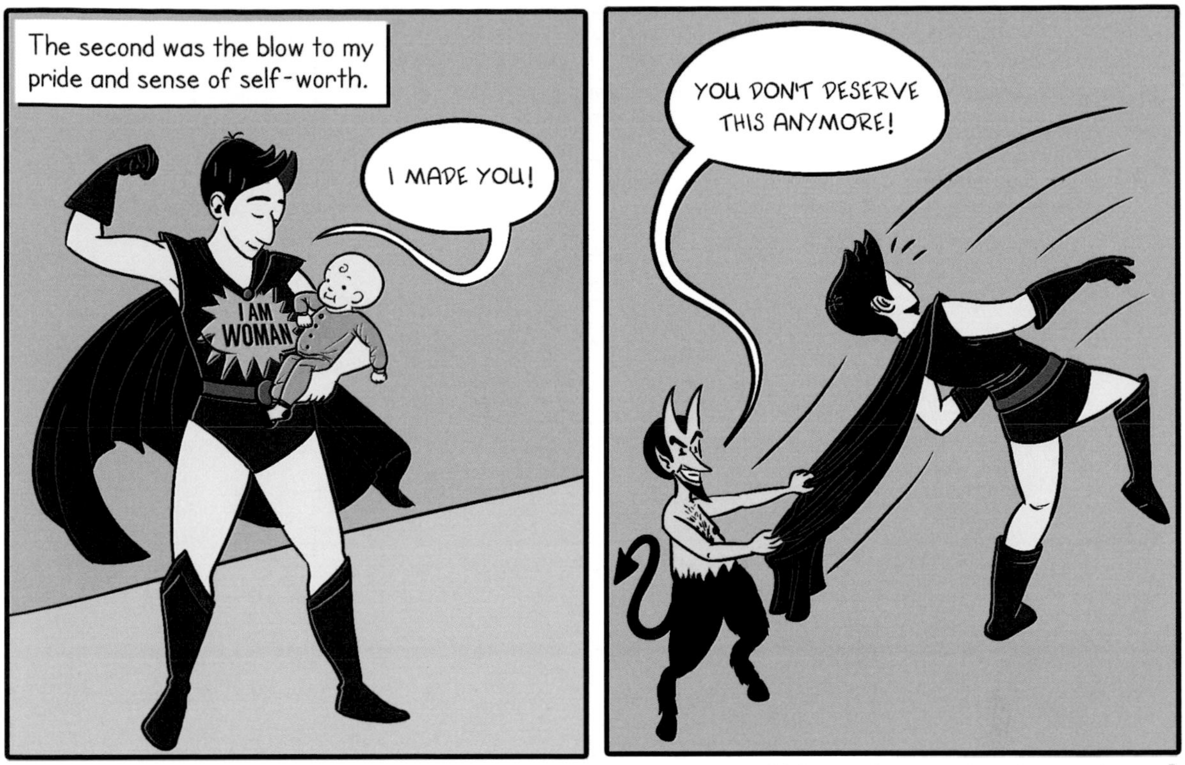
The second was the blow to my pride and sense of self-worth.
I MADE YOU!
I AM WOMAN
YOU DON'T DESERVE THIS ANYMORE!

It was a process, but I got over it (mostly). What helped was some "fake it till you make it" attitude, some counselling, and my introduction to epigenetics, which says that the environment influences the expression of genes without actually changing the physical DNA sequence. In other words, amongst other things, a baby can inherit traits from its mother whether or not they are biologically related.

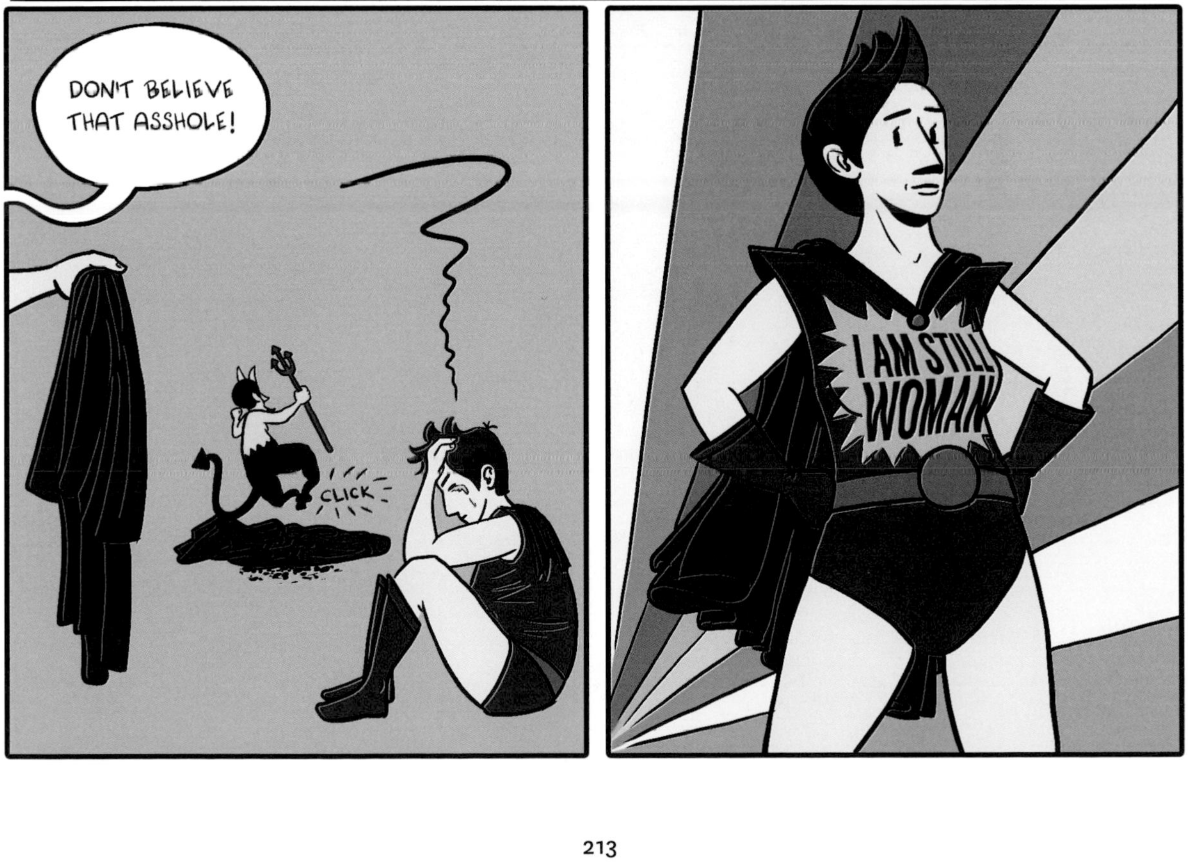
DON'T BELIEVE THAT ASSHOLE!
CLICK
I AM STILL WOMAN

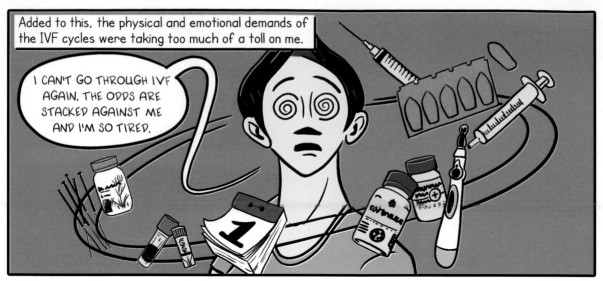

Added to this, the physical and emotional demands of the IVF cycles were taking too much of a toll on me.

I CAN'T GO THROUGH IVF AGAIN. THE ODDS ARE STACKED AGAINST ME AND I'M SO TIRED.

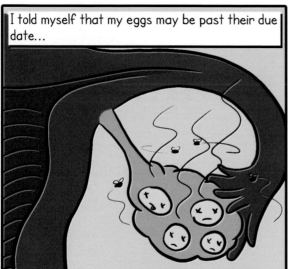

I told myself that my eggs may be past their due date...

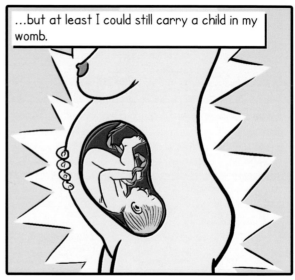

...but at least I could still carry a child in my womb.

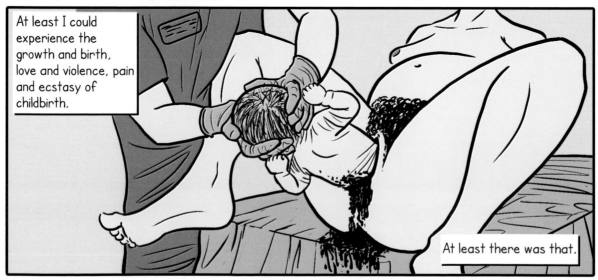

At least I could experience the growth and birth, love and violence, pain and ecstasy of childbirth.

At least there was that.

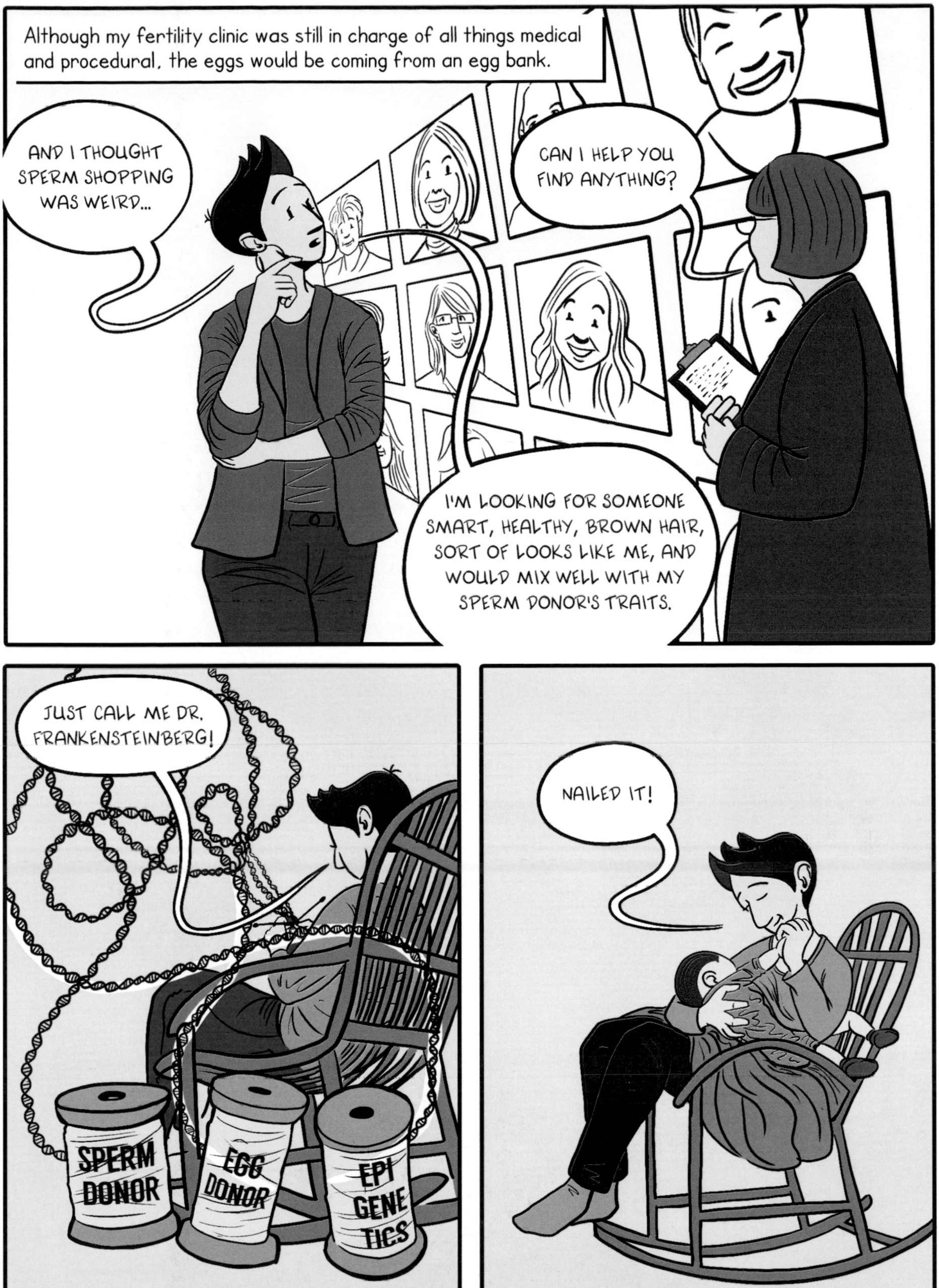
Although my fertility clinic was still in charge of all things medical and procedural, the eggs would be coming from an egg bank.
AND I THOUGHT SPERM SHOPPING WAS WEIRD...
CAN I HELP YOU FIND ANYTHING?
I'M LOOKING FOR SOMEONE SMART, HEALTHY, BROWN HAIR, SORT OF LOOKS LIKE ME, AND WOULD MIX WELL WITH MY SPERM DONOR'S TRAITS.
JUST CALL ME DR. FRANKENSTEINBERG!
SPERM DONOR
EGG DONOR
EPI GENE TICS
NAILED IT!

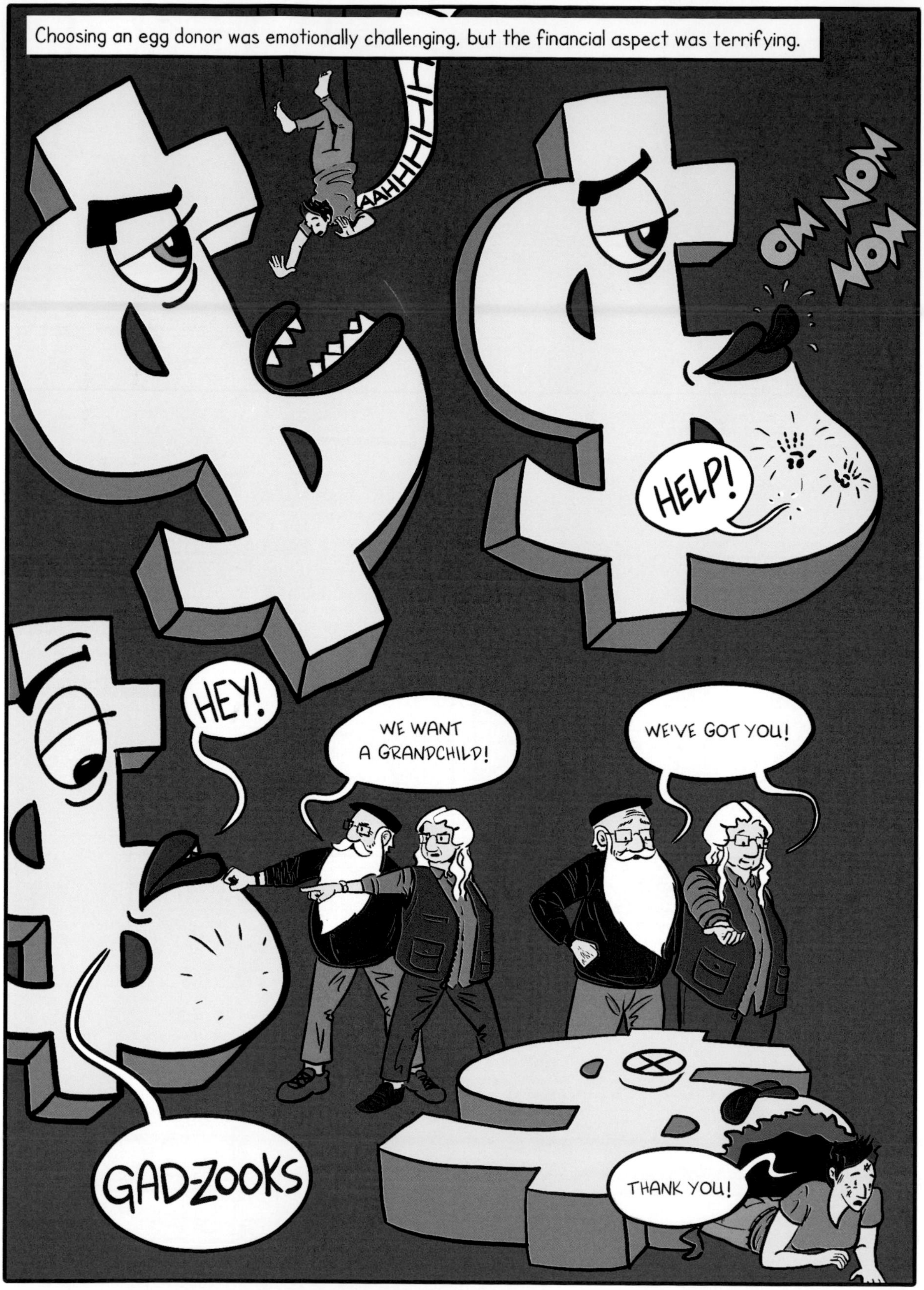
Choosing an egg donor was emotionally challenging, but the financial aspect was terrifying.
AAHHHHHHH
OM NOM NOM
HELP!
HEY!
WE WANT A GRANDCHILD!
WE'VE GOT YOU!
GAD-ZOOKS
THANK YOU!

A few things helped me reconcile myself to the cost of donor eggs.

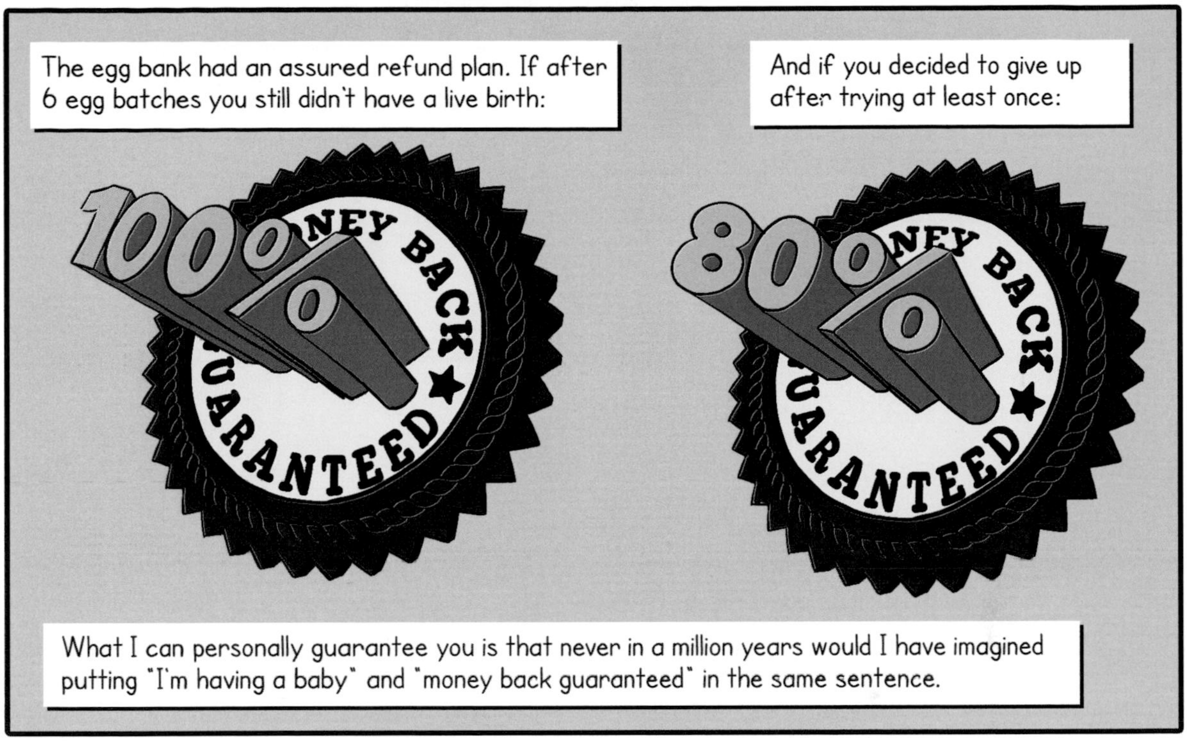
The egg bank had an assured refund plan. If after 6 egg batches you still didn't have a live birth:
100% MONEY BACK ★ GUARANTEED
And if you decided to give up after trying at least once:
80% MONEY BACK ★ GUARANTEED
What I can personally guarantee you is that never in a million years would I have imagined putting "I'm having a baby" and "money back guaranteed" in the same sentence.

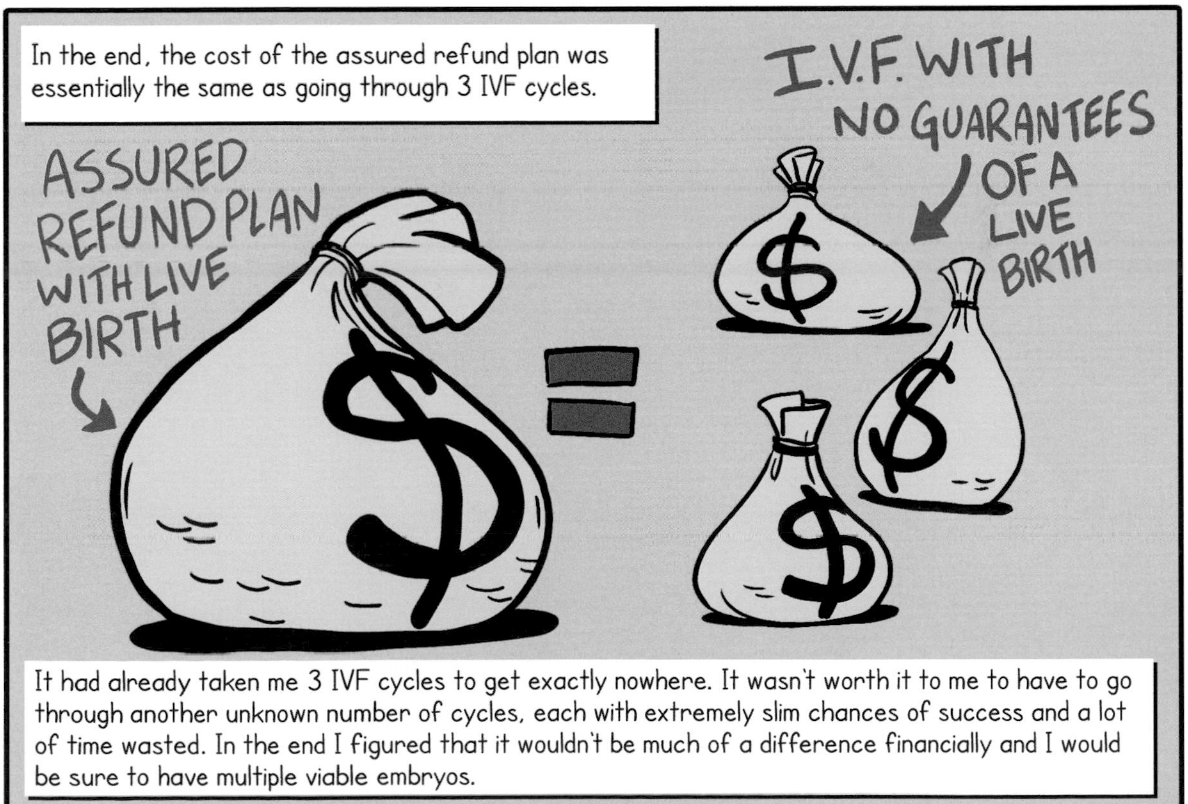
In the end, the cost of the assured refund plan was essentially the same as going through 3 IVF cycles.
ASSURED REFUND PLAN WITH LIVE BIRTH
I.V.F. WITH NO GUARANTEES OF A LIVE BIRTH
It had already taken me 3 IVF cycles to get exactly nowhere. It wasn't worth it to me to have to go through another unknown number of cycles, each with extremely slim chances of success and a lot of time wasted. In the end I figured that it wouldn't be much of a difference financially and I would be sure to have multiple viable embryos.

When it came time to wire money to the egg bank, I was in a state of paralyzed agitation. After hours of procrastination, I realized I couldn't do it alone. Not only was spending such a vast sum scary, but it marked the point of no return. Once the money was sent, that was it for my biology.

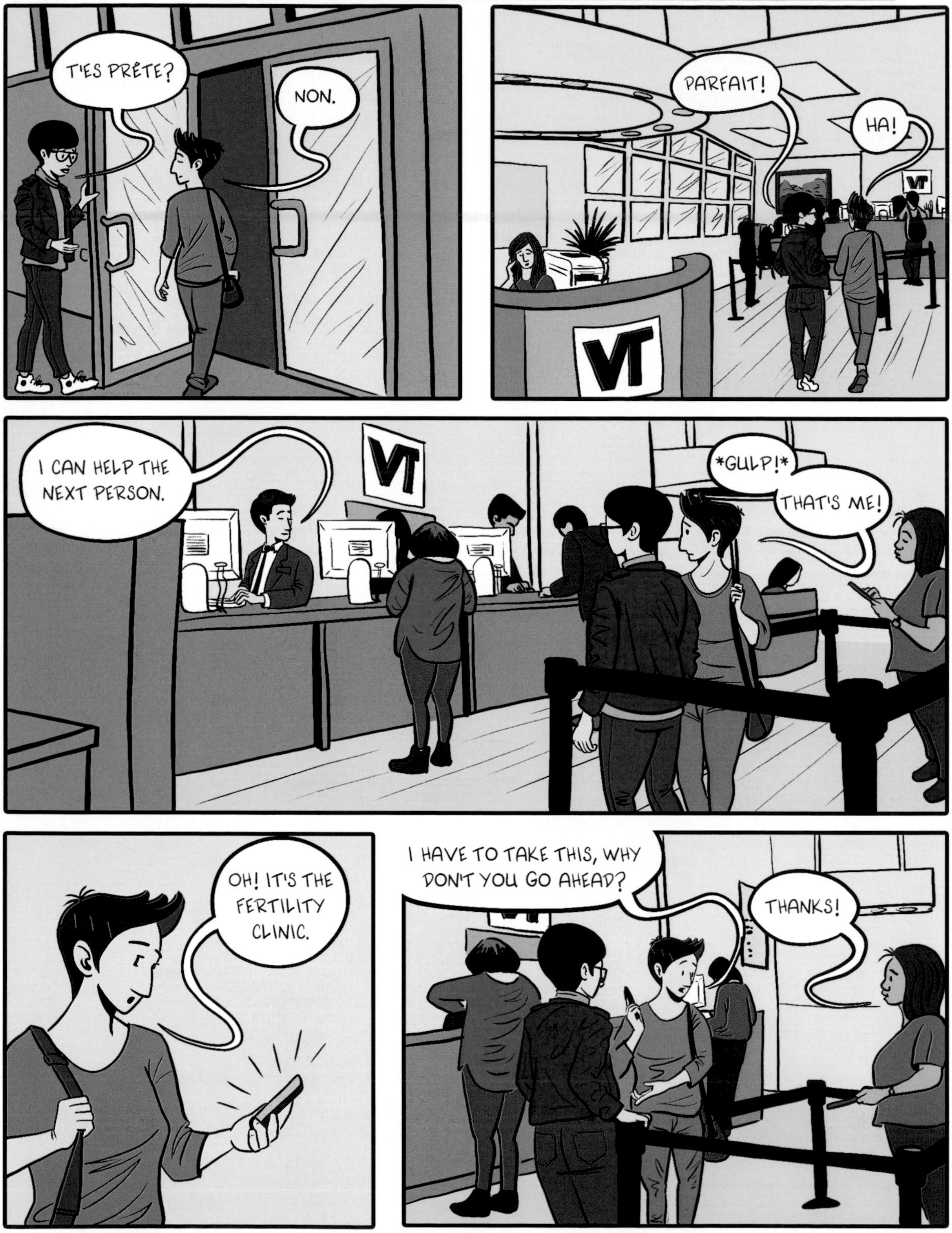

T'ES PRÊTE?
NON.
PARFAIT!
HA!
VT
VT
I CAN HELP THE NEXT PERSON.
GULP!
THAT'S ME!
OH! IT'S THE FERTILITY CLINIC.
I HAVE TO TAKE THIS, WHY DON'T YOU GO AHEAD?
THANKS!

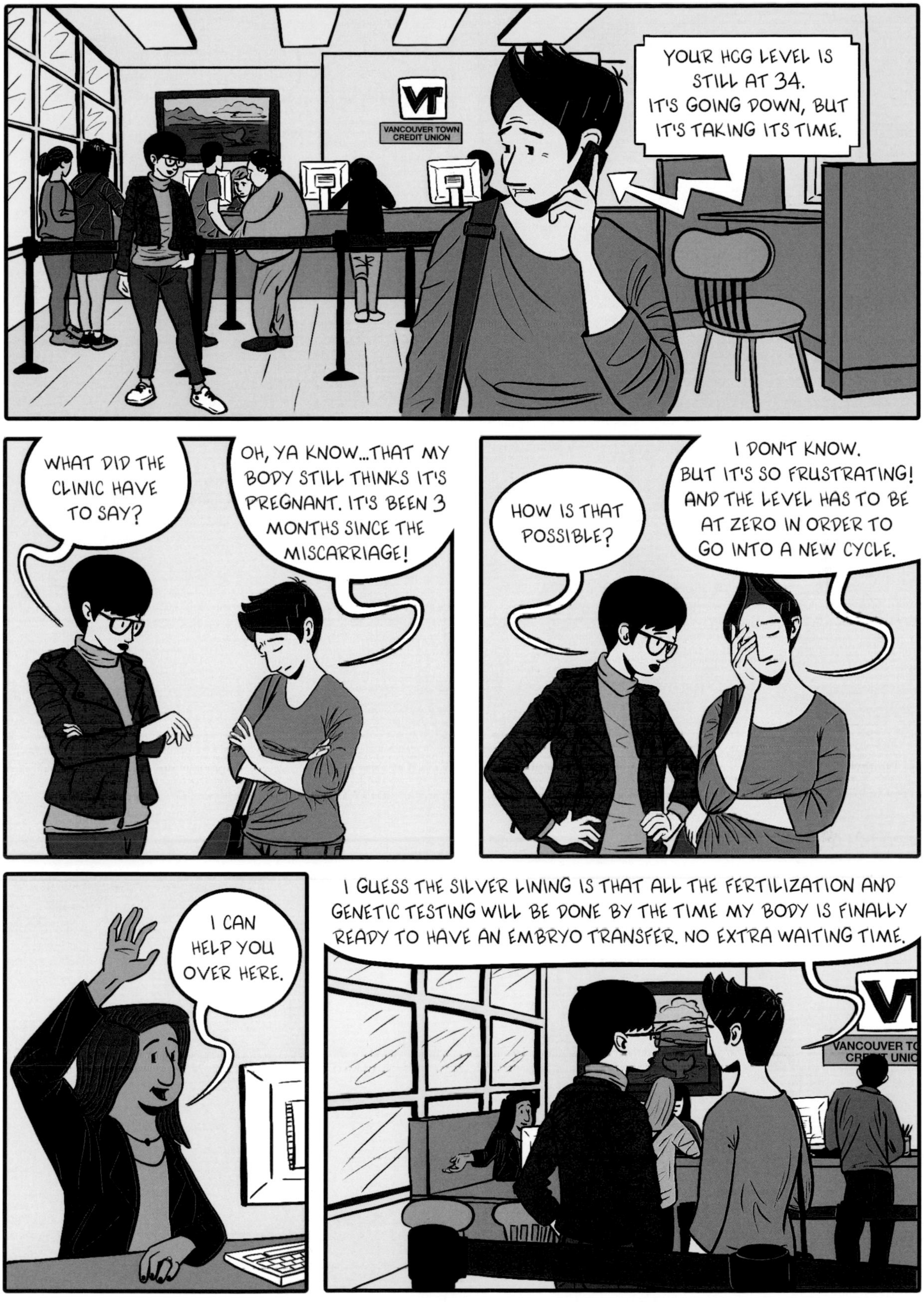

VANCOUVER TOWN CREDIT UNION
YOUR HCG LEVEL IS STILL AT 34. IT'S GOING DOWN, BUT IT'S TAKING ITS TIME.
WHAT DID THE CLINIC HAVE TO SAY?
OH, YA KNOW...THAT MY BODY STILL THINKS IT'S PREGNANT. IT'S BEEN 3 MONTHS SINCE THE MISCARRIAGE!
HOW IS THAT POSSIBLE?
I DON'T KNOW. BUT IT'S SO FRUSTRATING! AND THE LEVEL HAS TO BE AT ZERO IN ORDER TO GO INTO A NEW CYCLE.
I CAN HELP YOU OVER HERE.
I GUESS THE SILVER LINING IS THAT ALL THE FERTILIZATION AND GENETIC TESTING WILL BE DONE BY THE TIME MY BODY IS FINALLY READY TO HAVE AN EMBRYO TRANSFER. NO EXTRA WAITING TIME.

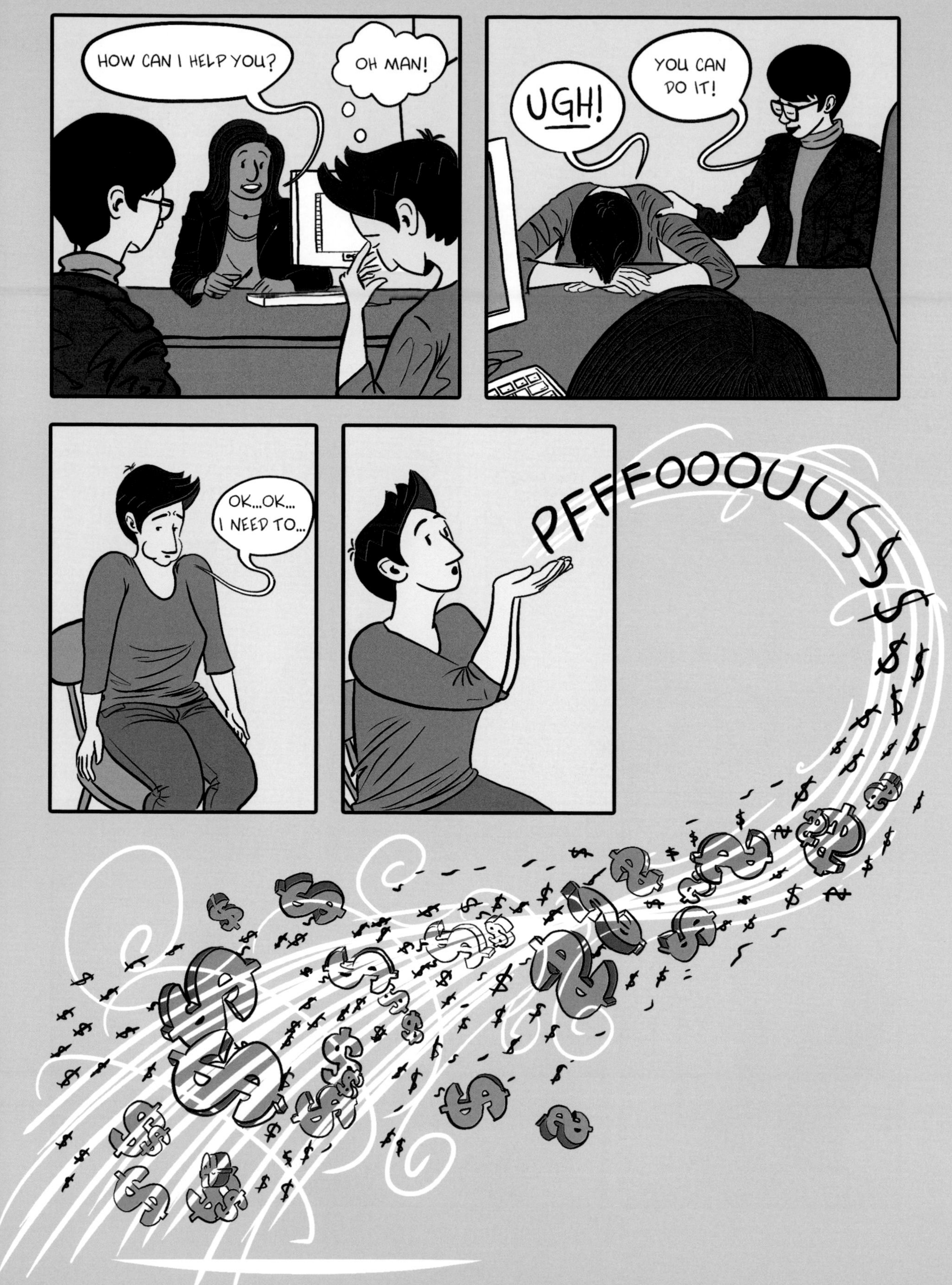
HOW CAN I HELP YOU?
OH MAN!
UGH!
YOU CAN DO IT!
OK...OK... I NEED TO...
PFFFOOOUUSS

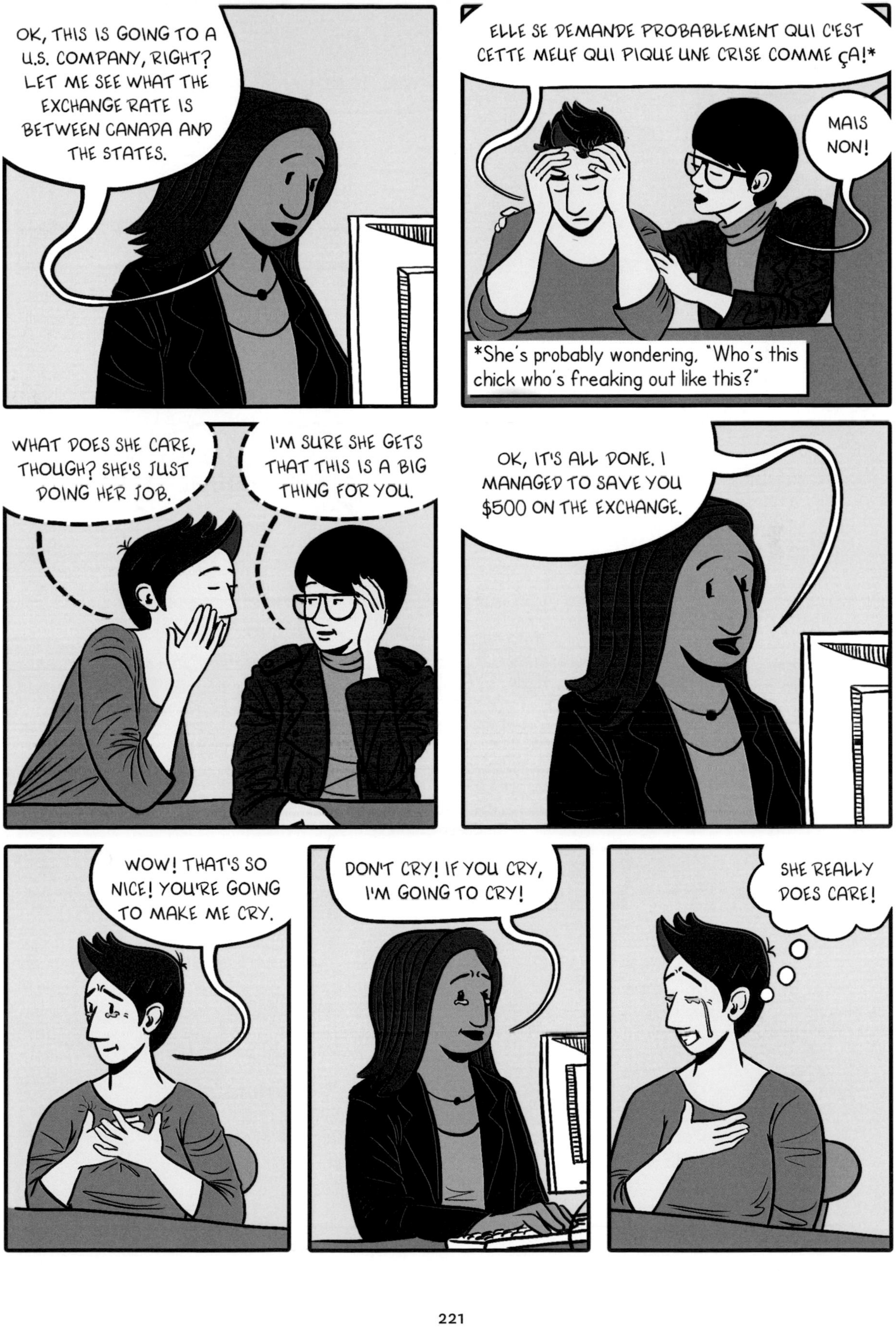
OK, THIS IS GOING TO A U.S. COMPANY, RIGHT? LET ME SEE WHAT THE EXCHANGE RATE IS BETWEEN CANADA AND THE STATES.
ELLE SE DEMANDE PROBABLEMENT QUI C'EST CETTE MEUF QUI PIQUE UNE CRISE COMME ÇA!*
MAIS NON!
*She's probably wondering, "Who's this chick who's freaking out like this?"
WHAT DOES SHE CARE, THOUGH? SHE'S JUST DOING HER JOB.
I'M SURE SHE GETS THAT THIS IS A BIG THING FOR YOU.
OK, IT'S ALL DONE. I MANAGED TO SAVE YOU $500 ON THE EXCHANGE.
WOW! THAT'S SO NICE! YOU'RE GOING TO MAKE ME CRY.
DON'T CRY! IF YOU CRY, I'M GOING TO CRY!
SHE REALLY DOES CARE!

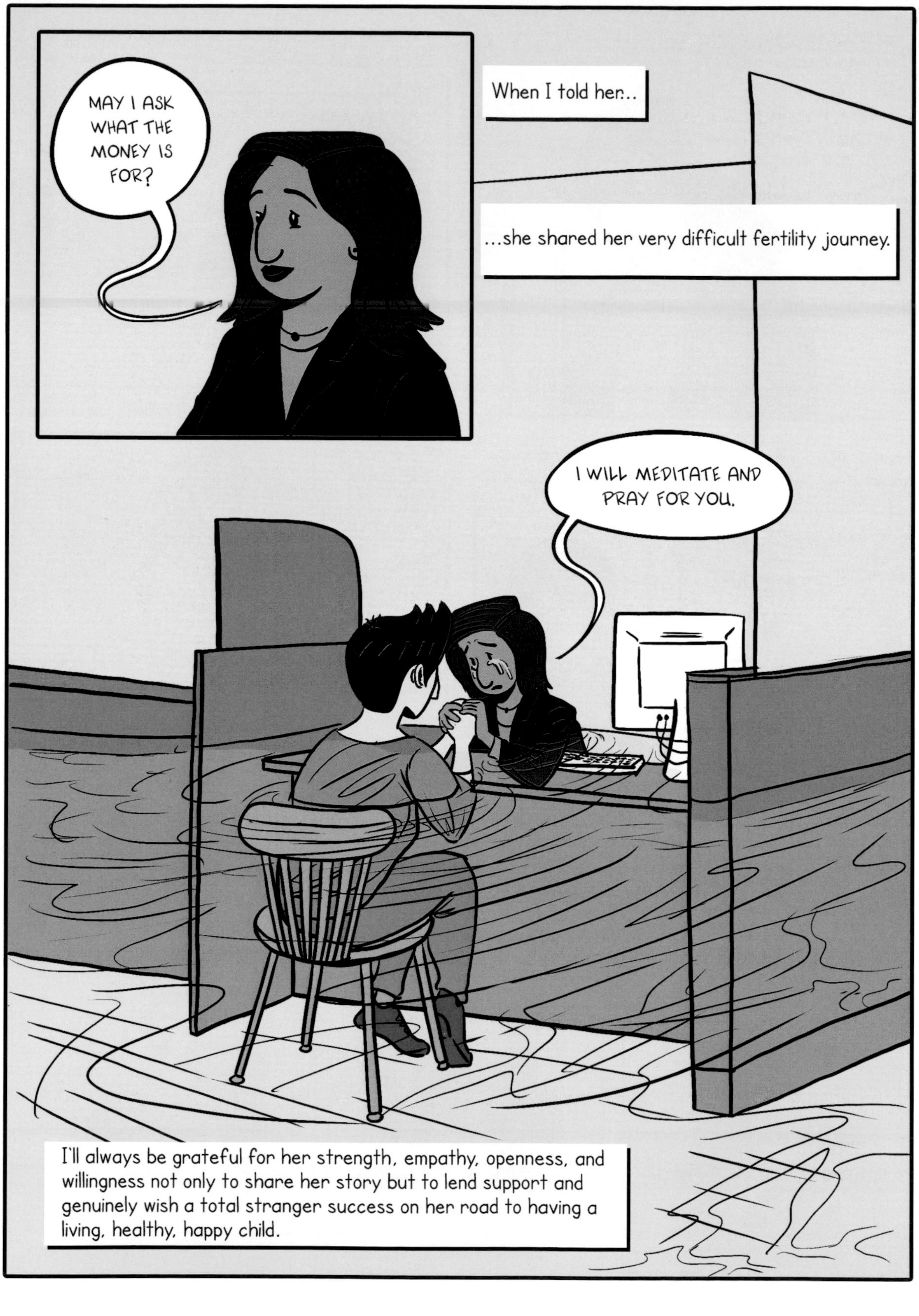
MAY I ASK WHAT THE MONEY IS FOR?
When I told her...
...she shared her very difficult fertility journey.
I WILL MEDITATE AND PRAY FOR YOU.
I'll always be grateful for her strength, empathy, openness, and willingness not only to share her story but to lend support and genuinely wish a total stranger success on her road to having a living, healthy, happy child.

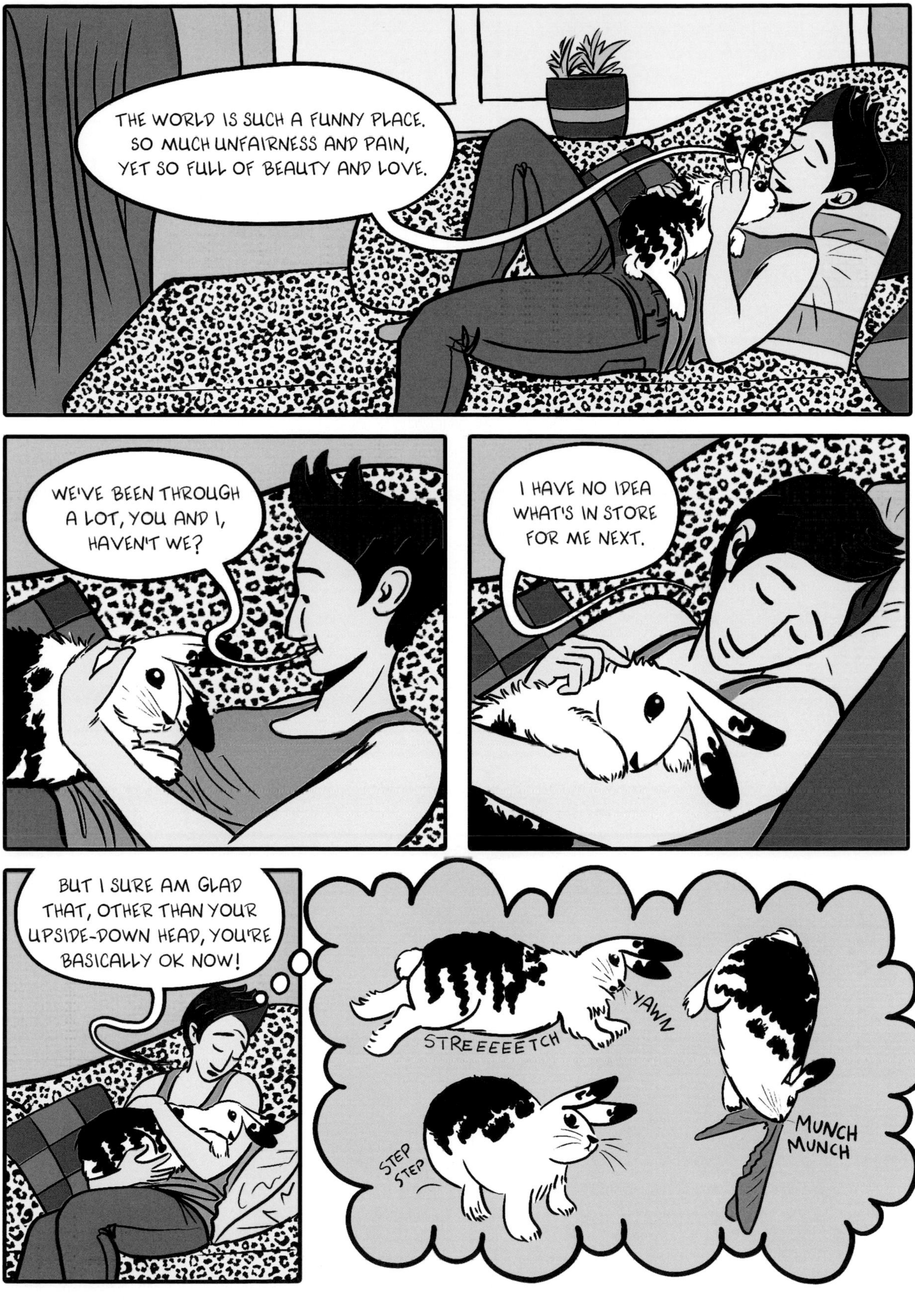
THE WORLD IS SUCH A FUNNY PLACE. SO MUCH UNFAIRNESS AND PAIN, YET SO FULL OF BEAUTY AND LOVE.
WE'VE BEEN THROUGH A LOT, YOU AND I, HAVEN'T WE?
I HAVE NO IDEA WHAT'S IN STORE FOR ME NEXT.
BUT I SURE AM GLAD THAT, OTHER THAN YOUR UPSIDE-DOWN HEAD, YOU'RE BASICALLY OK NOW!
STREEEEEETCH
YAWN
MUNCH MUNCH
STEP STEP

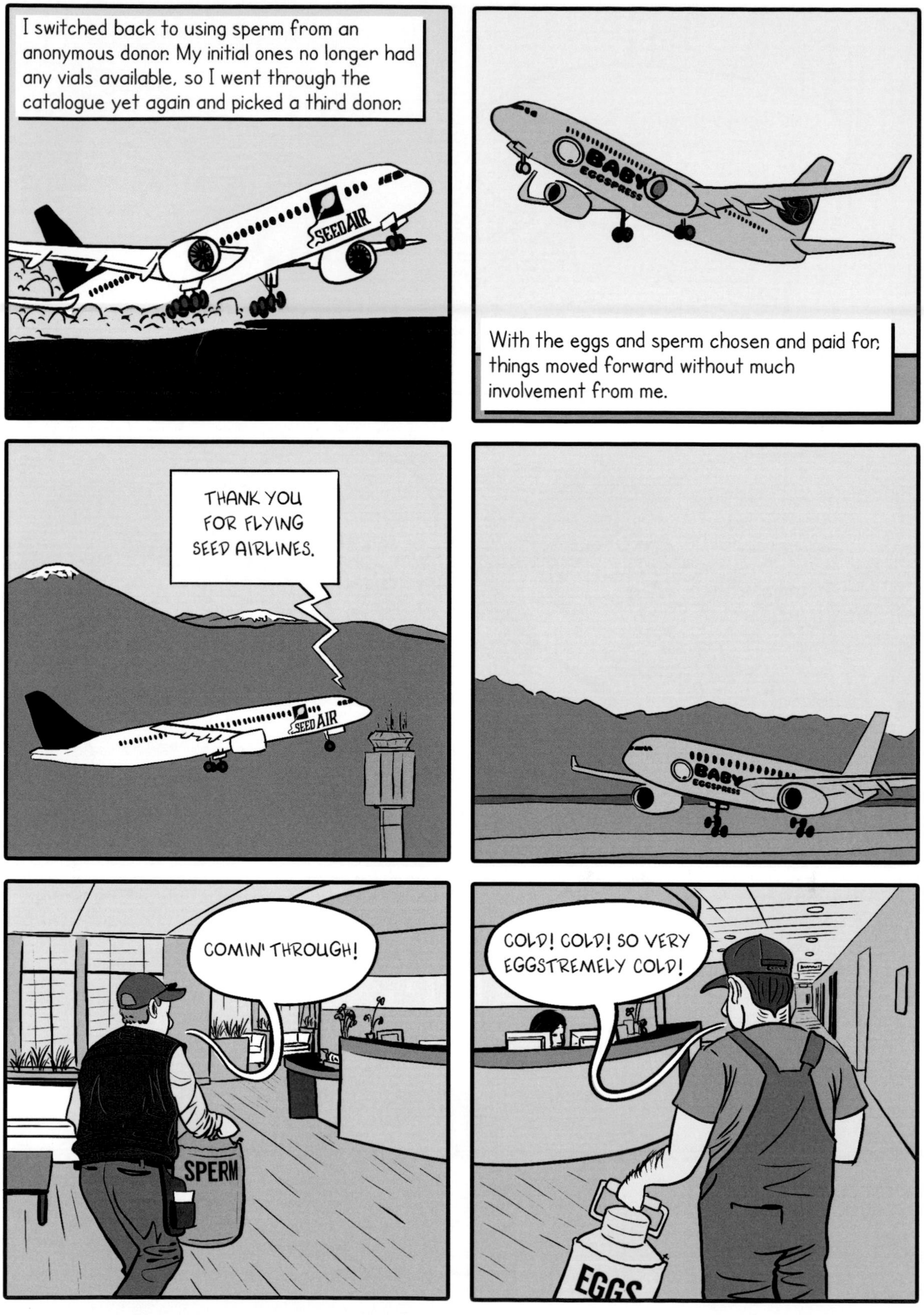
I switched back to using sperm from an anonymous donor. My initial ones no longer had any vials available, so I went through the catalogue yet again and picked a third donor.
SEEDAIR
BABY EGGSPRESS
With the eggs and sperm chosen and paid for, things moved forward without much involvement from me.
THANK YOU FOR FLYING SEED AIRLINES.
SEED AIR
BABY EGGSPRESS
COMIN' THROUGH!
SPERM
COLD! COLD! SO VERY EGGSTREMELY COLD!
EGGS

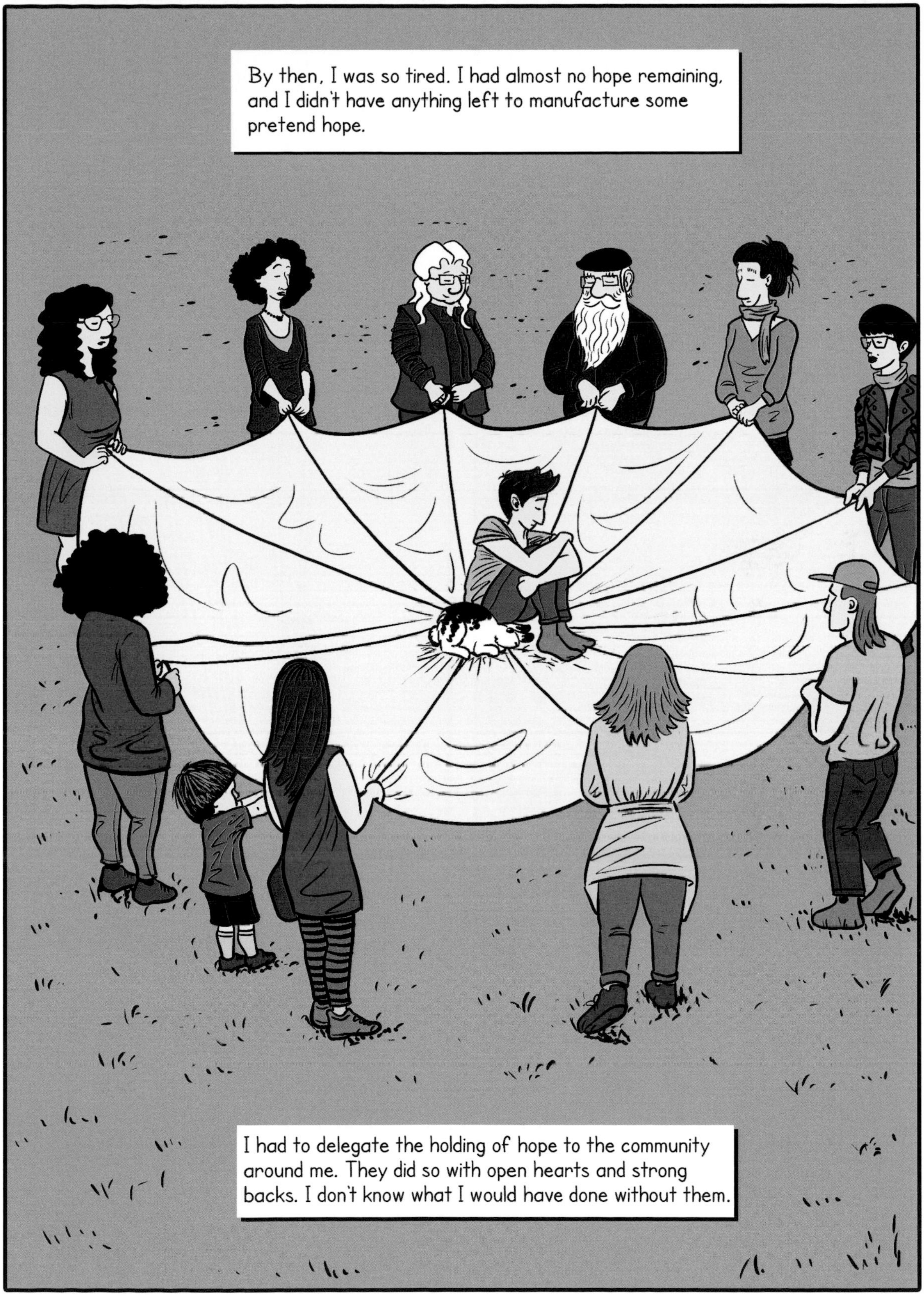
By then, I was so tired. I had almost no hope remaining, and I didn't have anything left to manufacture some pretend hope.
I had to delegate the holding of hope to the community around me. They did so with open hearts and strong backs. I don't know what I would have done without them.

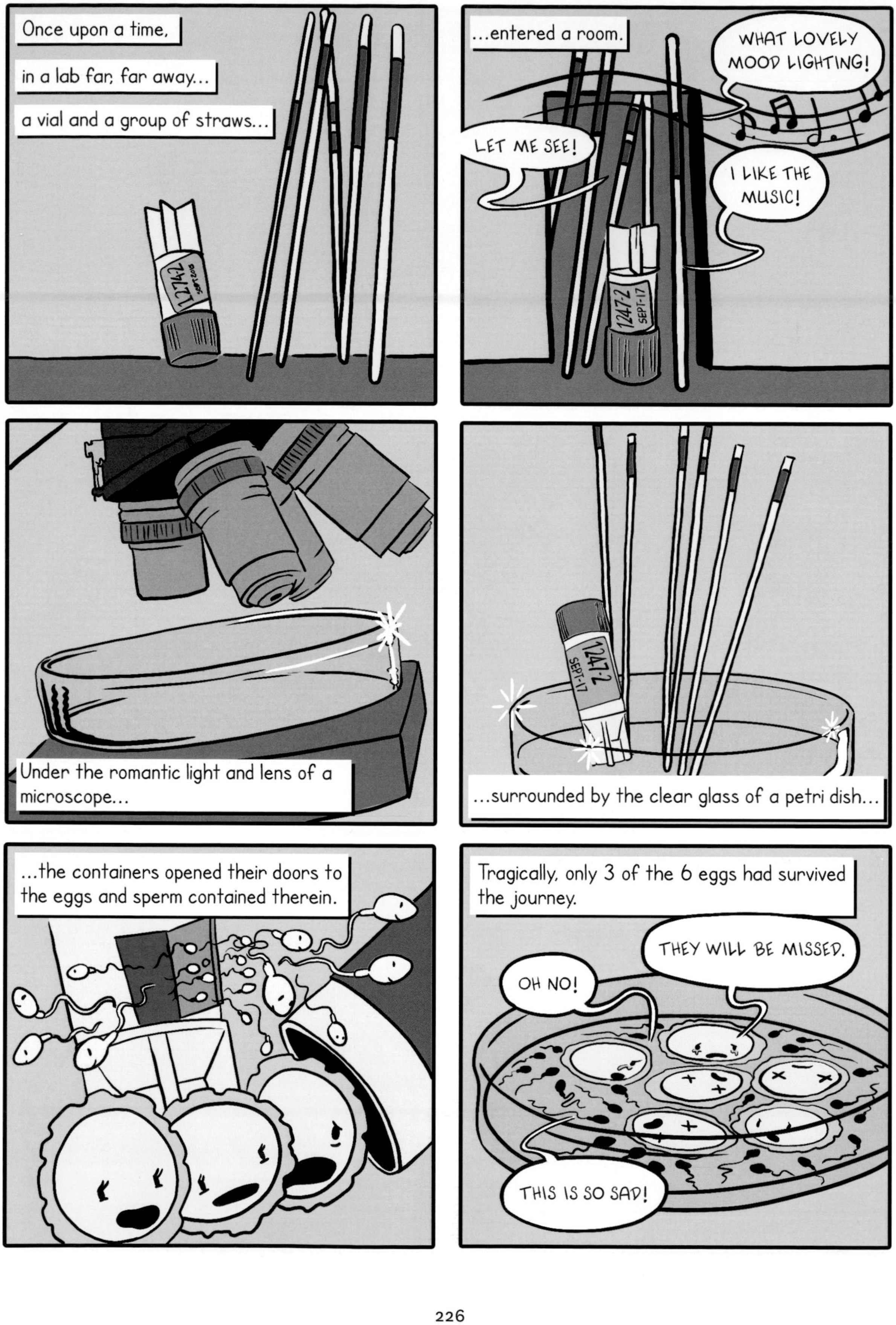

Once upon a time,
in a lab far, far away...
a vial and a group of straws...
1274-2 SEPT 2015
...entered a room.
WHAT LOVELY MOOD LIGHTING!
LET ME SEE!
I LIKE THE MUSIC!
1247-2 SEPT-17
Under the romantic light and lens of a microscope...
1247-2 SEPT-17
...surrounded by the clear glass of a petri dish...
...the containers opened their doors to the eggs and sperm contained therein.
Tragically, only 3 of the 6 eggs had survived the journey.
OH NO!
THEY WILL BE MISSED.
THIS IS SO SAD!

LET'S HONOUR THEM WITH A DANCE.
GOOD IDEA!
The 3 remaining eggs danced the night away with their spermy partners...
...growing and thriving as one.
By the third day, 2 were too exhausted to go on.
MUST...SLEEP...
By the sixth day, the remaining egg-now-blastocyst was ready for a rest.
I NEED AN ICE PACK FOR MY FEET!
I CAN HELP YOU WITH THAT.
FIRST, THOUGH, WE'LL TAKE A QUICK BIOPSY TO SEND TO THE LAB AND MAKE SURE YOU'RE HEALTHY.
OW! THAT PINCHES!
SLEEP WELL! AND WHEN YOU WAKE UP, WE'LL HOPEFULLY HAVE A BRAND NEW BALLROOM FOR YOU TO DANCE IN!
Weeks later...
GOOD NEWS! YOU'RE HEALTHY AND THE NEW BALLROOM IS READY. TIME TO START DANCING AGAIN!
AMAZING!
YOUR LIMO TO THE NEW BALLROOM...
OOO! TRAVELLING IN STYLE!

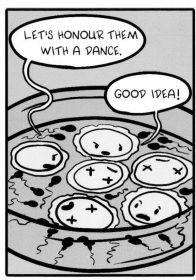

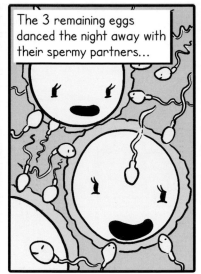

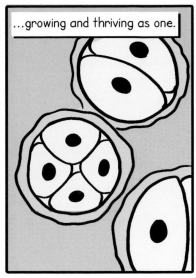

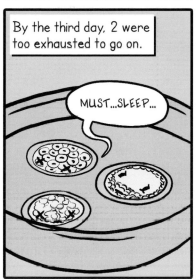

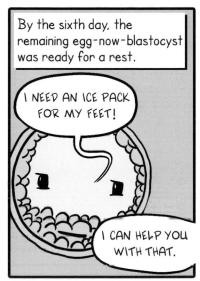

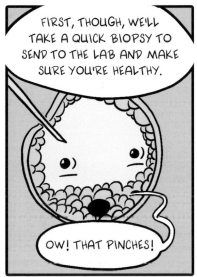

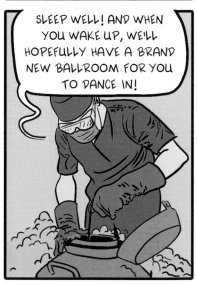

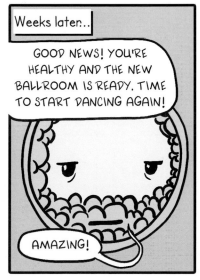

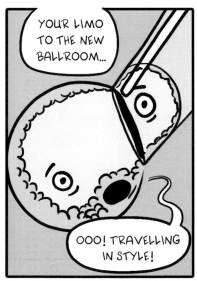

WHAT A SMOOTH RIDE!
ENTERING A TUNNEL! HOLD YOUR BREATH!
IT'S A BIT DARK IN HERE, BUT IT'S NICE.
MAKES ME WANT TO SNUGGLE RATHER THAN DANCE.
BUT I DO NEED TO EXERCISE AFTER BEING FROZEN FOR SO LONG...
9 days later.
CONGRATULATIONS! YOU'RE PREGNANT! YOUR HCG LEVEL IS AT 105.
THAT'S LOW COMPARED WITH MY OTHER PREGNANCIES.
DON'T WORRY, IT'S A GOOD NUMBER.
A few days later.
I DON'T KNOW WHAT'S WRONG WITH ME. I FEEL SO SLUGGISH. I NEED TO STOP FOR A MINUTE.
ZZZZZZZZZ

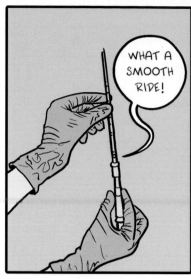

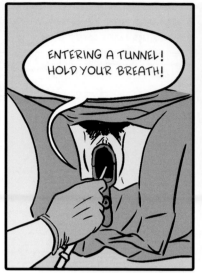

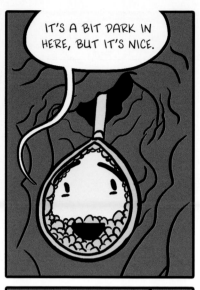

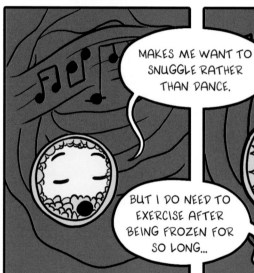

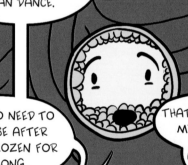

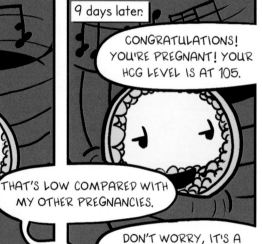

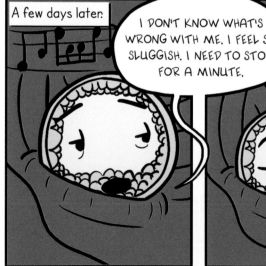

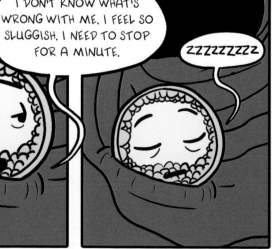

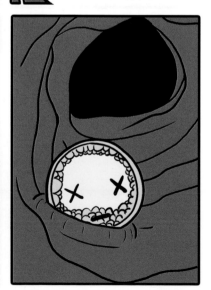

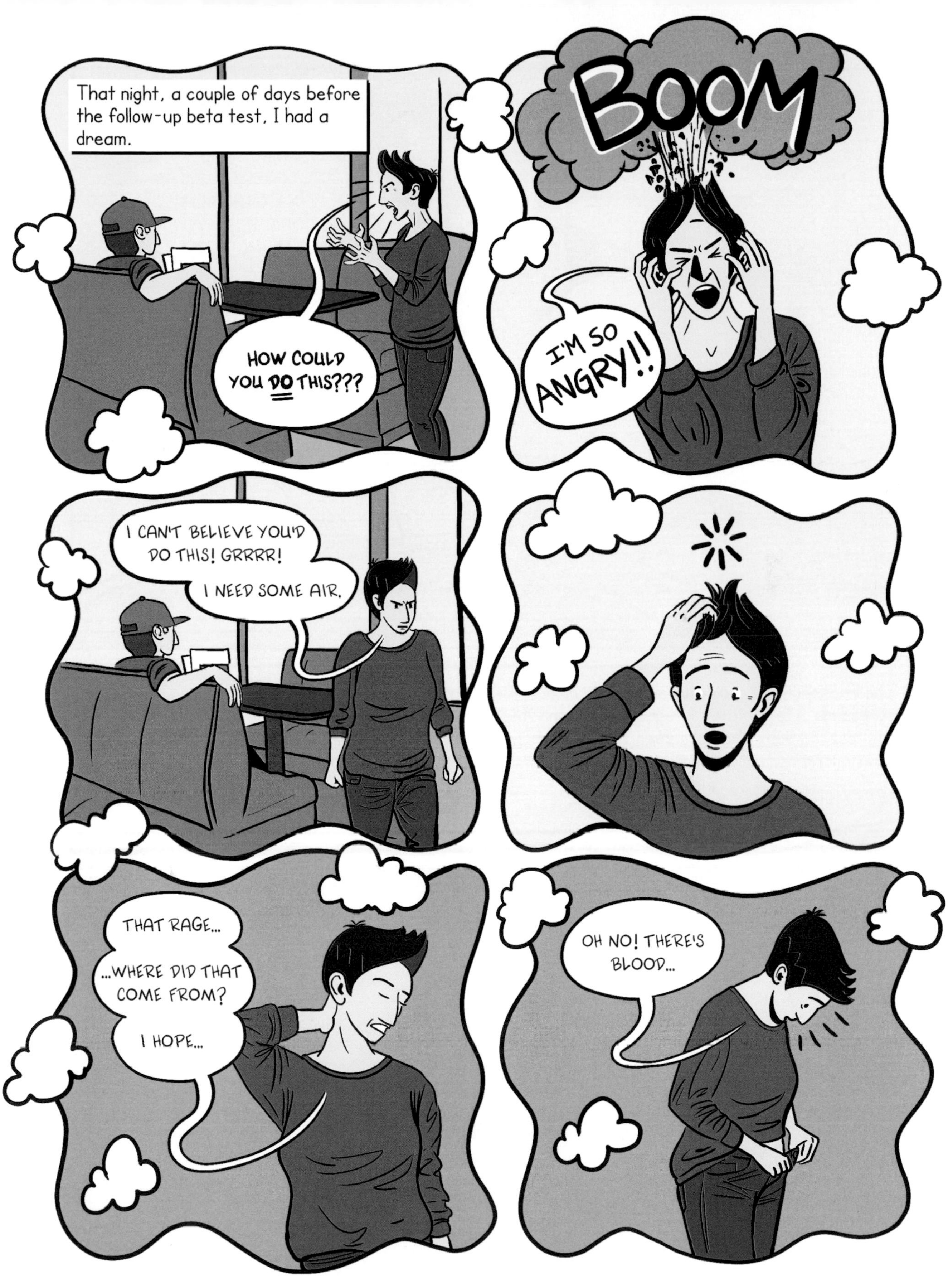
That night, a couple of days before the follow-up beta test, I had a dream.
HOW COULD YOU DO THIS???
BOOM
I'M SO ANGRY!!
I CAN'T BELIEVE YOU'D DO THIS! GRRRR!
I NEED SOME AIR.
THAT RAGE...
...WHERE DID THAT COME FROM?
I HOPE...
OH NO! THERE'S BLOOD...

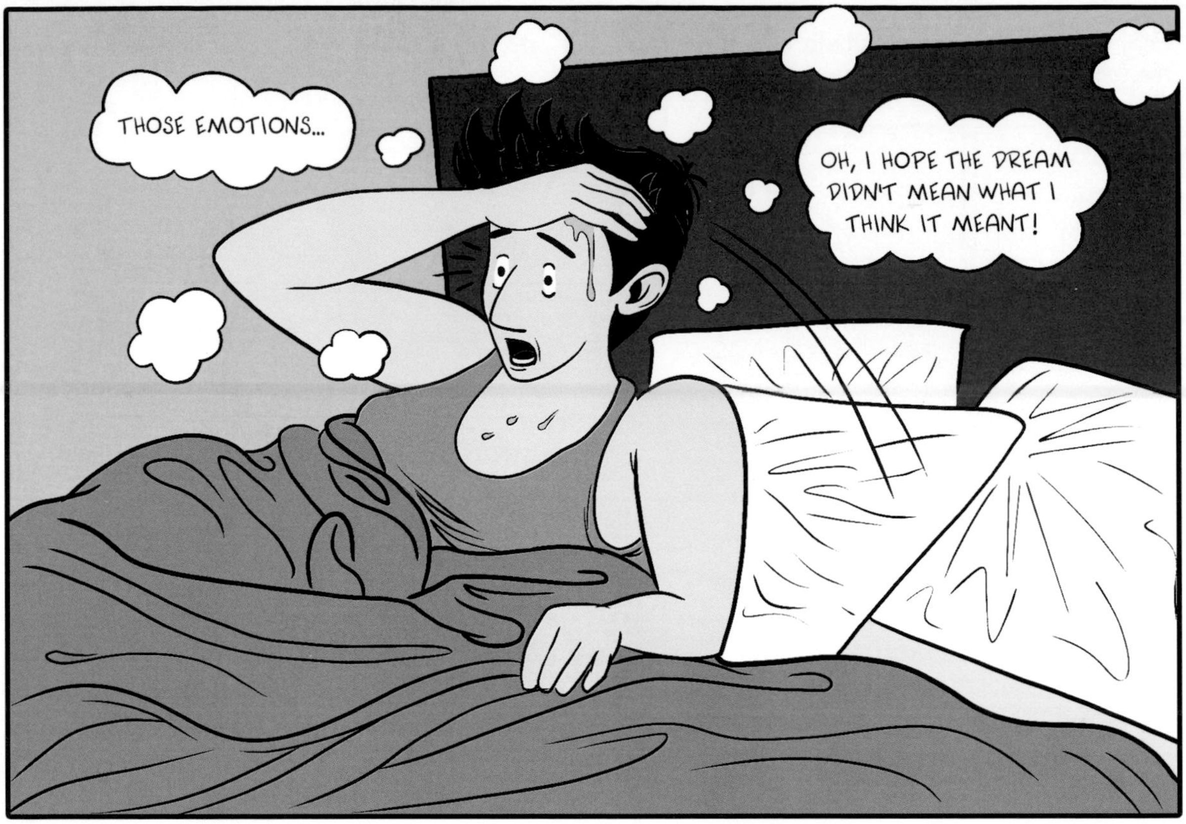
THOSE EMOTIONS...
OH, I HOPE THE DREAM DIDN'T MEAN WHAT I THINK IT MEANT!

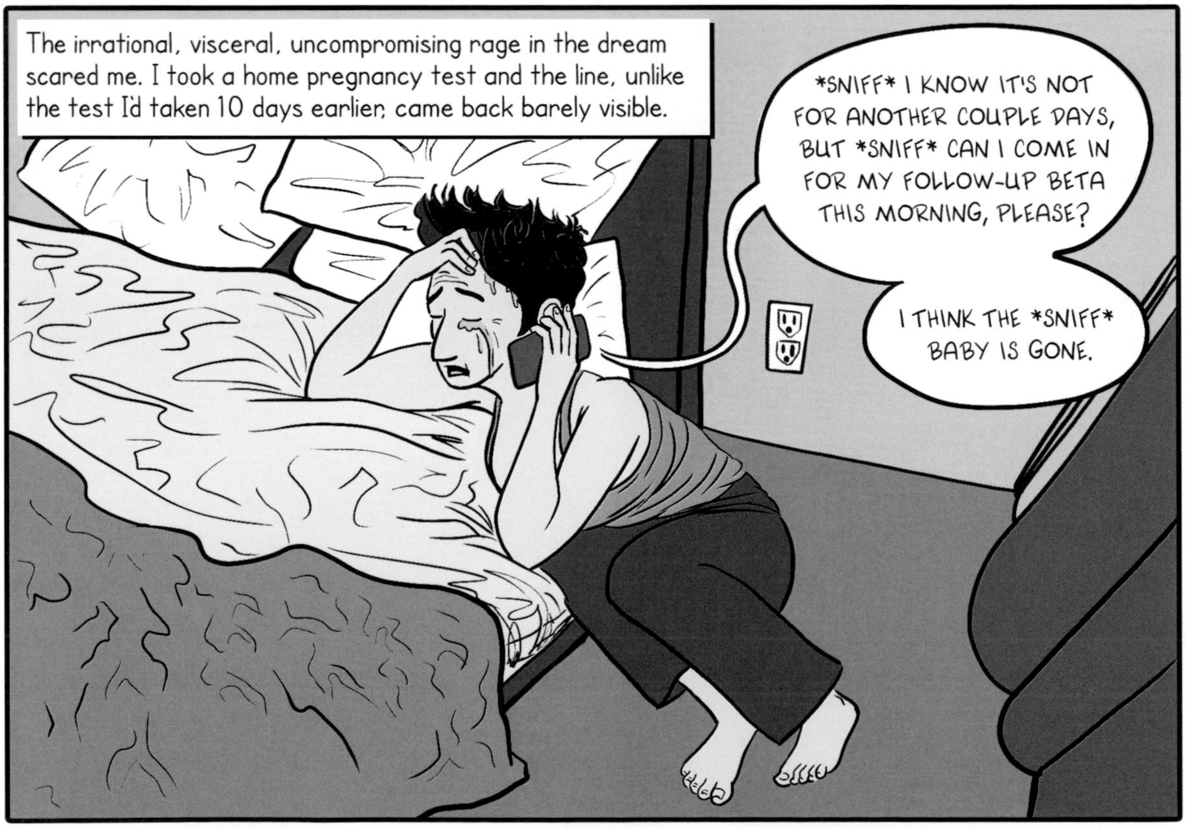
The irrational, visceral, uncompromising rage in the dream scared me. I took a home pregnancy test and the line, unlike the test I'd taken 10 days earlier, came back barely visible.
SNIFF I KNOW IT'S NOT FOR ANOTHER COUPLE DAYS, BUT *SNIFF* CAN I COME IN FOR MY FOLLOW-UP BETA THIS MORNING, PLEASE?
I THINK THE *SNIFF* BABY IS GONE.

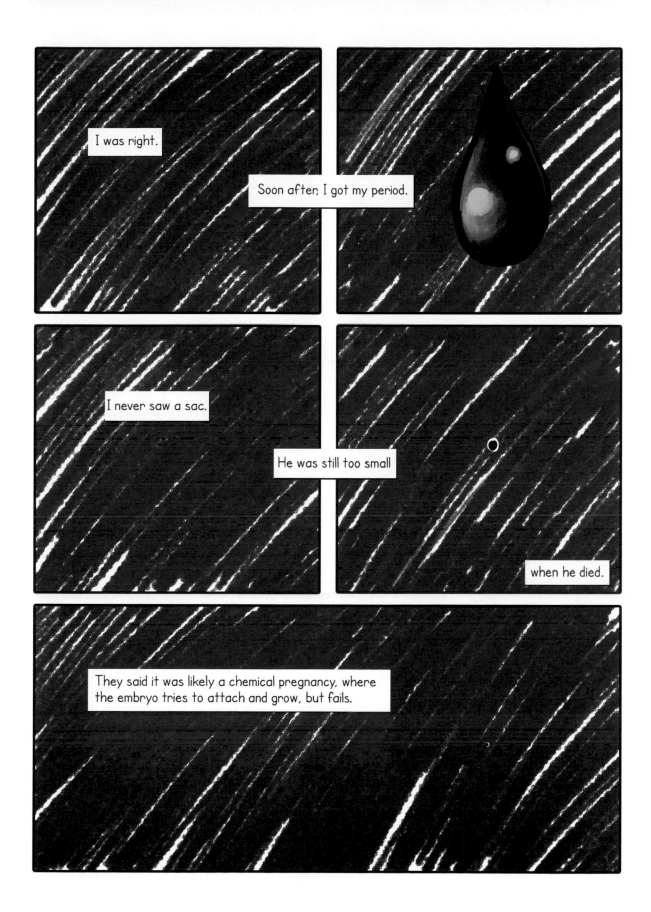

I was right.

Soon after, I got my period.

I never saw a sac.

He was still too small

when he died.

They said it was likely a chemical pregnancy, where the embryo tries to attach and grow, but fails.

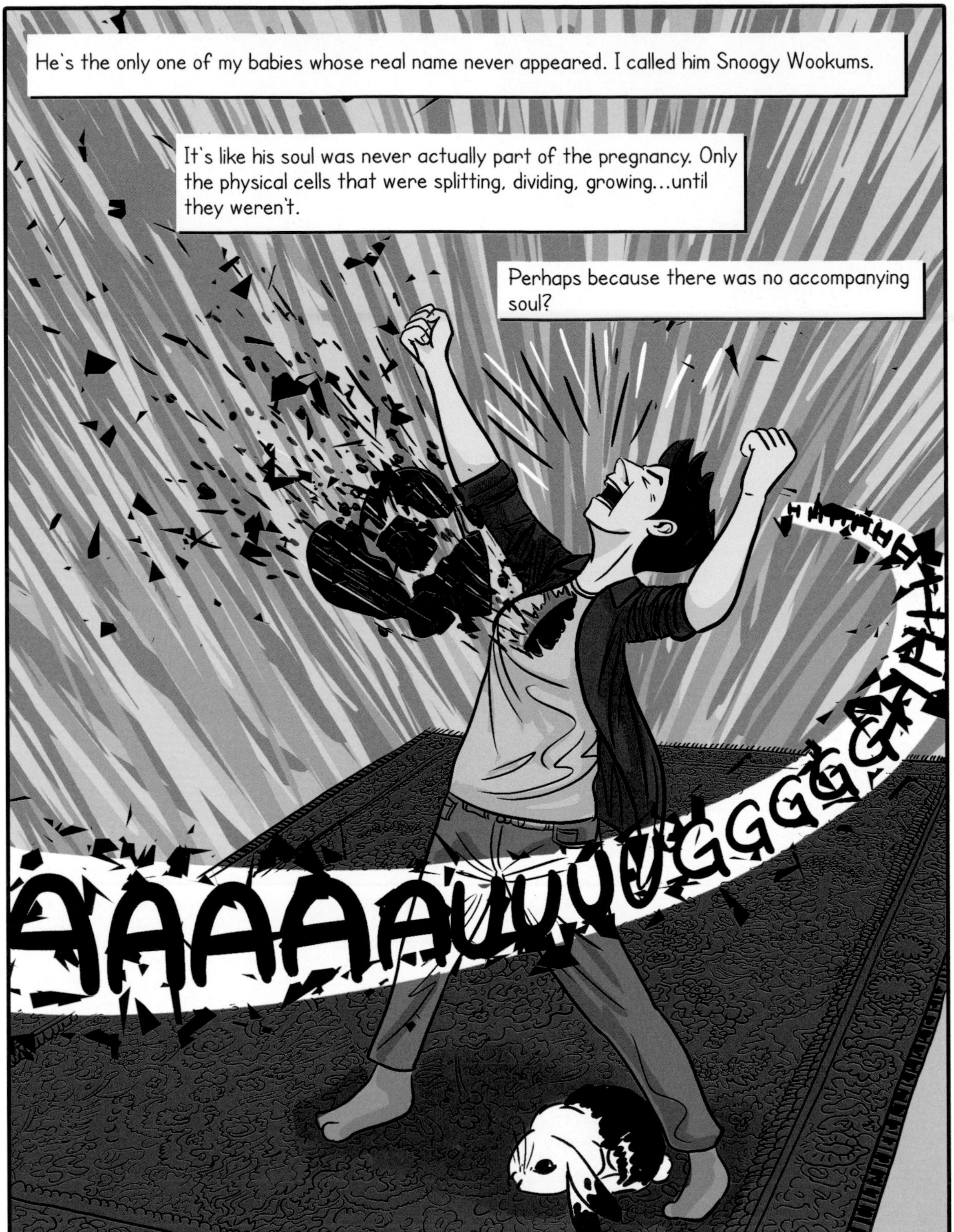
He's the only one of my babies whose real name never appeared. I called him Snoogy Wookums.
It's like his soul was never actually part of the pregnancy. Only the physical cells that were splitting, dividing, growing...until they weren't.
Perhaps because there was no accompanying soul?
AAAAAAUUUUGGGGGG
A very unexpected thing happened after the miscarriage.

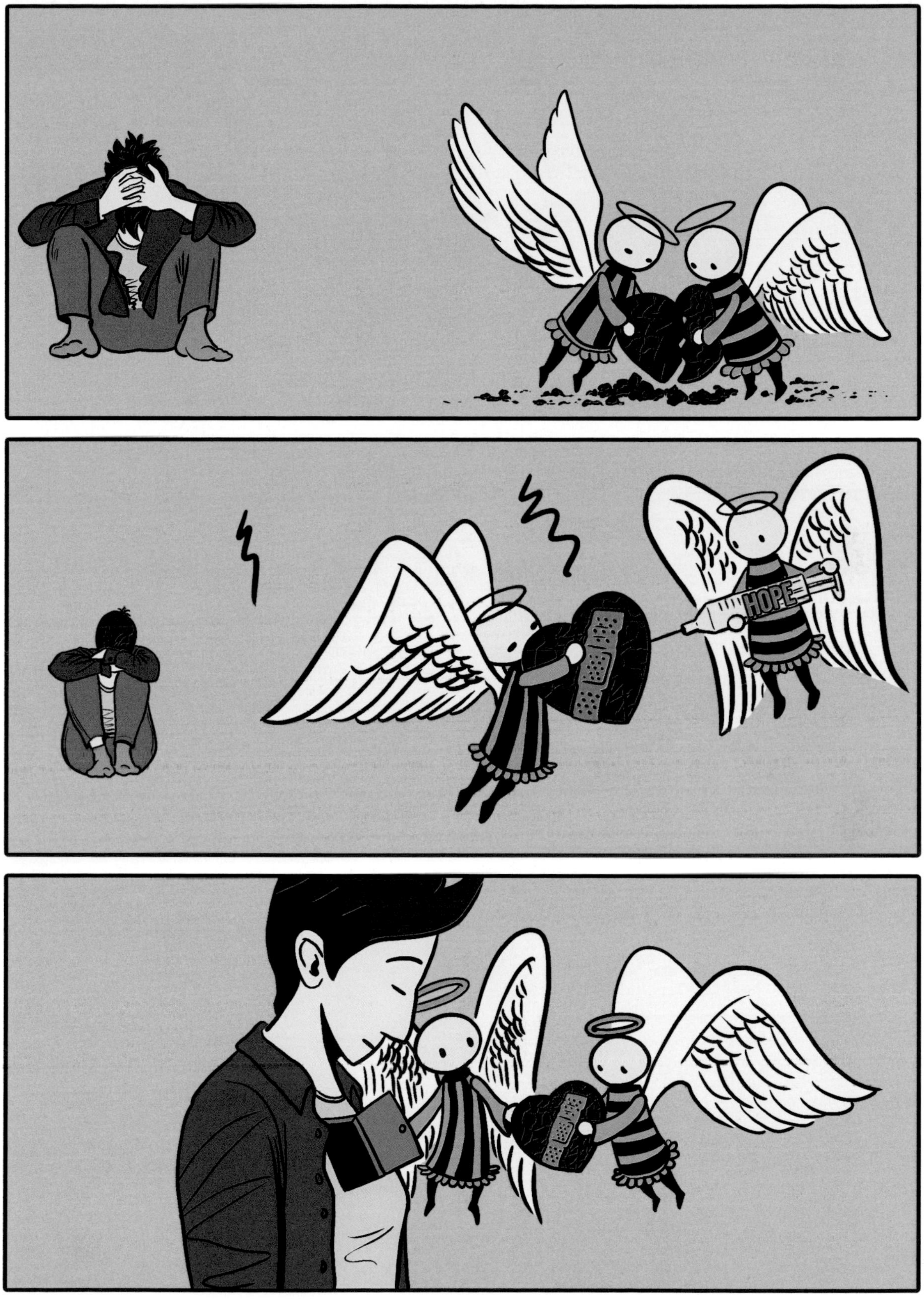
HOPE

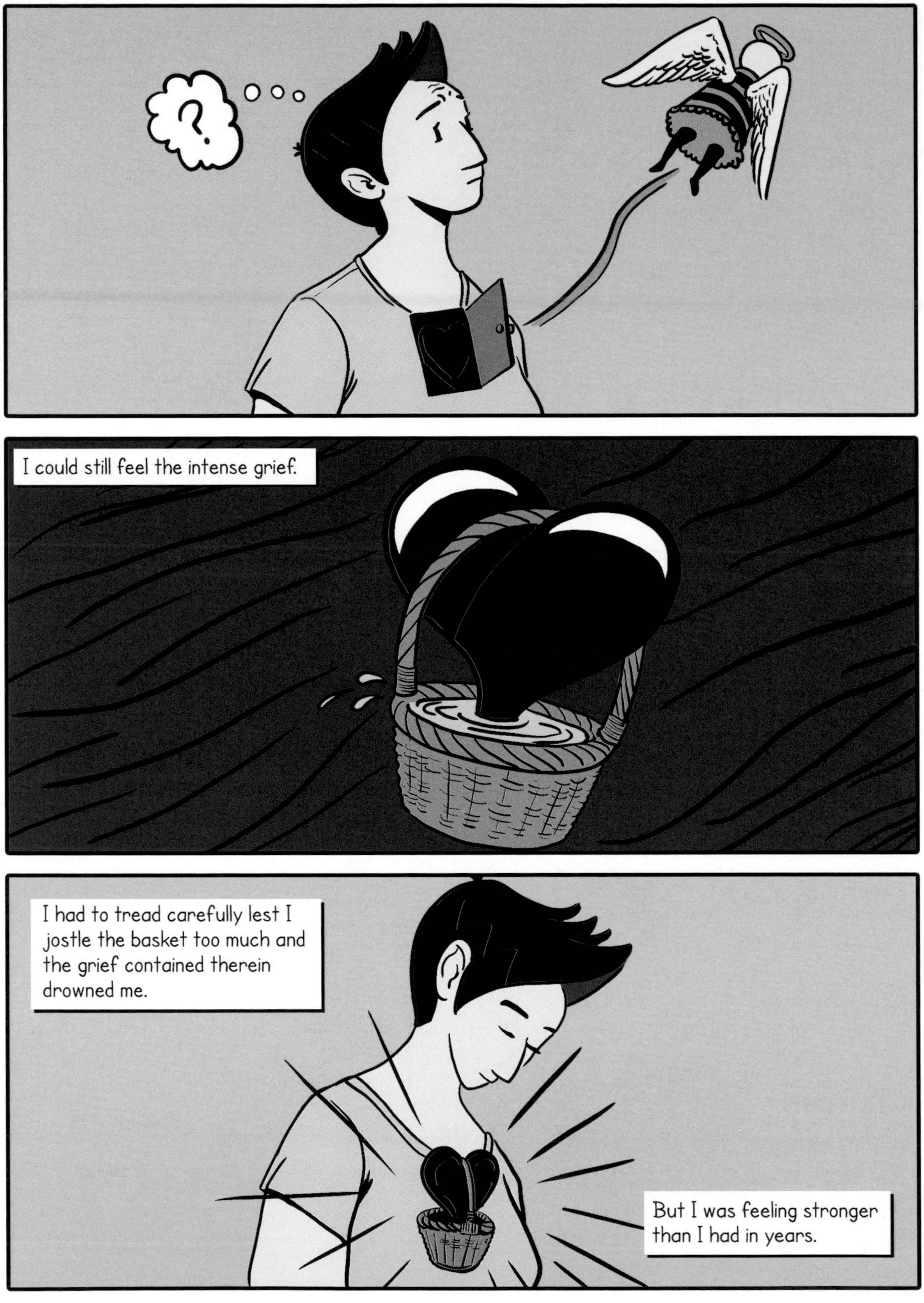
?
I could still feel the intense grief.
I had to tread carefully lest I jostle the basket too much and the grief contained therein drowned me.
But I was feeling stronger than I had in years.

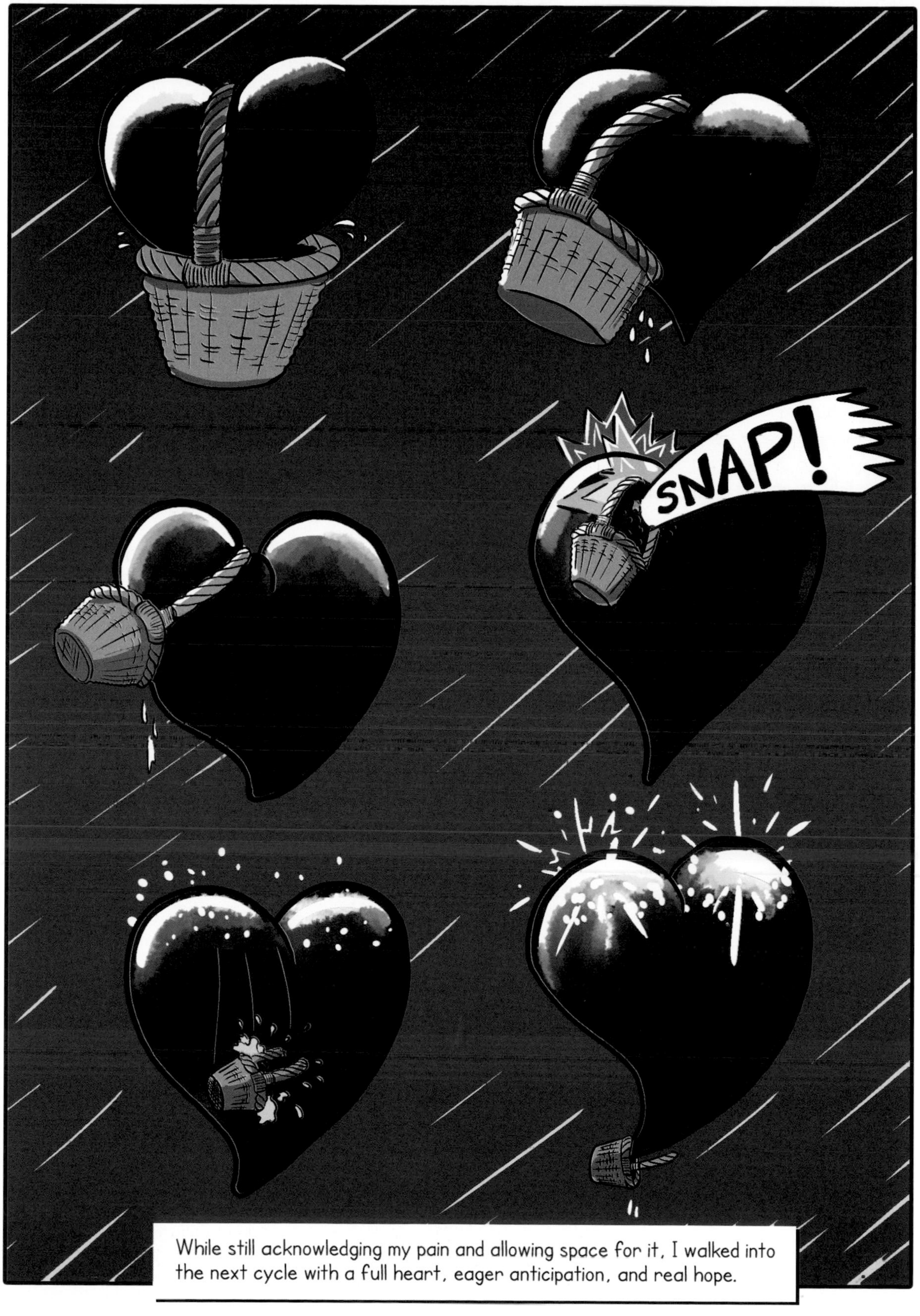
SNAP!

While still acknowledging my pain and allowing space for it, I walked into the next cycle with a full heart, eager anticipation, and real hope.

Chapter 7

Isaac and Abegail

DO YOU THINK SHE'LL EVER FIND US?
I HOPE SO!

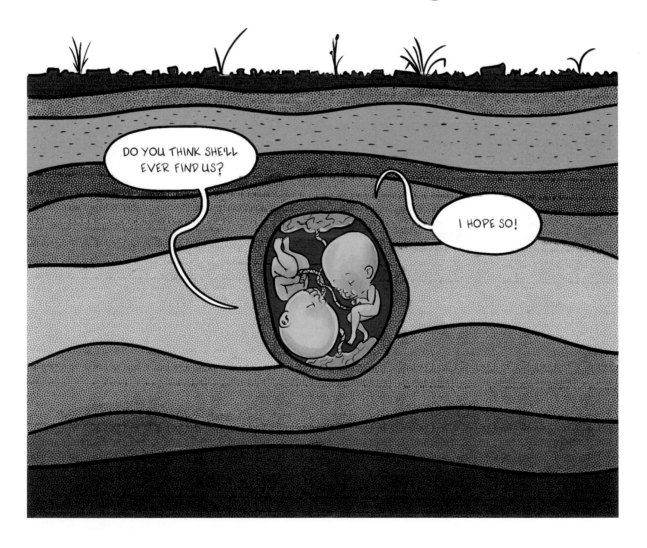

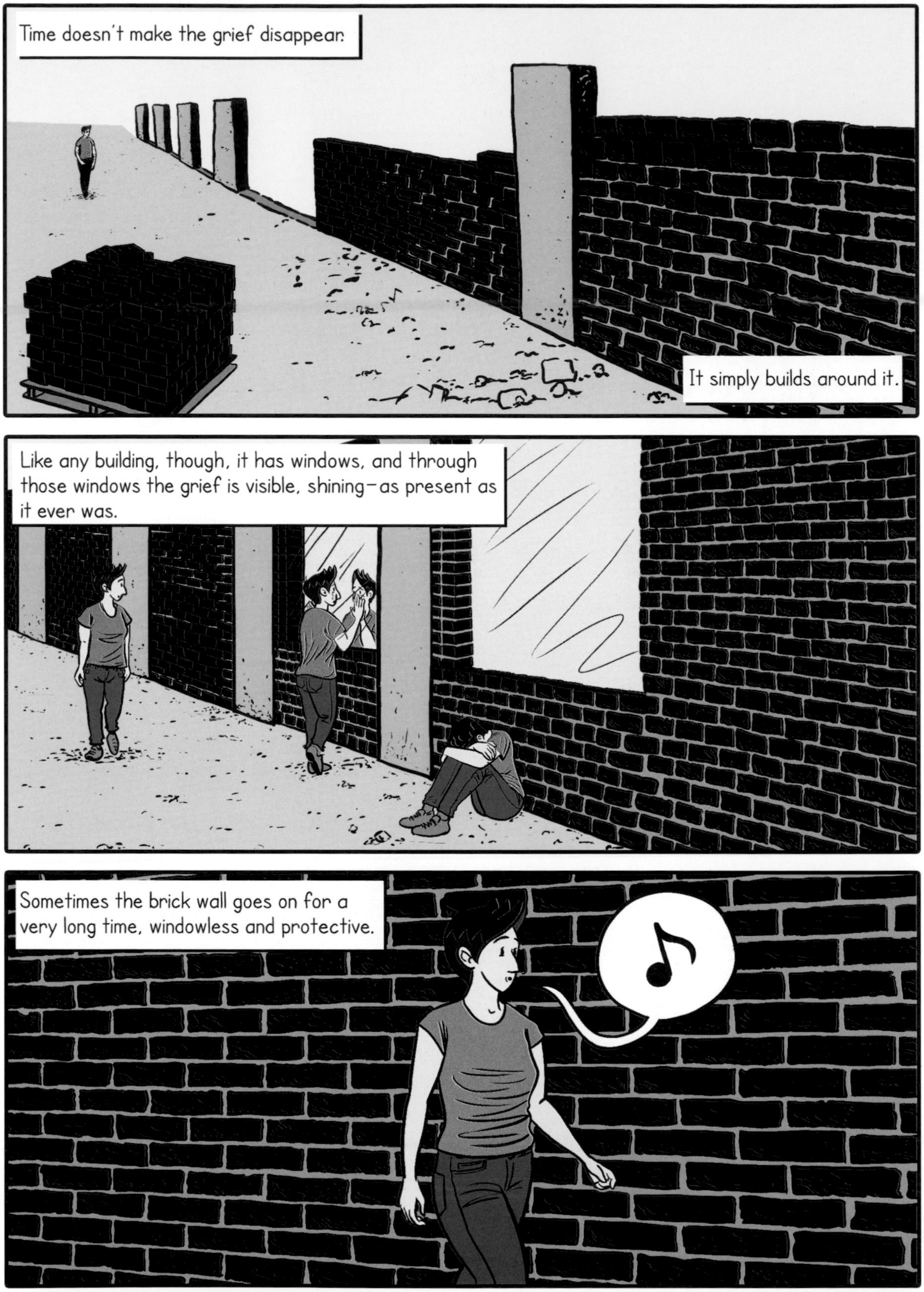

Time doesn't make the grief disappear.
It simply builds around it.
Like any building, though, it has windows, and through those windows the grief is visible, shining—as present as it ever was.
Sometimes the brick wall goes on for a very long time, windowless and protective.
♪

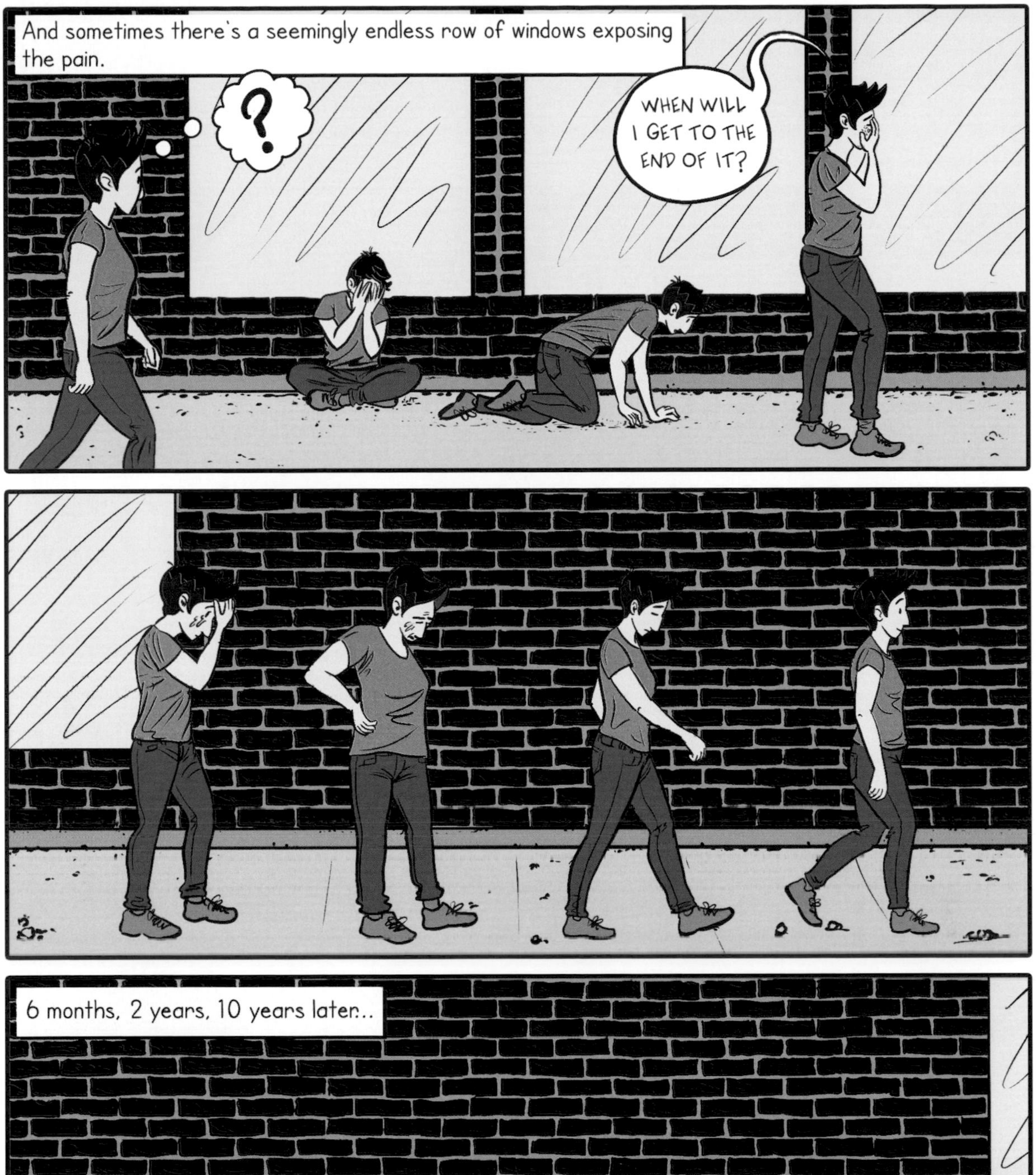
And sometimes there's a seemingly endless row of windows exposing the pain.
?
WHEN WILL I GET TO THE END OF IT?
6 months, 2 years, 10 years later..
Until you die.

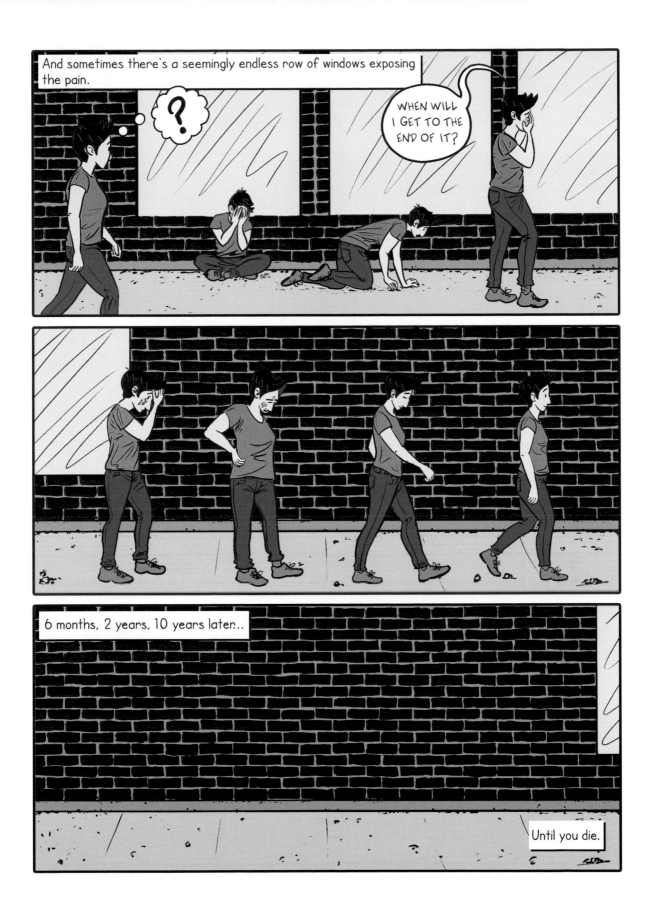

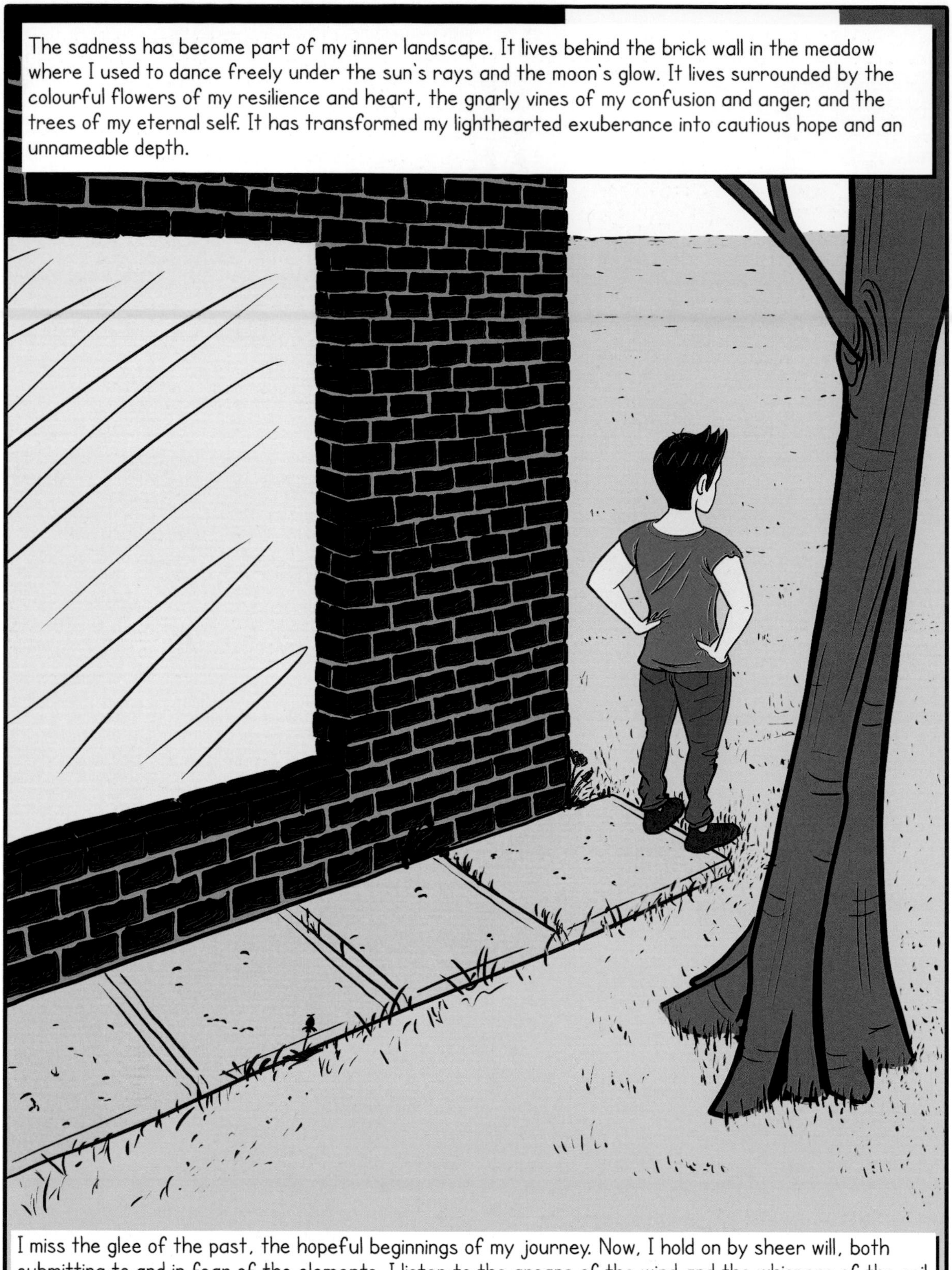
The sadness has become part of my inner landscape. It lives behind the brick wall in the meadow where I used to dance freely under the sun's rays and the moon's glow. It lives surrounded by the colourful flowers of my resilience and heart, the gnarly vines of my confusion and anger, and the trees of my eternal self. It has transformed my lighthearted exuberance into cautious hope and an unnameable depth.
I miss the glee of the past, the hopeful beginnings of my journey. Now, I hold on by sheer will, both submitting to and in fear of the elements. I listen to the groans of the wind and the whispers of the soil and hope that I am enough.

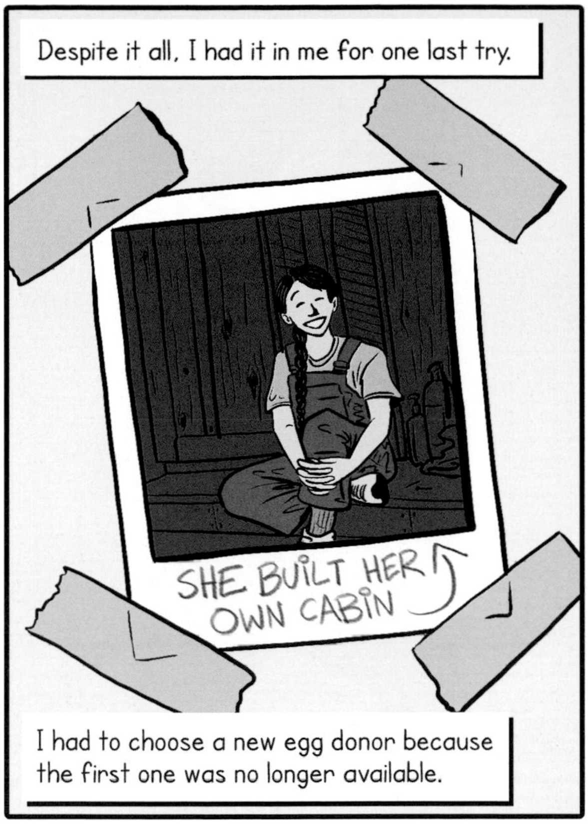
Despite it all, I had it in me for one last try.
SHE BUILT HER OWN CABIN
I had to choose a new egg donor because the first one was no longer available.

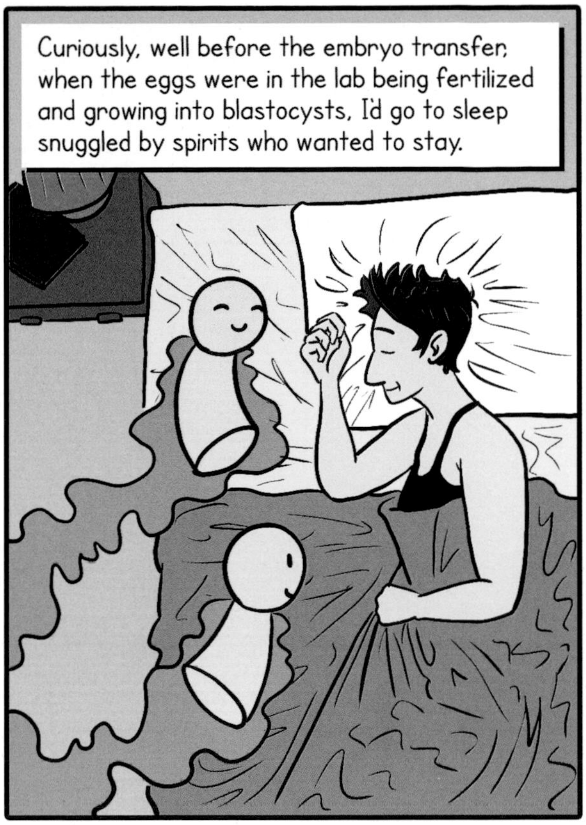
Curiously, well before the embryo transfer, when the eggs were in the lab being fertilized and growing into blastocysts, I'd go to sleep snuggled by spirits who wanted to stay.

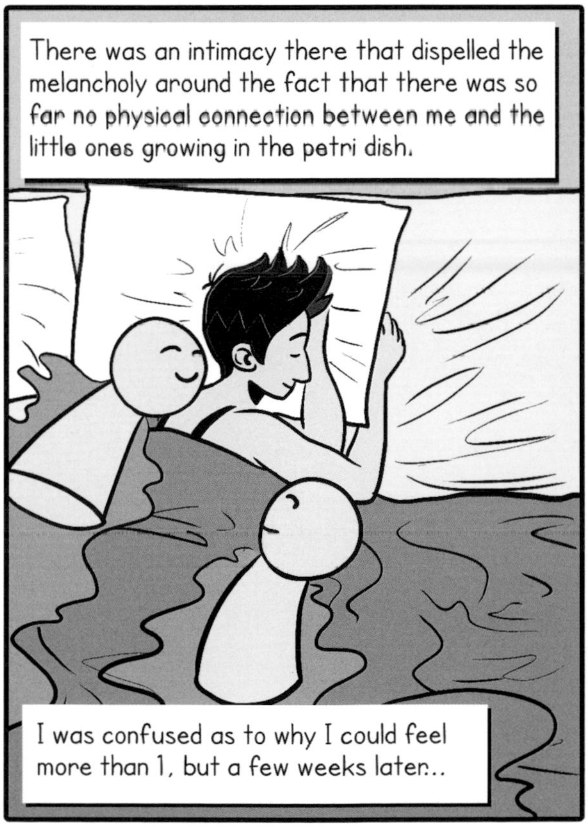
There was an intimacy there that dispelled the melancholy around the fact that there was so far no physical connection between me and the little ones growing in the petri dish.
I was confused as to why I could feel more than 1, but a few weeks later..

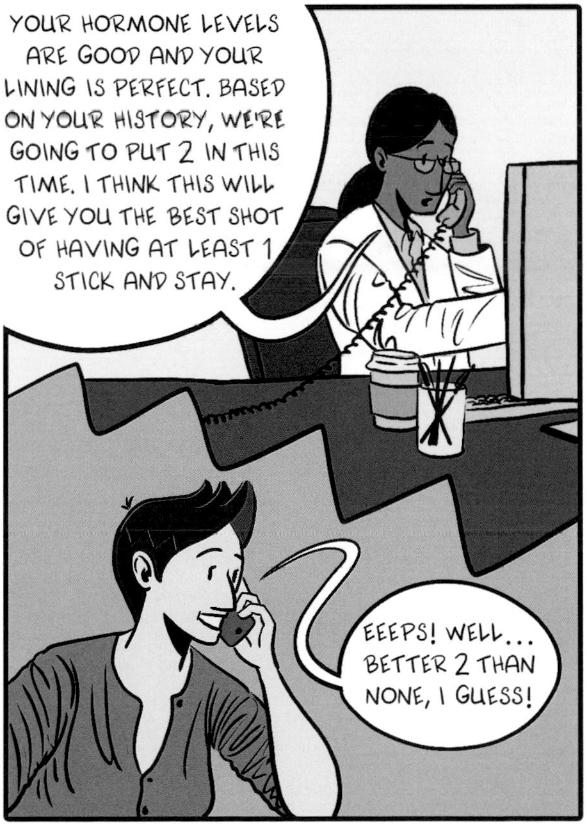
YOUR HORMONE LEVELS ARE GOOD AND YOUR LINING IS PERFECT. BASED ON YOUR HISTORY, WE'RE GOING TO PUT 2 IN THIS TIME. I THINK THIS WILL GIVE YOU THE BEST SHOT OF HAVING AT LEAST 1 STICK AND STAY.
EEEPS! WELL... BETTER 2 THAN NONE, I GUESS!

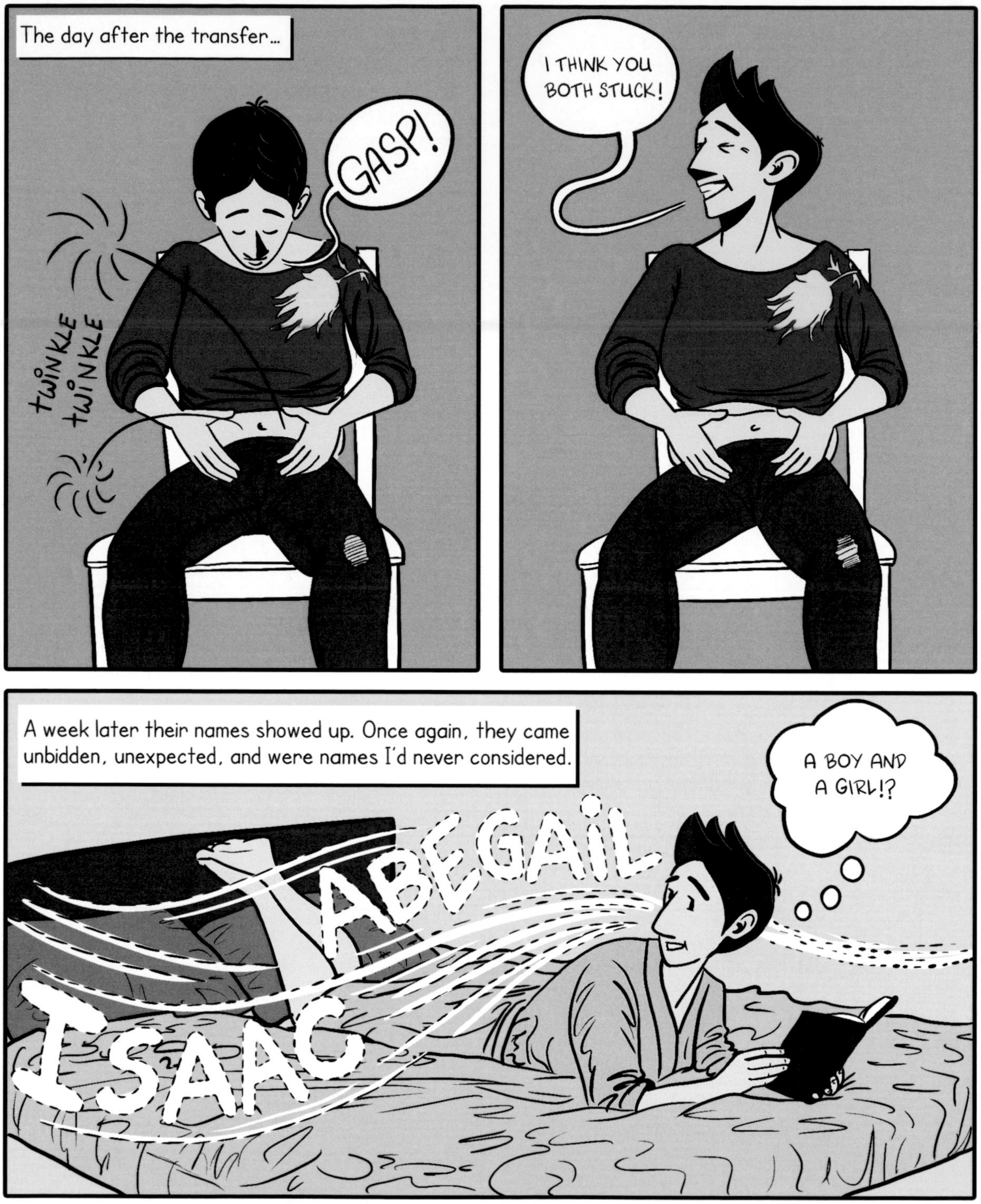
The day after the transfer...
TWINKLE TWINKLE
GASP!
I THINK YOU BOTH STUCK!
A week later their names showed up. Once again, they came unbidden, unexpected, and were names I'd never considered.
A BOY AND A GIRL!?
ABEGAIL
ISAAC

Amazingly, my intuition was proven right time and time again. The blood test a week later confirmed I was pregnant. The ultrasound 6 weeks after that showed that I was indeed carrying twins. The genetic counsellor who phoned me weeks later told me that it was a boy and a girl!

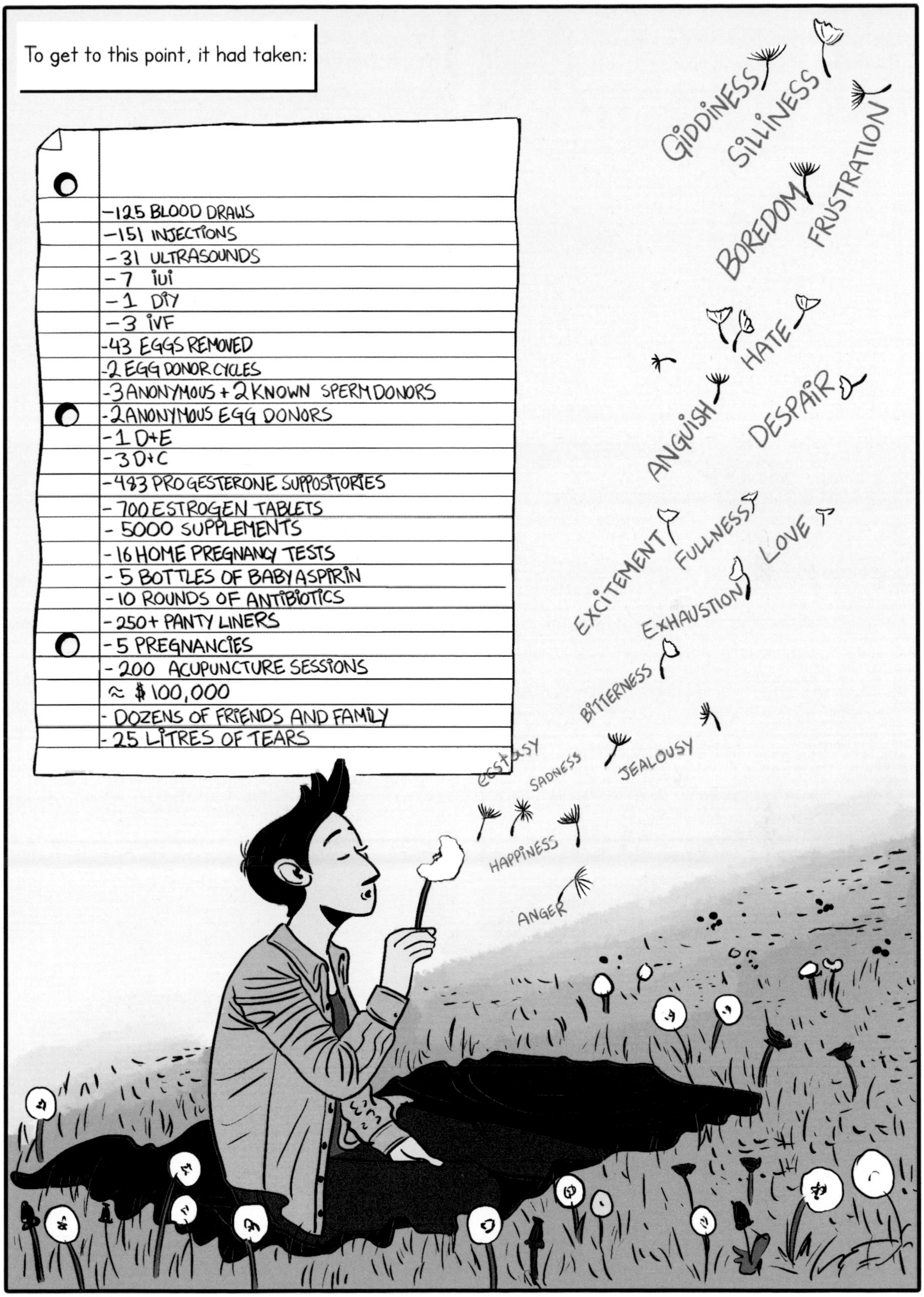
To get to this point, it had taken:
-125 BLOOD DRAWS
-151 INJECTIONS
-31 ULTRASOUNDS
-7 IUI
-1 DIY
-3 IVF
-43 EGGS REMOVED
-2 EGG DONOR CYCLES
-3 ANONYMOUS + 2 KNOWN SPERM DONORS
-2 ANONYMOUS EGG DONORS
-1 D+E
-3 D+C
-483 PROGESTERONE SUPPOSITORIES
-700 ESTROGEN TABLETS
-5000 SUPPLEMENTS
-16 HOME PREGNANCY TESTS
-5 BOTTLES OF BABY ASPIRIN
-10 ROUNDS OF ANTIBIOTICS
-250+ PANTY LINERS
-5 PREGNANCIES
-200 ACUPUNCTURE SESSIONS
≈ $100,000
- DOZENS OF FRIENDS AND FAMILY
- 25 LITRES OF TEARS
GIDDINESS
SILLINESS
FRUSTRATION
BOREDOM
HATE
DESPAIR
ANGUISH
EXCITEMENT
FULLNESS
LOVE
EXHAUSTION
BITTERNESS
ecstasy
SADNESS
JEALOUSY
HAPPINESS
ANGER

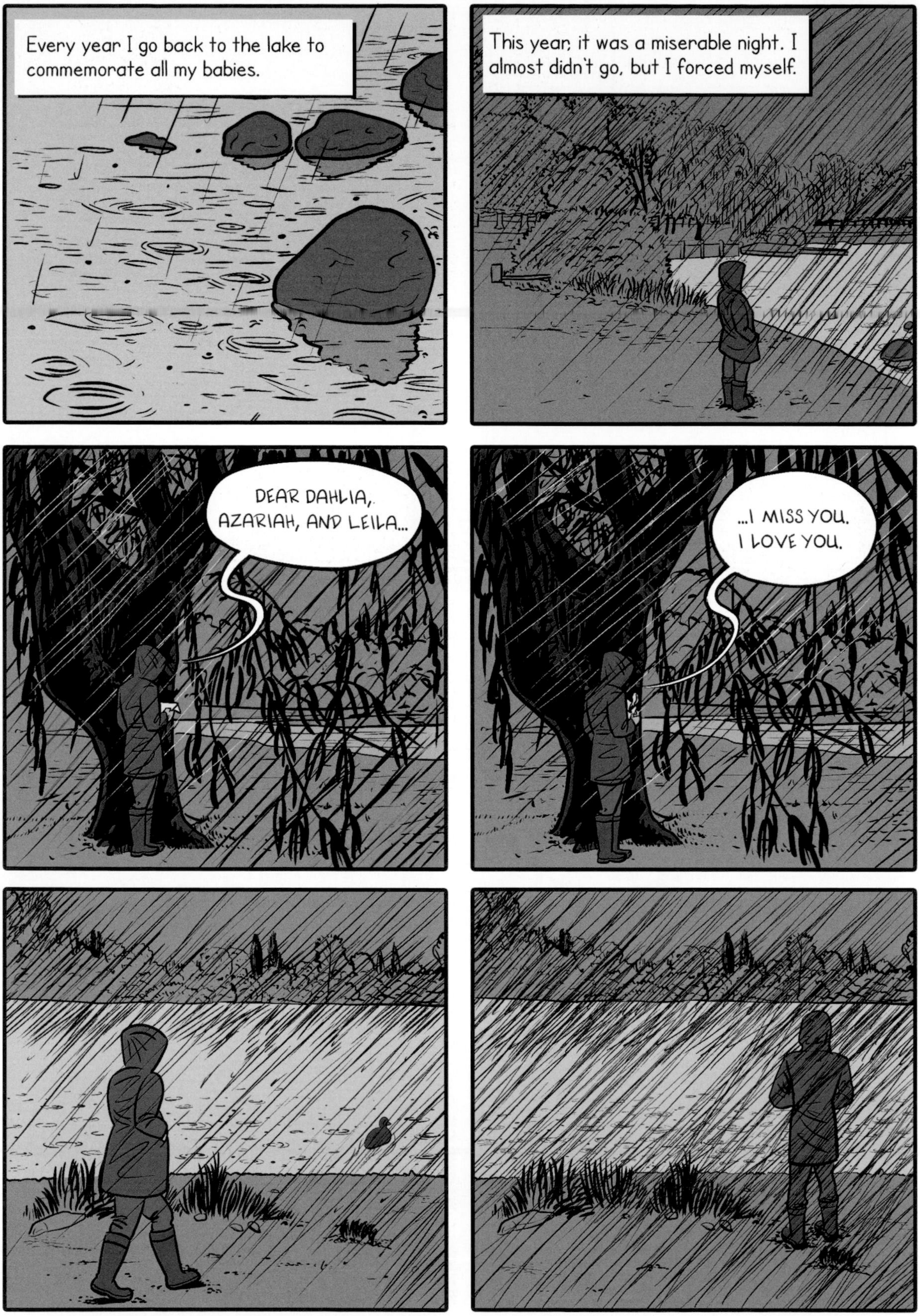
Every year I go back to the lake to commemorate all my babies.
This year, it was a miserable night. I almost didn't go, but I forced myself.
DEAR DAHLIA, AZARIAH, AND LEILA...
...I MISS YOU. I LOVE YOU.

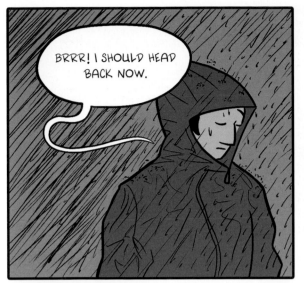

BRRR! I SHOULD HEAD BACK NOW.

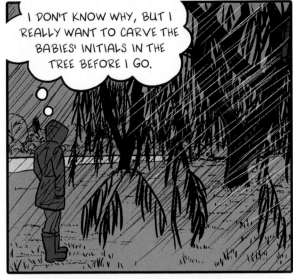

I DON'T KNOW WHY, BUT I REALLY WANT TO CARVE THE BABIES' INITIALS IN THE TREE BEFORE I GO.

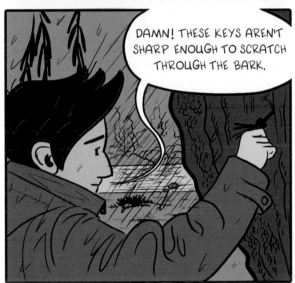

DAMN! THESE KEYS AREN'T SHARP ENOUGH TO SCRATCH THROUGH THE BARK.

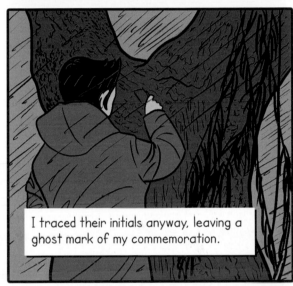

I traced their initials anyway, leaving a ghost mark of my commemoration.

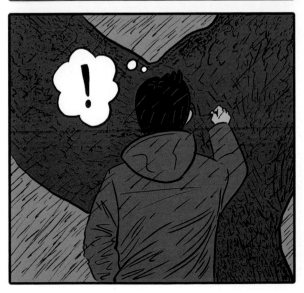

!

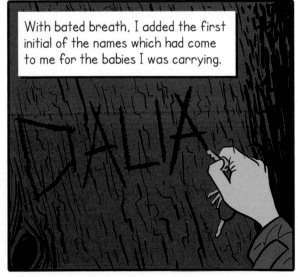

With bated breath, I added the first initial of the names which had come to me for the babies I was carrying.

DALIA

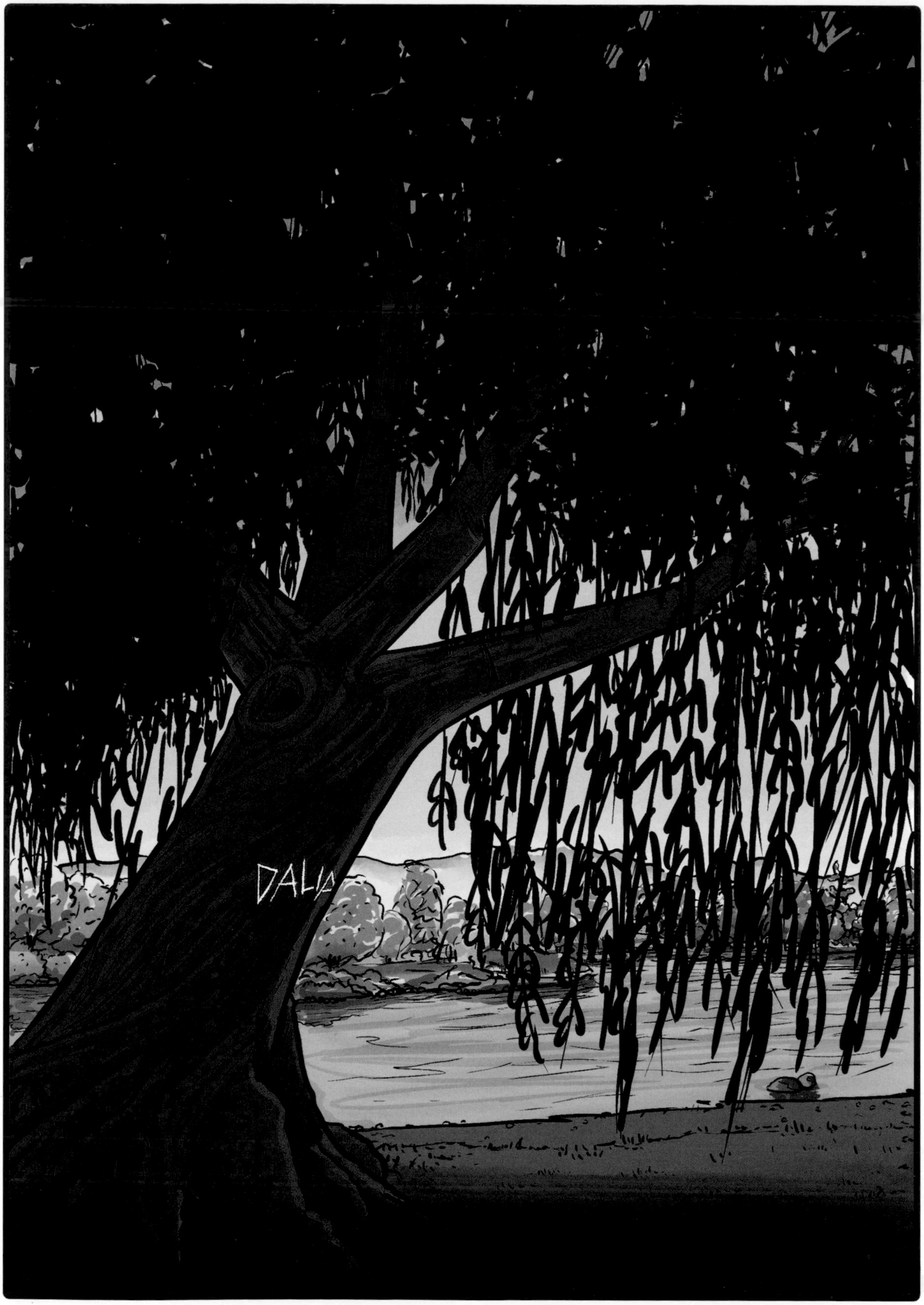
DALIA

Although when spelled with an "h", Dahlia is a type of flower; without the "h," it means "destiny" or "fate."

YEAR FIVE

APRIL 2018–NOVEMBER 2018

Epilogue

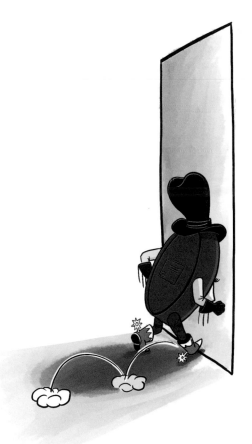

On November 10, 2018, Isaac and Abegail were born.

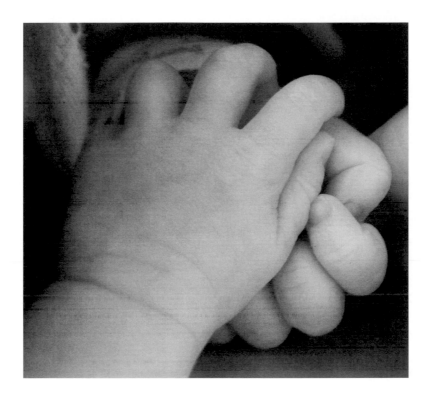

I am the luckiest woman on earth.

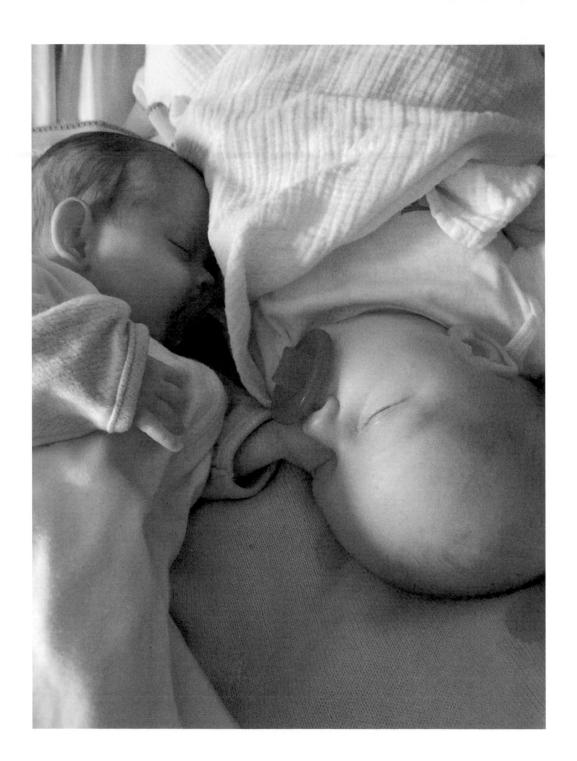

Acknowledgements

My eternal gratitude goes to my family and friends who have stuck by me and supported me through the years. You have fished me out of the depths of hell and celebrated with me in times of joy.

Lani Brunn, you have accompanied me to countless appointments in my baby-making quest. I don't know what I would have done without your humour, compassion, grace, and love.

To my parents, Danny Steinberg and Claudine Pommier, thank you for your never-ending support and enthusiasm, both for the creation of my little humans and the creation of this book. I couldn't ask for better parents.

Thank you, Gabrielle Steinberg, for sticking so many needles in me, bringing me back to health more than once, and being there during some seriously hard moments (I hope the welts from my fingernails have healed).

Thank you, Naomi Steinberg, for cheering me on in this journey.

To my grandmother, Esther Steinberg, with your sage advice, careful words, and sparkly eyes, thank you for being such an integral part of this journey and for being the guardian angel to my angel babies.

To Ella VanGaya, Fred Morel, Meris Goodman, Meghan Goodman, Johanna Wetzel, Maya Alonso, Lindsey McEwan, Jean-Michel Le Gal, Damon Morris, Maryam Nabavi, and Rielle Capler—thank you for being there, lending an ear, poking me in the butt with needles, providing warm hugs, taking me to or from the clinic or hospital, going on walks, helping me keep my hope alive, and otherwise providing invaluable support.

To Alex Danard, thank you not only for being there as a friend, but for providing such valuable feedback on the manuscript.

To Christache, thank you for taking on such a daunting project! Your drawing skills and insightful input have brought the book to a whole other level of awesome.

To Even Oldridge, thank you for lending me your Wacom tablet for the colouring process. It was a lifesaver!

To everyone at Olive Fertility Centre, especially Dr. Taylor, Dr. Nakhuda, Dr. Tallon, all the nurses, Kirin Sidhu, Gladys Lundgren, and Wendy Baker... Well, that was a slog, wasn't it! Thank you for not giving up, and for being so encouraging. Thank you also for allowing me to photograph and videotape my journey. The footage proved invaluable in the writing of this book. Thank you to Leah Tannock for checking the manuscript to make sure I got all the medical stuff right.

To Susan Cormier and Bryant Ross from C.R. Apiary, and Sujatha Ranatunge—I'll forever be grateful for your kindness. I will always remember how a single, seemingly small gesture can impact a person for a lifetime.

To Felicia Chang, Lani Brunn (again), Keith Terrillon, and Ella VanGaya (also again), thank you for documenting so much of my journey and the mini-interviews we did before or after procedures. Your questions were invaluable, insightful, and thoughtful.

To Josie Chang, much gratitude for allowing me to include part of your story in this book.

To Cora Beitel and Stephanie Dow, thank you for being there in the hope and the despair.

To Pascal Pillot-Bruhat, I am so grateful for the hours you spent hanging out with my littles while I plugged away at the book. Your help and support was invaluable.

Thank you to Trena White at Page Two for immediately believing in the project, and for everyone on the team—Trena, Amanda Lewis, Rony Ganon, Peter Cocking, Caela Moffet, and Annemarie Tempelman-Kluit—for your hard work and enthusiasm about the book.

And finally, Sherbert. Sherbert, my goofus piranha-bunny, my snuggly, funny, demanding animal. Your courage and strength in your own healing journey were an inspiration. I am grateful and awed that you ended up in my life. The universe works in mysterious ways!

I hope I didn't forget anyone, but if I did, I apologize and THANK YOU!

FINANCIAL BACKERS

A humongous thank you to the many, many, MANY people who contributed to our Indiegogo fundraiser. You contributed over $11,000 to help make this book a reality. Your support and belief in the book mean the world to me.

THE FOLLOWING INDIVIDUALS CONTRIBUTED $250 OR MORE TO THE CAMPAIGN

Claudine Pommier + Daniel Steinberg
Eliot Steinberg + Rachel Wiener
Yacov Steinberg + Savione Dgany
Maria Lorenzi
Sasha Vilner
Thomas Woods + Lydia Lovison
Joyce Ozier

For a complete list of donors, please visit www.cataloguebabynovel.com.

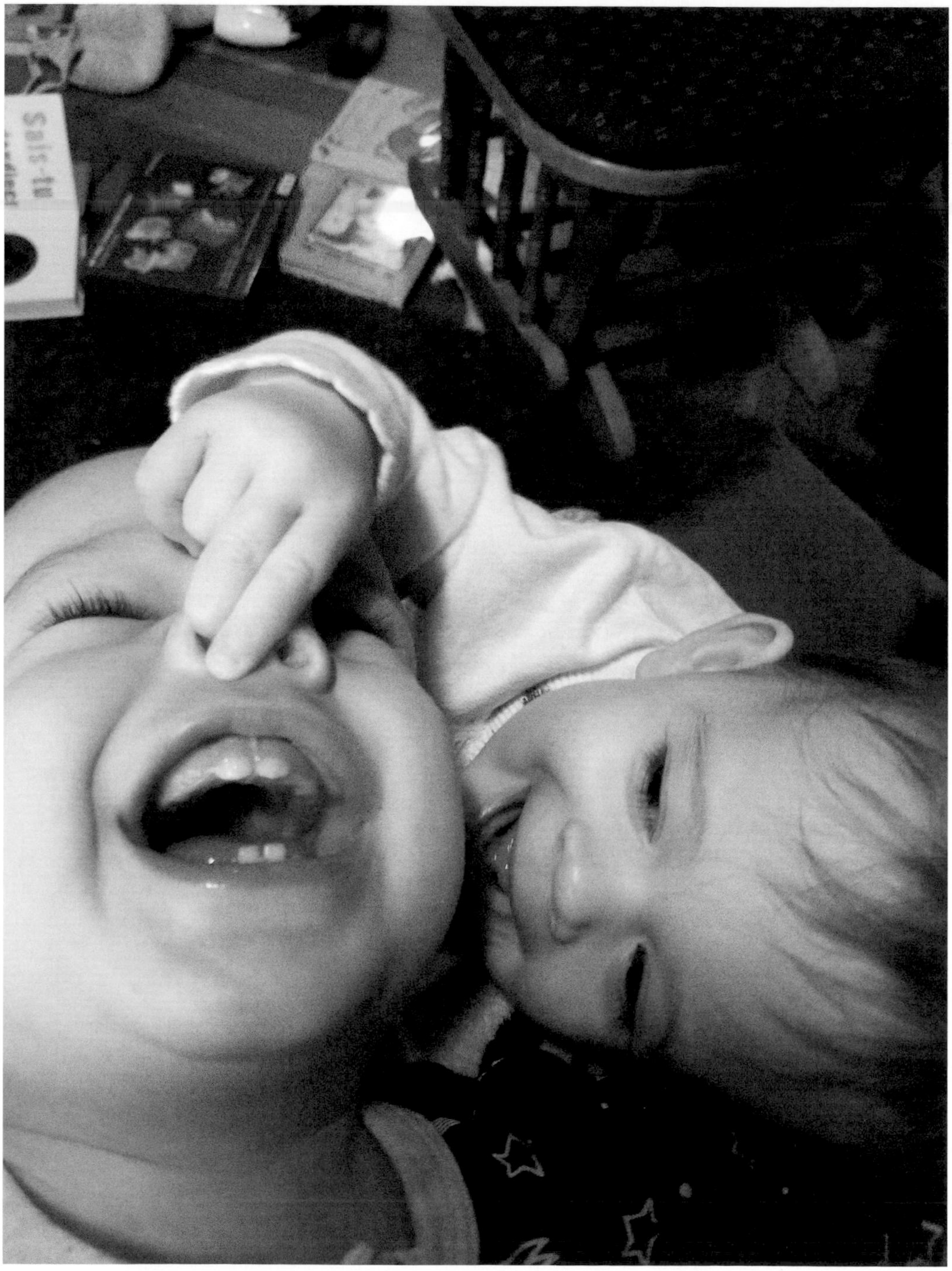
Sais-tu

Glossary

Please keep in mind that these definitions relate to how the terms are used in the context of this book. For example, many of the hormones mentioned in the glossary also have several other functions not directly related to my story.

AMH: Anti-Müllerian hormone (AMH) is a protein released by the ovaries and is related to the development of follicles in the ovary. The level of AMH in a woman's blood is generally a good indicator of her ovarian reserve (whether or not she has a good number of eggs).

Amnio: Amniocentesis (amnio) is the sampling of amniotic fluid using a hollow needle inserted into the uterus during pregnancy, to screen for developmental abnormalities in a fetus. Unlike the NIPT or SIPS test, results are considered accurate enough to be diagnostic.

Blastocyst: The cluster of cells that are contained in a hollow structure and that are formed after fertilization. The inner cells become the embryo and the outer layer of cells becomes the placenta.

D+C: Dilation and curettage (D+C) is a procedure to remove tissue from inside the uterus. Doctors perform dilation and curettage to diagnose and treat certain uterine conditions, such as heavy bleeding, or to clear the uterine lining after a miscarriage or abortion.

D+E: Dilation and evacuation (D+E), also sometimes called dilation and extraction, is the dilation of the cervix and surgical evacuation of the contents of the uterus when a pregnancy is further along.

Estrogen: A hormone crucial to a woman's reproductive function and cycle. Amongst other things, it helps stimulate the growth of the follicles, and enhances the uterine lining in preparation for pregnancy.

Fallopian tube: The tube that leads from the ovary to the uterus, down which the egg travels once released from its follicle in the ovary. It is generally in the Fallopian tube that the sperm will meet the egg and begin the fertilization process.

Follicle: A small sac that hopefully contains an egg. At ovulation, the follicle bursts and releases the egg, which will then travel down the Fallopian tube.

hCG: Human chorionic gonadotropin (hCG) is a hormone produced by the placenta after the implantation of an embryo. Because there is no detectable amount of hCG in the body when a person is not pregnant, the presence of hCG is used in pregnancy tests (both home kits and blood tests) to signal a pregnancy.

HSG: Hysterosalpingogram (HSG) is an imaging test that is used to examine the cavity of the uterus and Fallopian tubes to check for problems such as blockages. In a hysterosalpingogram, dye (called "contrast material") is injected via a tube inserted through the vagina into the uterus.

Hysteroscopy: The insertion of a tiny camera into the uterus via the vagina to determine the health of the uterus (e.g., the presence of cysts, polyps, scarring, or products of conception, or to try to find the reason for heavy bleeding).

Intralipid IV: Intralipid is a fat emulsion comprising soya bean oil, egg phospholipids, and glycerine that has been shown to have immunosuppressive properties. It is sometimes used post–embryo transfer to discourage the body from rejecting the embryo.

IUI: Intra-uterine insemination (IUI) is a fertility treatment whereby sperm is placed directly into a woman's uterus. The goal of IUI is to increase the number of sperm that reach the Fallopian tubes and then, hopefully, to fertilize an egg.

IVF: In vitro fertilization (IVF) is a medical procedure whereby eggs are retrieved from a woman's ovaries and subsequently fertilized in a lab and grown to a day 3–6 blastocyst. The blastocyst is then either transferred back into the woman's uterus or frozen for future transfer.

Laminaria: The day before a termination procedure, laminaria are inserted into the cervix. Generally made of thin strips of sterile seaweed, they expand as they absorb the body's natural fluids and thus slowly enlarge the opening of the cervix.

LH: In women, the luteinizing hormone (LH) is associated with reproduction and ovulation. Detecting an LH surge indicates that the body is initiating an ovulation.

Misoprostol: A drug taken to induce uterine contractions, either to start labour or to induce an abortion.

NIPT: Non-invasive prenatal testing (NIPT), also known as Panorama, is a blood test to determine the likelihood that the fetus could be affected by chromosome abnormalities. It is said to be 99% accurate.

Progesterone: A steroid hormone that stimulates the uterus to prepare for pregnancy. Once implantation has occurred, it is secreted by the placenta to prevent rejection of the fetus.

SIPS test: Serum integrated prenatal screening (SIPS) tests the likelihood of a fetus having chromosomal abnormalities. It involves two blood tests (one at 12 weeks' gestation and another at 16–20 weeks) as well as an ultrasound to measure the nuchal fold of the fetus (the fold of skin at the back of the fetus's neck, seen in the second trimester). It has a supposed accuracy of 82–85%.

TTC: Trying To Conceive.

About the Author and Illustrator

MYRIAM STEINBERG is currently a writer. In her past life, she was a visual artist and event organizer. For 11 years, she was the brains and brawn of the In the House Festival, which brought live performances of all kinds into people's living rooms and backyards throughout her hometown of Vancouver, Canada. Myriam was nominated for the YWCA Women of Distinction Award for her work on the festival. *Catalogue Baby* is her first book. www.cataloguebabynovel.com | @catalogue_baby

Born in Bristol, England, **CHRISTOPHER D. ROSS (CHRISTACHE)** currently works as an illustrator, writer, actor, and youth instructor in British Columbia, Canada. He lives with his cats, Wally and Morris, and his partner, Jill, whose love and support throughout the process of drawing this book have been indispensable and to whom he is eternally grateful. He previously illustrated the children's book *Some Bunny Loves You*. This is his first graphic novel. To see more of Christache's work, please visit him online at www.christache.com or on Instagram at @christachedraws.

The Rilke excerpt on page 133 is from Rainer Maria Rilke, *Letters to a Young Poet*, translated by Reginald Snell. New York: Dover, 2019.

Cataloguing in publication information is available from Library and Archives Canada.
ISBN 978-1-989603-64-2 (paperback)
ISBN 978-1-77458-015-8 (ebook)

Page Two
www.pagetwo.com

Edited by Amanda Lewis
Copyedited by John Sweet
Proofread by Alison Strobel
Cover design by Jennifer Lum and Christache
Printed and bound in Canada by Friesens
Distributed in Canada by Raincoast Books
Distributed in the US and internationally by Publishers Group West, a division of Ingram

21 22 23 24 25 5 4 3 2 1

www.cataloguebabynovel.com

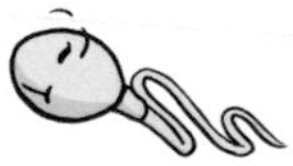